ATLAS *of*

MEDICAL-SURGICAL NURSING

Prepared by

Janice Tazbir RN, MS, CS, CCRN
Associate Professor, School of Nursing
Purdue University Calumet, Hammond, Indiana

Patricia Keresztes PhD, RN, CCRN
Assistant Professor of Nursing, Saint Mary's College
Notre Dame, Indiana

THOMSON
★
DELMAR LEARNING

Atlas of Medical-Surgical Nursing
Prepared by Janice Tazbir and Patricia Keresztes

Vice President, Health Care Business Unit:
William Brottmiller

Director of Learning Solutions:
Matthew Kane

Acquisitions Editor:
Tamara Caruso

Senior Product Manager:
Patricia Gaworecki

Editorial Assistant:
Jennifer Waters

Marketing Director:
Jennifer McAvey

Marketing Channel Manager:
Michele McTighe

Marketing Coordinator:
Chelsey Iaquinta

Production Director:
Carolyn Miller

Senior Art Director:
Jack Pendleton

Content Project Manager:
Katie Wachtl

For permission to use material from this text or product, contact us by
Tel (800) 730-2214
Fax (800) 730-2215
www.thomsonrights.com

Library of Congress Cataloging-in-Publication Data
ISBN 1-4180-0958-X

Tazbir, Janice.
  Atlas of medical-surgical nursing / prepared by Janice Tazbir, Patricia Keresztes.
    p. ; cm.
  ISBN 1-4180-0958-X
  1. Nursing–Atlases. 2. Surgical nursing–Atlases. I. Keresztes, Patricia. II. Title.
  [DNLM: 1. Perioperative Nursing–Atlases. WY 17 T248a 2008]
  RT57 T39 2008
  610.73022'3–dc22
                                                2007033683

NOTICE TO THE READER

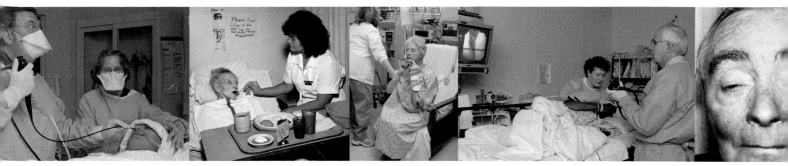

Dedications

Thanks go to my past, present and future nursing students who inspire and challenge me daily. Most importantly, thanks to my family: Johnny, Jade and Joule, they are the air I breathe.

Janice

My special thanks to my sister Mary and my parents, Bob and Loretta, without whom I could not have written this book. As always, a special thank you to my Mom who has always been my strength and inspiration.

Patricia

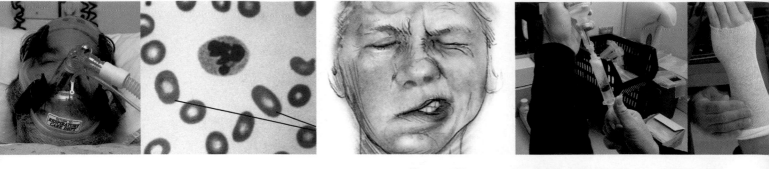

CONTENTS

Part 1 Diseases and Disorders   1

A

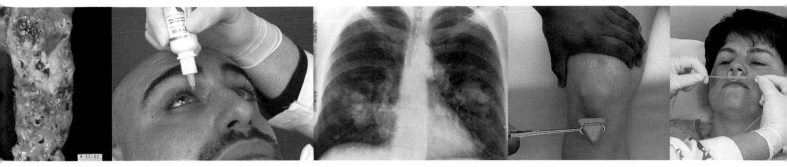

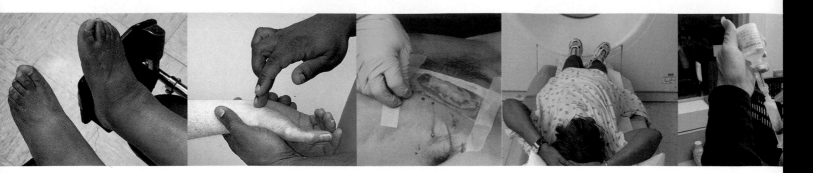

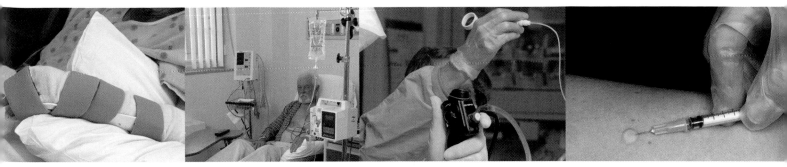

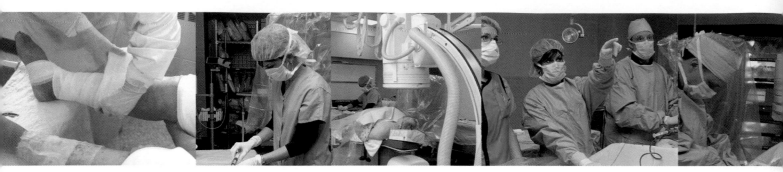

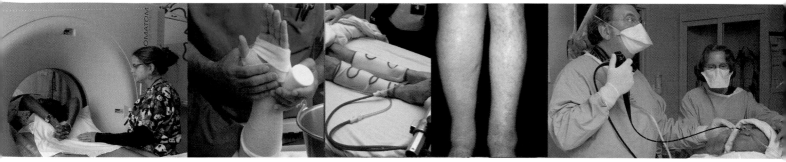

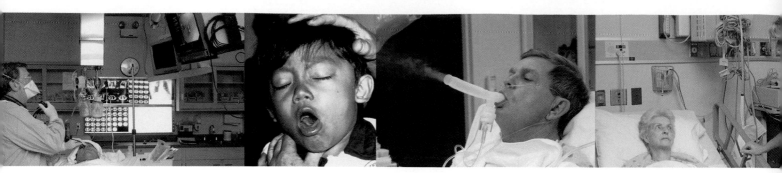

Preface

"A picture is worth a thousand words"

The first edition of the *Atlas of Medical-Surgical Nursing* is designed to visually represent, describe and explain diseases, disorders and procedures in medical-surgical nursing practice. It is a hands-on reference text that is intended for student nurses, practicing nurses, and as a teaching tool for patients. *Atlas of Medical-Surgical Nursing* is the book that should be in every nursing school library and nursing unit next to the drug reference guide and the medical dictionary. It helps answer the questions: "what is it, what does it look like, and what I look for?"

Conceptual Approach

The concept for the *Atlas of Medical-Surgical Nursing* arose from a need to enhance and refresh medical-surgical nursing knowledge by providing a visual reference text. Intended to complement the textbooks used in today's nursing classrooms, this text provides a visual experience that allows the reader to quickly absorb difficult concepts that translate into effective nursing care. As students and frequently as practitioners, nurses have not had the opportunity to witness a particular disease or procedure. Even though nurses have cared for many patients with a certain disease or observed certain procedures, most patients have not. Taking the book inside the patient's room and showing them what an angiogram or peptic ulcer looks like helps to reduce patient anxiety by promoting effective patient teaching.

It also provides an easy to use and understand instructional tool for practitioners and patients in any care setting. In addition, there is a full color visually appealing design with images and captions that engages the reader in a user friendly way. The Nursing Process framework is used

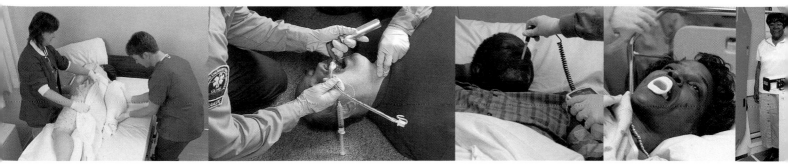

effectively to organize key information for each topic. In addition, *Nursing Considerations* are also included to facilitate critical thinking, an essential aspect in fostering caring, ethical and responsible professional practice.

Organization

The book is divided into two sections covering 125 topics in medical-surgical nursing care. Section I is focused on diseases and disorders, while Section II addresses procedures and treatments. Each section is alphabetically organized for ease of use. Topics for this text were chosen to complement medical-surgical nursing textbooks that are not always able to visually represent all the content they cover and to provide the ideal companion for the visual learning. Additionally, each topic begins within the framework of the Nursing Process; defining the condition, identifying the key assessments to look for in patients, planning and implementation points to assist in guiding care, evaluations and outcomes to monitor effectiveness, and finally nursing considerations essential for implementing care.

At the heart of the book are the images. With over 525 high quality, full color photographs and drawings, these images with rich captions "tell the story" of each topic in the text. This allows the reader to "see" the disease or procedure and gain a visual as well as conceptual understanding of the topic.

The *Atlas of Medical-Surgical Nursing* is the newest offering in Delmar Learning's continuing commitment to help bridge the gap between theory and application buy providing readers with the information, knowledge and skills that support today's nursing practice.

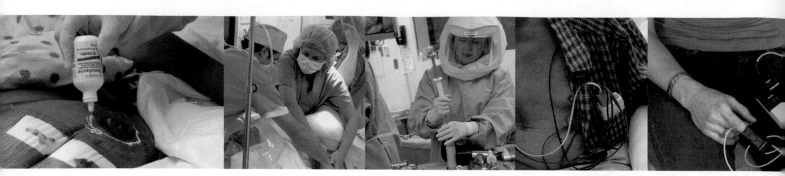

Acknowledgments

Publishing a text, especially the first of its kind, is a team effort and we are thankful for all that were involved in the process. Our gratitude and respect goes to Patricia Gaworecki, Product Manager and editor; the one with all the answers. She helped us "see" this book and kept us on task with the visual element of this challenging text. Her editing was insightful and on the mark, her humor was much appreciated. Further thanks go to Katie Wachtl, Content Project Manager and the person responsible for turning our piles of pages and pictures into a book. Her artistry is realized.

Janice Tazbir and Patricia Keresztes

Delmar Learning would also like to thank the administration, staff and patients at the St. Vincent Health System in Little Rock, Arkansas who allowed us to take many of the photographs that appear in this text.

PART **1**

DISEASES & DISORDERS

ACNE

Acne is a disease of the sebaceous gland and hair follicle. Acne develops when sebaceous glands become overactive and the oil secreted becomes trapped in the pores. It occurs in 80% of all teenagers but can affect people well into adulthood.

Assessment

- Pimples
- Whiteheads and blackheads
- Rash
- Scarring

Planning and Implementation

- Hygiene habits
- Wash affected area with warm water and mild soap
- Topical ointments such as Retin A, Benzyl Peroxide and topical antibiotics

Evaluation and Outcomes

The patient will:

- Understand need for adequate hygiene
- Identify appropriate topical medications for use
- Maintain body image

Nursing Considerations

- Teach the patient to avoid topical exposure to oils, grease, cocoa butter.

- Inform the patient that it may take 4-6 weeks for treatment to show results.

- Teach patients that foods do not cause acne.

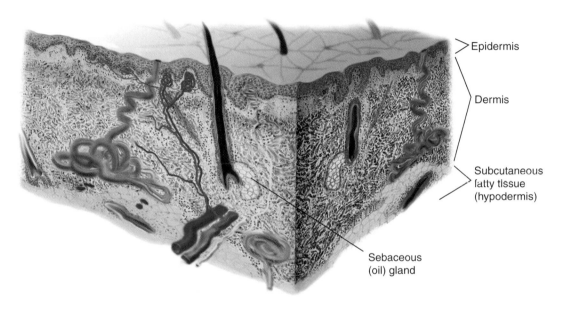

Epidermis

Dermis

Subcutaneous fatty tissue (hypodermis)

Sebaceous (oil) gland

The sebaceous gland is located in the dermal layer of the skin. Overactivity of this gland causes acne.

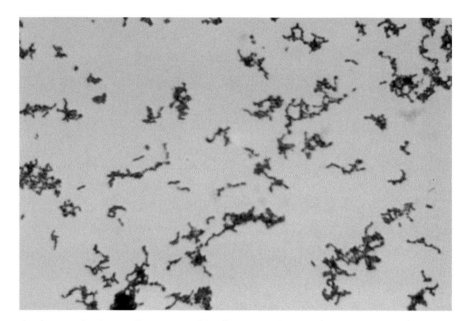

A microscopic picture of a gram positive bacterium Propionibacterium acnes that resides in the sebaceous glands and is a causative agent for acne.

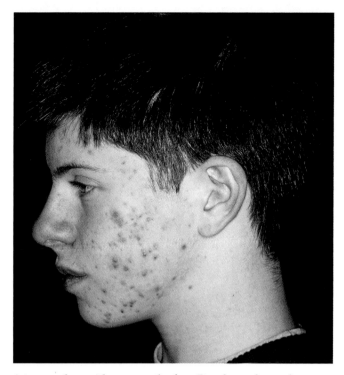

A teenage boy with acne on the face. Papules and pustules (areas of infection) can be seen. This will require treatment with antibiotics. (Courtesy of Viewing Medicine)

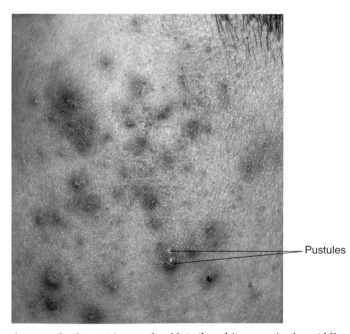

Pustules

Acne on the face with pustules. Note the white areas in the middle that are the infected areas. This will require treatment with antibiotics. (Courtesy of Viewing Medicine)

ACUTE PULMONARY EDEMA

Acute pulmonary edema is the sudden accumulation of fluid within the lungs due to leakage from the pulmonary capillaries into the alveoli. It is typically seen in patients with congestive heart failure.

Assessment

- Shortness of breath
- Lung sounds with rales
- Low oxygen levels (hypoxia)
- Pink, frothy sputum
- Jugular venous distention

Planning and Implementation

- Lung sounds
- Arterial blood gases
- Oxygen saturation level
- Supplemental oxygen therapy
- Strict intake and output measurements (I&O)

Evaluation and Outcome

The patient will:

- Experience no shortness of breath
- Have clear breath sounds
- Maintain normal arterial blood gas values
- Oxygenate adequately on room air

Nursing Considerations

- Therapy for acute pulmonary edema consists of diuretics, ACE inhibitors, and morphine sulfate.

- Patients should be taught to report a weight gain of three pounds in one week, swelling of the ankles or legs, or shortness of breath.

- Patients should be instructed to adhere to a sodium restricted diet.

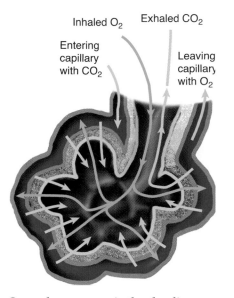

Inhaled O_2

Exhaled CO_2

Entering capillary with CO_2

Leaving capillary with O_2

Gas exchange occurs in the alveoli. Pulmonary edema inhibits this process, leading to hypoxia.

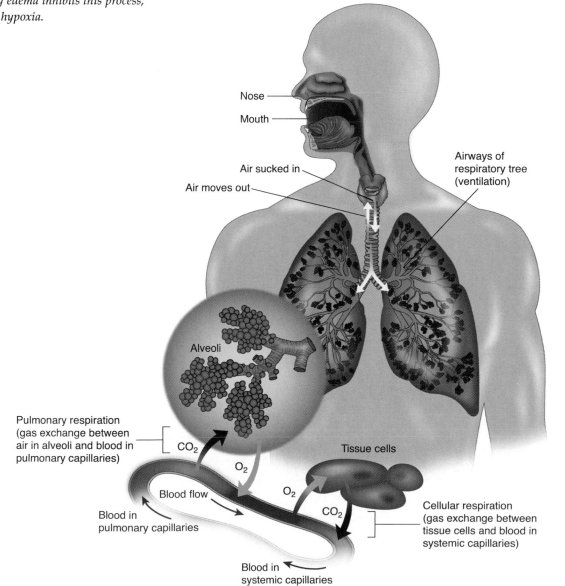

Nose

Mouth

Air sucked in

Air moves out

Airways of respiratory tree (ventilation)

Alveoli

Pulmonary respiration (gas exchange between air in alveoli and blood in pulmonary capillaries)

CO_2

O_2

Tissue cells

O_2

CO_2

Blood flow

Cellular respiration (gas exchange between tissue cells and blood in systemic capillaries)

Blood in pulmonary capillaries

Blood in systemic capillaries

In pulmonary respiration there is gas exchange between the blood and the alveoli. In cellular respiration there is gas exchange between the arterial blood and the tissues. Lack of oxygen in the arterial blood from pulmonary edema leads to a lack of oxygen available to the tissues.

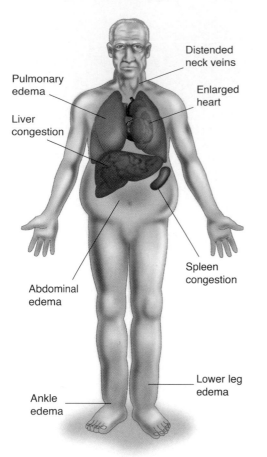

Pulmonary edema

Liver congestion

Abdominal edema

Ankle edema

Distended neck veins

Enlarged heart

Spleen congestion

Lower leg edema

Congestive heart failure is a common cause of pulmonary edema. Patients with congestive heart failure may also have liver congestion, ascites, peripheral edema, and jugular venous distention.

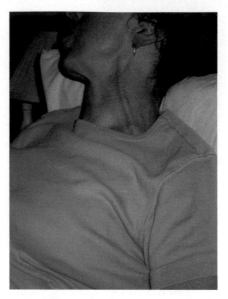

Patients with pulmonary edema also have a fluid volume overload. Fluid volume overload is an increase in intravascular volume. The nurse needs to assess for jugular venous distention, as shown in this picture, a key assessment. Both conditions are treated with diuretics to remove excess fluid.

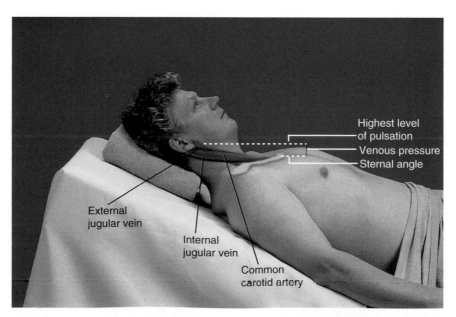

Highest level of pulsation
Venous pressure
Sternal angle

External jugular vein

Internal jugular vein

Common carotid artery

In assessing for jugular venous distention, the head of the bed should be at 30 degrees.

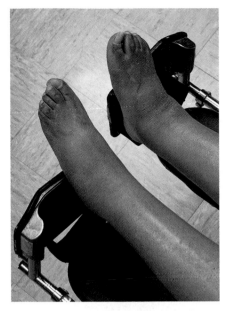

The nurse should assess the patient with pulmonary edema for signs of peripheral edema, usually in the feet and ankles. Patients should elevate their feet to help decrease the swelling. Diuretics are also given to remove excess fluid causing the swelling.

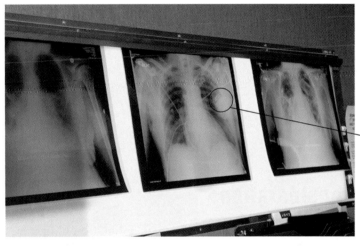

'Patchy' areas of edema

This chest X-ray is from a patient diagnosed with pulmonary edema. Note the appearance of patchy white areas over the lung fields. This is the area of edema of fluid in the lung.

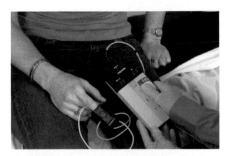

Obtaining a pulse oximetry reading is key for a patient with pulmonary edema.

ACUTE RESPIRATORY DISTRESS SYNDROME (ARDS)

Acute respiratory distress syndrome (ARDS) is a non-cardiac pulmonary edema characterized by alveolar injury resulting in increased permeability to plasma and inflammatory cells, leading to refractory hypoxemia. Synonyms include adult respiratory distress syndrome, shock lung, wet lung, capillary leak syndrome, and adult hyaline membrane disease. The mortality rate is 30-40%.

Assessment

- Dyspnea
- Hypoxia
- Rales
- Tachypnea

Planning and Implementation

- Supplemental oxygen
- Continuous oxygen saturation monitoring
- Elevate head of bed
- Assess lung sounds

Evaluation and Outcomes

The patient will:

- Oxygenate adequately on room air
- Have clear breath sounds
- Have no shortness of breath
- Have a normal respiratory rate

Nursing Considerations

- ARDS occurs secondary to aspiration, sepsis, inhalation injury, trauma, multiple blood transfusions, and pancreatitis.

- Prone positioning may be utilized in therapy to help with mobilization of fluids and improvement in gas exchange.

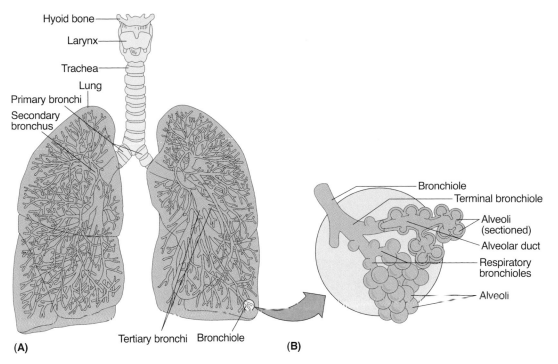

(A)

(B)

The normal anatomy of the lung. The alveoli are the terminal units of the lung where gas exchange occurs. In acute respiratory distress syndrome, fluid leaks from the vascular space into the alveoli, inhibiting gas exchange and leading to hypoxia.

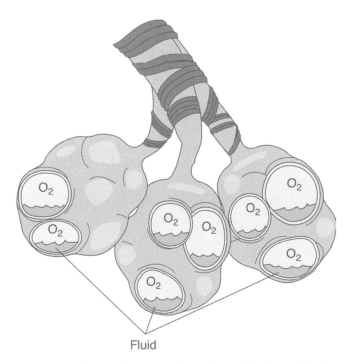

Fluid

In acute respiratory distress syndrome, there is leakage of fluid into the alveoli, causing hypoxia. The fluid leaks from the vascular space into the alveoli. The leakage of fluid inhibits movement of oxygen into the blood. The patient may experience shortness of breath, hypoxia, and cyanosis.

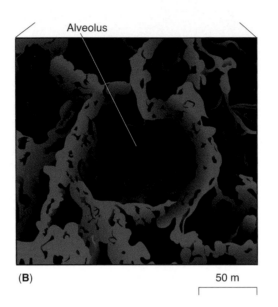

(B)

50 m

The normal anatomy of the alveoli showing a microscopic view of the alveoli. Lack of gas exchange from leakage of fluid into the alveoli in acute respiratory distress syndrome leads to hypoxia.

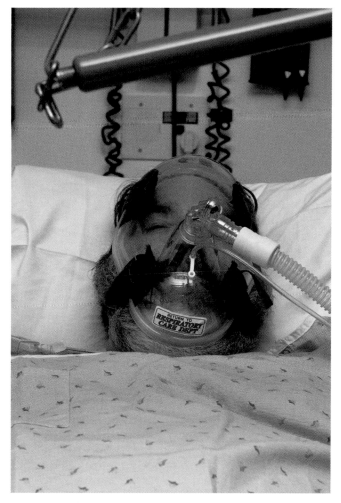

A treatment for acute respiratory distress syndrome includes using a BiPap mask. A BiPap mask exerts a positive pressure on the airways, keeping the alveoli open and helping to increase gas exchange. This mask is uncomfortable for patients and may cause tissue breakdown on the bridge of the nose.

ACQUIRED IMMUNODEFICIENCY SYNDROME/HUMAN IMMUNODEFICIENCY VIRUS (AIDS/HIV)

Acquired immunodeficiency syndrome (AIDS) is a fatal disease that leads to the destruction of the immune system. Human Immunodeficiency Virus (HIV) is a retrovirus infection that replicates rapidly, destroys CD4 T cells, and renders the body at risk for opportunistic infections. The virus spreads through unsafe sexual contact, and parenteral (blood) and perinatal exposure.

Assessments

- Leukopenia
- Fever
- Neurological changes
- Nausea/vomiting/diarrhea
- Weight loss

Planning and Implementation

- Neutropenic precautions
- Signs and symptoms of infection
- Pain relief
- Nutrition
- Neurologic assessments

Evaluation and Outcomes

The patient will:

- Verbalize need to comply with medication regimen
- Maintain adequate nutritional intake
- Be free of infection
- Maintain self-esteem

Nursing Considerations

- Elderly patients have a depressed immune system which may increase the risk for acquiring the HIV infection.

- The CD4 cell count is used as a guide to determine immune system function. A CD4 cell count of <500 implies a compromised immune system.

- Opportunistic infections occur with a CD4 cell count <200 and include toxoplasmosis, candidiasis, Mycobacterium avium complex (MAC), histoplasmosis, Kaposi's sarcoma, pneumocystis carinii pneumonia, and herpes.

- Patients need to be instructed on the side effects of medications and the need to comply with the medication regimen.

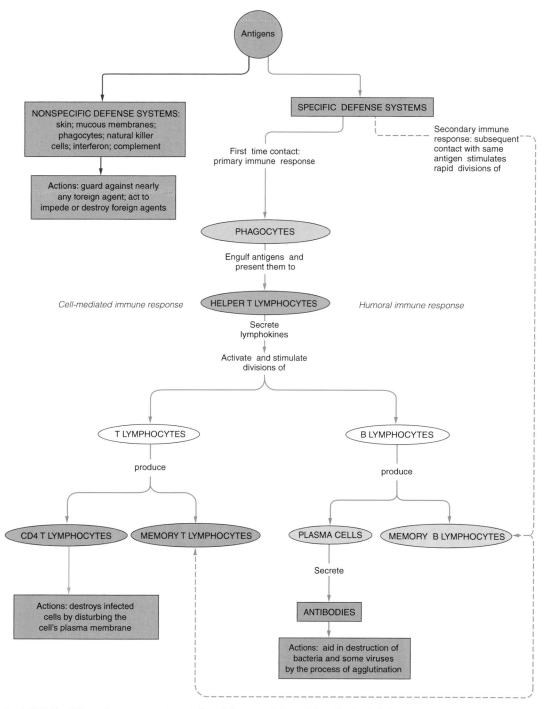

In AIDS the T lymphocytes are targeted and destroyed, impairing the body's immune system. Specifically, it is the CD4 T lymphocytes that are destroyed.

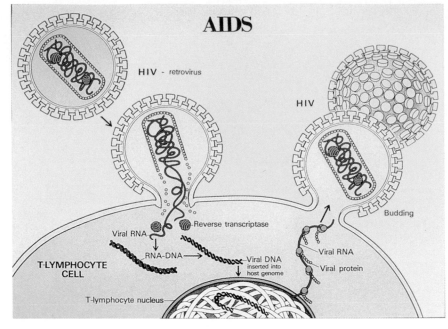

Human Immunodeficiency Virus is a retrovirus. This virus enters the T lymphocyte and alters the RNA of the normal T lymphocyte. The inability of the body to produce normal T lymphocytes compromises the immune system. (Courtesy of the National Cancer Institute)

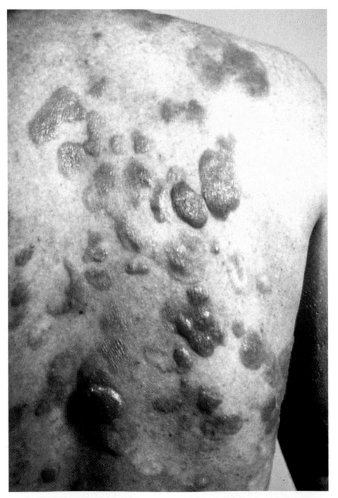

Patients with AIDS are at risk for developing Kaposi's sarcoma. Kaposi's sarcoma is commonly caused by the herpes virus. The skin lesions are very painful. (Courtesy of the National Cancer Institute)

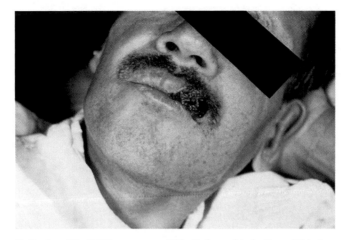

Patients with AIDS are susceptible to fungal infections. This is a lesion caused from histoplasmosis due to the compromised immune system. (Courtesy of the Centers for Disease Control)

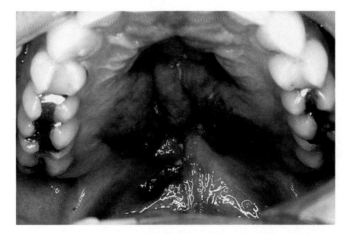

Kaposi's sarcoma can also cause lesions in the mouth. These lesions are very painful and frequent oral care is needed. (Courtesy of the Centers for Disease Control)

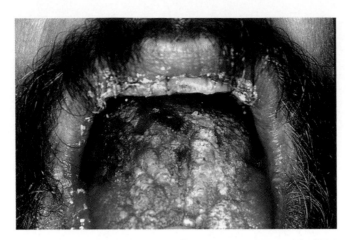

*Oral candidiasis, thrush, commonly occurs in patients with AIDS.
This is a fungal infection caused by a depressed immune system.
Frequent oral care needs to be done as thrush alters taste and
leads to altered oral intake. (Courtesy Centers for Disease Control)*

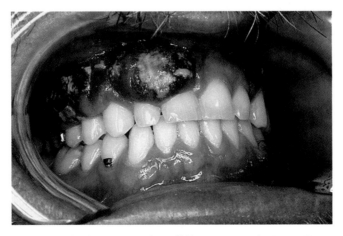

*In the mouth, this is an oral candidiasis on top of a Kaposi's
sarcoma lesion. Oral care is of prime concern, as this is very
painful and leads to altered taste sensation and decreased
nutritional intake. (Courtesy of the Centers for Disease Control)*

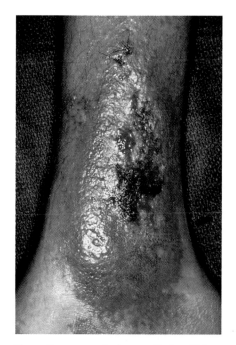

Kaposi's sarcoma lesion on the leg. This wound needs to assessed for infection and be kept clean due to the depressed immune system in the AIDS patient. (Courtesy of the Centers for Disease Control)

AMPUTATION

Amputation is the removal of a limb or portion of the limb. Amputations can occur traumatically or surgically.

Assessment

- Pulses
- Color and temperature
- Sensation
- Pain

Planning and Implementation

- Provide pain relief
- Inspect for signs of infection
- Assess distal pulses
- Appropriate dressing of the stump

Evaluation and Outcomes

The patient will:

- Verbalize relief of pain
- Be free of infection
- Maintain body image
- Identify prosthesis application and care

Nursing Considerations

➤ Nurses need to be aware that patients may experience phantom pain at the amputation site.

➤ Teach patients to examine the skin where the prosthesis fits for signs of skin breakdown.

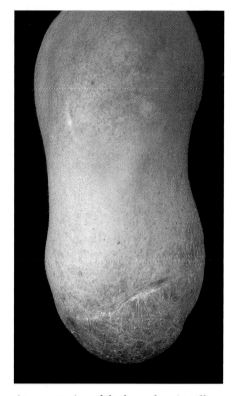

An amputation of the lower leg. A well-healed scar is visible at the base of the stump. (Courtesy of Viewing Medicine)

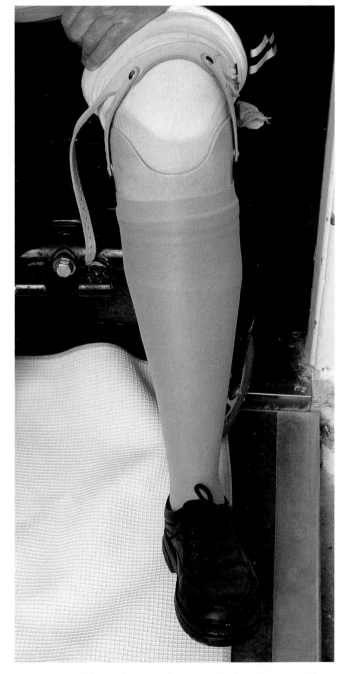

An amputated leg with a prosthesis attached to the stump. The prosthesis needs to be properly fitted or it may result in skin breakdown at the site of the stump. (Courtesy of Viewing Medicine)

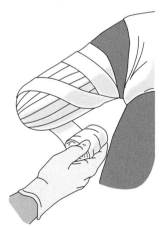

The amputated limb must be dressed appropriately. When dressing an amputated stump, the nurse should use circular turns when wrapping the stump.

ANAPHYLAXIS

Anaphylaxis is a severe, life-threatening allergic reaction resulting in bronchoconstriction and hypotension. Histamine and other substances are released, causing smooth muscle contraction, vascular dilation, edema, and airway obstruction. Anaphylaxis triggers include food (e.g., peanuts), medications (e.g., penicillin), insect venom (e.g., bee stings), and latex products.

Assessments

- Hypotension
- Wheezes and stridor
- Tachycardia
- Generalized itching

Planning and Implementation

- Lung sounds
- Patency of airway
- Vital signs
- Supplemental oxygen

Evaluation and Outcomes

The patient will:

- Maintain airway
- Maintain adequate oxygenation
- Maintain adequate blood pressure
- Identify drug/food allergies

Nursing Considerations

- Teach the patient that he/she may carry their own emergency syringe of epinephrine (EpiPen kit) in case of an anaphylactic reaction.

- Teach the patient to wear a Medic Alert identification bracelet.

- Teach the patient to avoid contact with allergens.

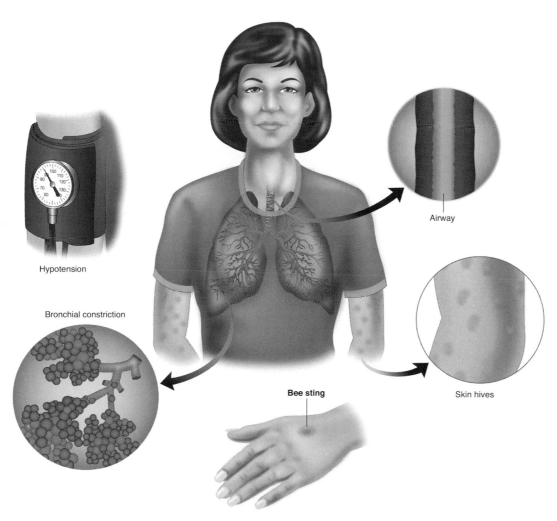

Hypotension

Bronchial constriction

Airway

Skin hives

Bee sting

An anaphylactic reaction is a life-threatening emergency which stems from an allergic reaction to such things as medications, bee stings, or foods. Patients develop an allergic response from contact with a substance or antigen that causes the body to produce antibodies in response to the antigen. Death may result from hypotension and/or bronchial constriction. Maintaining an adequate airway is the prime focus of the nurse.

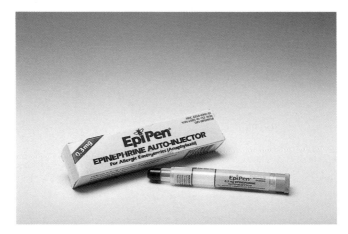

After injection, epinephrine will reverse the effects of the allergic reaction, causing bronchodilation and increasing blood pressure. This response to epinephrine is similar to the fight or flight response.

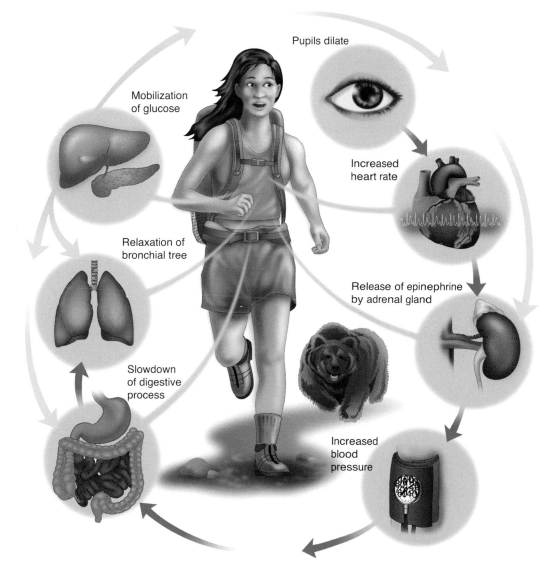

Pupils dilate

Mobilization of glucose

Increased heart rate

Relaxation of bronchial tree

Release of epinephrine by adrenal gland

Slowdown of digestive process

Increased blood pressure

Patients with allergies should be taught to wear a Medic Alert bracelet and carry a syringe of epinephrine that can be administered in emergency situations. Epinephrine will cause bronchodilation and increase blood pressure.

ANEMIA, IRON DEFICIENCY

Anemia is a decrease in the number of red blood cells or a decrease in the hemoglobin value. Anemia is more common in women and is often caused by a gastrointestinal bleed. Iron deficiency anemia results from a lack of adequate iron intake in the diet. It is also called microcytic, hypochromic anemia because the red blood cells are small with less color.

Assessments

- Fatigue
- Pallor
- Shortness of breath
- Palpitations

Planning and Implementation

- Monitor complete blood count
- Administer blood or blood products
- Space activities
- Nutritional intake

Evaluation and Outcomes

The patient will:

- Have a normal red blood cell count
- Have more energy
- Take in adequate amounts of dietary iron daily
- Complete activities of daily living without difficulty

Nursing Considerations

- There is a higher incidence in women and in pregnancy.

- Patients need to be instructed to increase intake of iron from sources such as organ meats, kidney beans, whole wheat grains and cereals, green leafy vegetables, and egg yolks.

- Patients should be instructed that iron supplements may cause dark, tarry stools, and stools may falsely hemetest positive.

- Iron is best absorbed with Vitamin C, and dairy products decrease absorption.

- Patients receiving intravenous iron must be closely observed for signs of reaction.

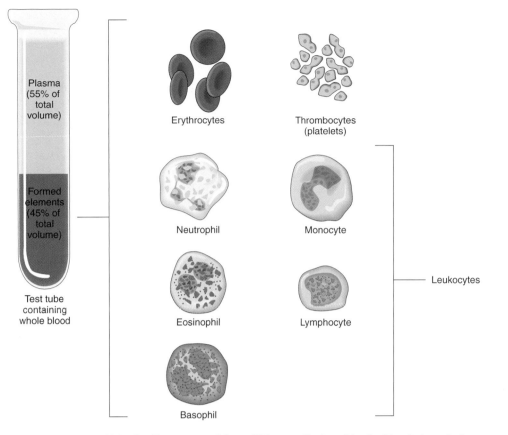

Erythrocytes, or red blood cells, are one of three different cells found in the blood. Anemia is a decrease in the amount of circulating red blood cells.

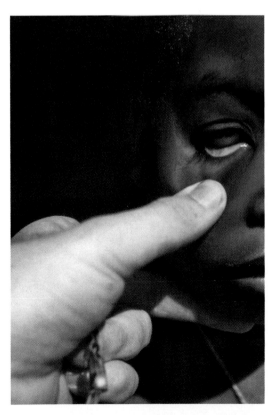

Red blood cells give tissues such as the conjunctive their typical pink or red coloring. A decrease in the number of circulating red blood cells in anemia leads to a pale coloring of tissues. (Courtesy of the Centers for Disease Control)

ANEMIA, PERNICIOUS

Anemia is a decrease in the numbers of red blood cells or a decrease in the hemoglobin value. Pernicious anemia is caused by inadequate absorption of Vitamin B12 due to a lack of intrinsic factor secreted by the stomach. This results in the presence of large, immature red blood cells called megaloblasts.

Assessment

- Fatigue
- Pallor
- Glossitis
- Shortness of breath
- Palpitations

Planning and Implementation

- Monitor complete blood count
- Administer blood or blood products
- Space activities
- Nutritional intake

Evaluation and Outcomes

The patient will:

- Have a normal red blood cell count
- Have more energy
- Replace Vitamin B12
- Complete activities of daily living without difficulty

Nursing Considerations

- Patients who have undergone gastric bypass surgery are at risk for the development of pernicious anemia due to a loss of intrinsic factor secreted by the stomach which allows for the absorption of Vitamin B12.

- Patients need to be instructed that they may need life-long therapy with parenteral B12.

- Patients should be instructed to eat foods high in Vitamin B12, such as animal proteins, egg whites, and dairy products.

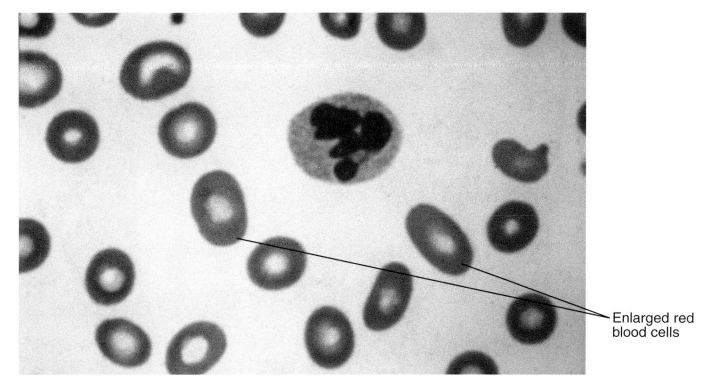

Enlarged red
blood cells

A slide of red blood cells from a patient with pernicious anemia. The red blood cells are large (megaloblasts) which is a hallmark sign of this type of anemia. Courtesy of Viewing Medicine

ANEMIA, SICKLE CELL

Anemia is a decrease in the numbers of red blood cells or a decrease in the hemoglobin value. Sickle cell anemia is a genetic blood dyscrasia due to the presence of hemoglobin S, an abnormal form of hemoglobin. Under low oxygen conditions, the abnormal hemoglobin deforms the red blood cells and causes the red blood cells to sickle in their shape. The sickled red blood cells cannot flow through the capillaries, leading to tissue hypoxia.

Assessment

- Fatigue
- Pallor
- Shortness of breath
- Pain
- History

Planning and Implementation

- Monitor complete blood count
- Administer blood or blood products
- Administer oxygen
- Decrease oxygen demands
- Pain management during crisis.

Evaluation and Outcomes

The patient will:

- Have a normal red blood cell count
- Have more energy
- Be pain free
- Complete activities of daily living without difficulty

Nursing Considerations

- Nurses should refer those diagnosed with sickle cell disease for genetic counseling.

- Nurses need to be aware that patients with sickle cell disease may develop tolerance to narcotics after many sickle cell crises and may require higher doses of narcotics to achieve pain relief.

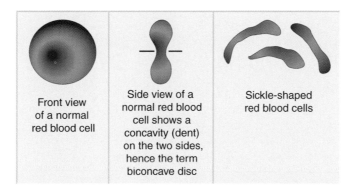

| Front view of a normal red blood cell | Side view of a normal red blood cell shows a concavity (dent) on the two sides, hence the term biconcave disc | Sickle-shaped red blood cells |

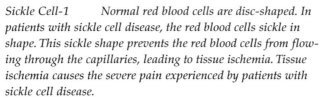

Sickle Cell-1   *Normal red blood cells are disc-shaped. In patients with sickle cell disease, the red blood cells sickle in shape. This sickle shape prevents the red blood cells from flowing through the capillaries, leading to tissue ischemia. Tissue ischemia causes the severe pain experienced by patients with sickle cell disease.*

Sickle Cell Anemia

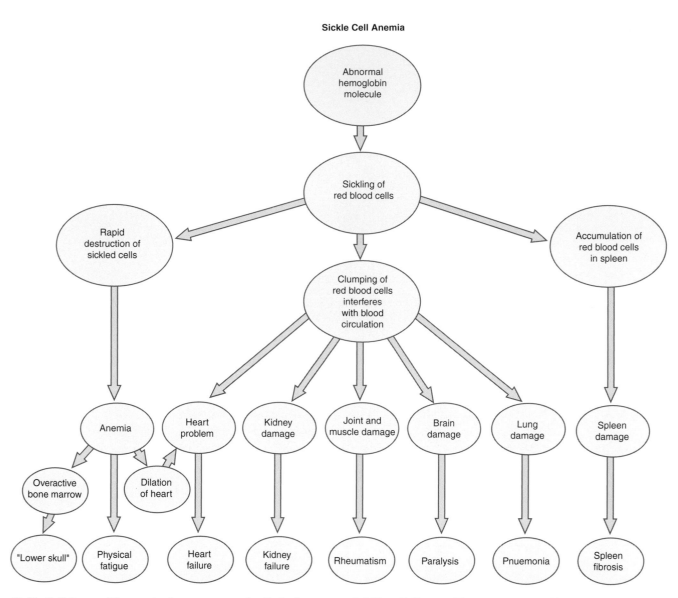

Sickle Cell-2   *The eventual consequences for the body system of sickle cell disease. The tissues are unable to get adequate oxygen and become ischemic. This leads to heart failure, kidney failure, arthritis, and paralysis.*

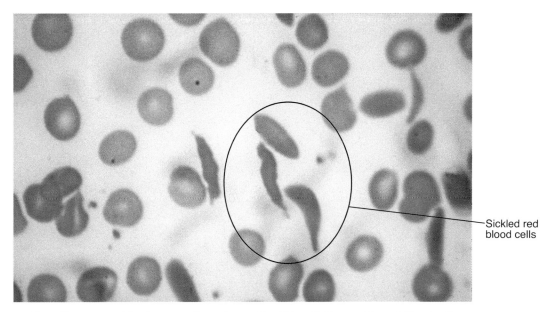

Sickled red
blood cells

Sickle Cell-3   *A blood smear of a patient with sickle cell disease. The red blood cells
should be round in shape. The sickled cells can clearly be seen. (Courtesy of Viewing Medicine)*

ANEURYSM, AORTIC

An aneurysm is a localized dilation or weakening of the artery. Aortic aneurysms may occur anywhere along the entire length of the aorta, but are most common in the abdominal aorta. The cause may be due to hypertension or atherosclerotic disease.

Assessment

- Hypotension
- Abdominal pain
- Back pain
- Pulsatile abdominal mass

Planning and Implementation

- Vital signs
- Urine output
- Peripheral pulses
- Motor/sensory function lower extremities

Evaluation and Outcomes

The patient will:

- Have stable vital signs
- Have adequate urine output
- Have palpable peripheral pulses
- Be pain free

Nursing Considerations

- Risk factors for development of an aortic aneurysm include male gender, hypertension, tobacco use, COPD, and connective tissue disease.

- Nurses need to monitor patients for motor and sensory function distal to the aneurysm, since neurological symptoms occur in 5% of patients as a result of spinal cord ischemia.

- The majority of patients present with no previous clinical manifestations.

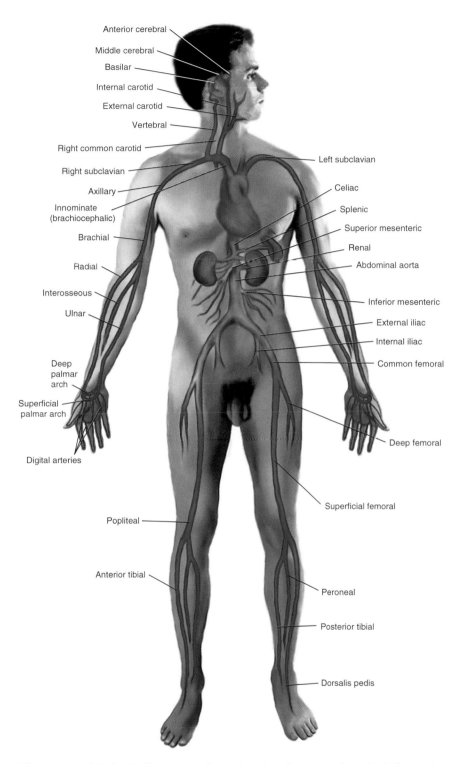

Anterior cerebral
Middle cerebral
Basilar
Internal carotid
External carotid
Vertebral
Right common carotid
Right subclavian
Axillary
Innominate (brachiocephalic)
Brachial
Radial
Interosseous
Ulnar
Deep palmar arch
Superficial palmar arch
Digital arteries
Popliteal
Anterior tibial

Left subclavian
Celiac
Splenic
Superior mesenteric
Renal
Abdominal aorta
Inferior mesenteric
External iliac
Internal iliac
Common femoral
Deep femoral
Superficial femoral
Peroneal
Posterior tibial
Dorsalis pedis

The arteries of the body. The aorta is the main artery that arises from the left ventricle. The part of the aorta above the diaphragm is the thoracic aorta. The abdominal artery starts below the level of the diaphragm. The majority of aortic aneurysms are in the abdominal aorta.

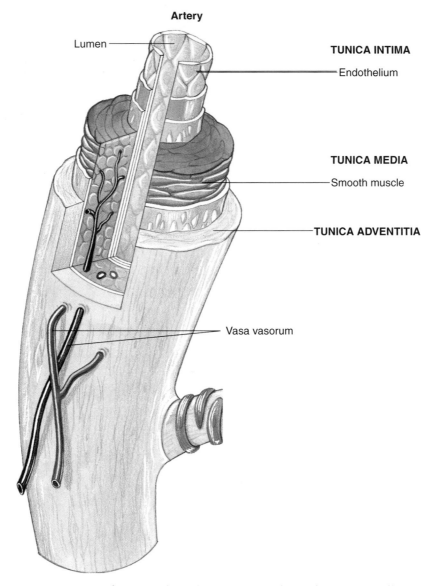

Artery

Lumen

TUNICA INTIMA

Endothelium

TUNICA MEDIA

Smooth muscle

TUNICA ADVENTITIA

Vasa vasorum

Aneurysms are a weakening in the wall of the artery. The weakening is usually in the middle layer of the artery or the tunica media. The weakening may be caused by genetics, hypertension, or hyperlipidemia.

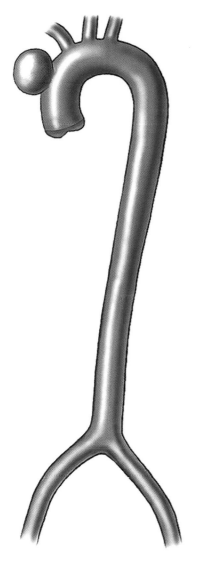

A saccular aneurysm, which is an outpouching of a segment of the aorta.

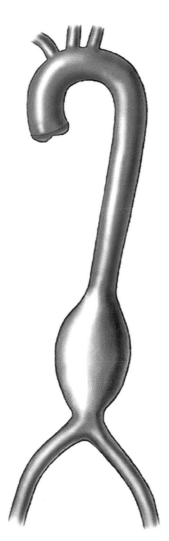

A fusiform aneurysm named for its spindle shape. The aneurysm involves all layers of the aorta.

A dissecting aneurysm, which indicates a tear in the aorta and bleeding into the layers of the aorta, causing the formation of a hematoma. If the tear goes through the entire layers of the aorta, there is massive blood loss with a poor prognosis. Patients will complain of severe back pain and present with tachycardia and hypotension.

ANEURYSM, CEREBRAL

An aneurysm is a localized dilation or weakening of the artery. Cerebral aneurysms may occur anywhere in the cerebral arterial circulation, and most commonly occur at bifurcations. Cerebral aneurysms can be congenital or acquired.

Assessments

- Severe headache
- Nausea and vomiting
- Seizures
- Loss of consciousness

Planning and Implementation

- Vital signs
- Neurological status
- Seizures
- Pain management

Evaluation and Outcomes

The patient will:

- Have stable vital signs
- Maintain neurological status
- Be free of pain
- Not experience seizures

Nursing Considerations

- Normal saline is the IV fluid most commonly used with neurological patients.

- Calcium channel blockers are used to prevent cerebral vasospasm.

- Cerebral aneurysms are most common in men age 40 and younger; more common in women age 40 and over.

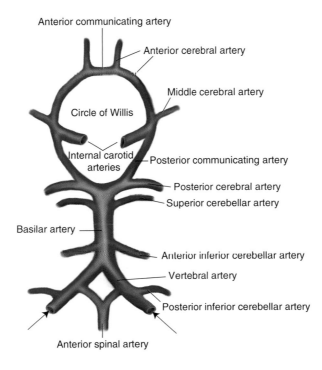

Anterior communicating artery

Anterior cerebral artery

Middle cerebral artery

Circle of Willis

Internal carotid arteries

Posterior communicating artery

Posterior cerebral artery

Superior cerebellar artery

Basilar artery

Anterior inferior cerebellar artery

Vertebral artery

Posterior inferior cerebellar artery

Anterior spinal artery

The arterial circulation of the brain. Cerebral aneurysms most commonly occur in the Circle of Willis and at the bifurcations of the arteries.

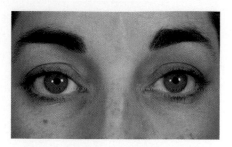

Assessing the pupils of patients with cerebral aneurysms is important for the nurse, because changes in pupil size or reaction is a sign of increased intracranial pressure. This illustrates constricted or narrow pupils.

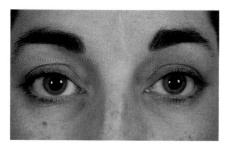

The pupils are dilated or large in size. Changes in pupil size or reaction indicate an increase in intracranial pressure.

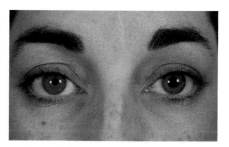

The pupils are unequal in size. This may indicate an increase in intracranial pressure.

ARTHRITIS, OSTEOARTHRITIS

Osteoarthritis is a non-inflammatory degenerative joint disease characterized by degeneration of the articular cartilage, hypertrophy of the bone at margins, and changes in the synovial membrane. The incidence of osteoarthritis increases with age, weight, and joint injury. Primary osteoarthritis refers to the development without any known reason, and secondary refers to the development of osteoarthritis with a known cause, such as a history of joint trauma or mechanical stressors (obesity or athletics).

Assessment

- Pain in joints
- Stiffness, especially in the morning
- Crepitus with range of motion
- Swelling of joints
- Limited movement

Planning and Implementation

- Range of motion
- Pain relief
- Anti-inflammatory medications
- Application of heat

Evaluation and Outcomes

The patient will:

- Be able to complete activities of daily living
- Maintain full range of motion in joints
- Be free of pain
- Understand medications

Nursing Considerations

- Implement safety precautions because joint pain and stiffness may cause an unsteady gait.

- Plan activities when osteoarthritis medications peak.

- Collaborate with physical therapy to encourage the use of assistive devices like gripper devices to minimize bending.

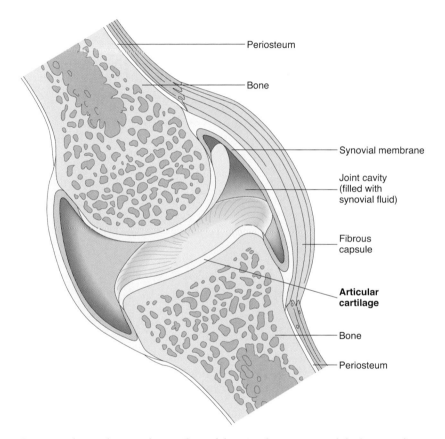

Periosteum

Bone

Synovial membrane

Joint cavity
(filled with
synovial fluid)

Fibrous
capsule

**Articular
cartilage**

Bone

Periosteum

In osteoarthritis, the articular cartilage of the joint degenerates and the bony surfaces rub against each other. This leads to stiffness and loss of movement in the joints.

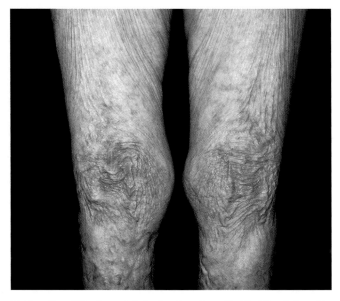

Deformity of the knee joints due to osteoarthritis. The deformity is present on the inner aspect of the knee. This is painful to patients and may limit mobility and range of motion. Courtesy of Viewing Medicine

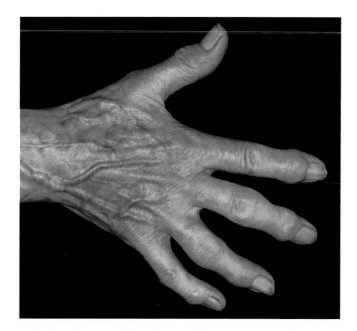

Heberden's nodes are visible on the last joint of the fingers. The joint is stiff and painful for the patient. Courtesy of Viewing Medicine

ARTHRITIS, RHEUMATOID

Rheumatoid arthritis is an autoimmune disease causing chronic inflammation of the joints, occurring around the joints and organs, including the kidneys and lungs. Patients may experience periods of remission and exacerbation. The joints most commonly affected are the wrists, knees, fingers, ankles, and feet.

Assessment

- Pain in joints
- Stiffness in the morning
- Swelling of joints
- Deformities of hands and feet

Planning and Implementation

- Range of motion
- Pain relief
- Pharmacologic therapy
- Application of heat

Evaluation and Outcomes

The patient will:

- Be able to complete activities of daily living
- Maintain full range of motion in joints
- Be free of pain
- Understand medication regimen
- Maintain body image

Nursing Considerations

- Nurses need to monitor for systemic effects of rheumatoid arthritis, including pericarditis, pulmonary fibrosis, pulmonary nodules, and pleurisy.

- Instruct the patient on the importance of rest and conservation of energy.

- Teach the patient about medication therapy including salicylates, NSAIDs, cytotoxic drugs, disease modifying agents, and gold therapy, and compliance with the therapy.

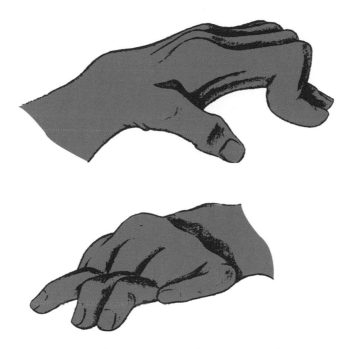

Rheumatoid arthritis causes chronic inflammation of the joint, leading to disfigurement of the joints. Joints are very painful, making it difficult for patients to complete their activities of daily living.

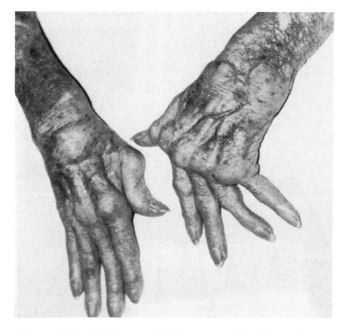

Rheumatoid arthritis causes disfigurement of the joints. A patient with joint deformities will have issues with an alteration of body image.

ASTHMA

Asthma is a chronic inflammatory disease of the airways, resulting in inflammation of the lining of the airways with increased mucus production. The cause is unknown but asthma often is "triggered" by certain factors such as allergens. Triggers include upper respiratory infections, gastroesophageal reflux disease, exercise, pollens, smoke, pollution, emotions, and menses.

Assessment

- Shortness of breath
- Chest tightness
- Wheezing
- Coughing

Planning and Implementation

- Bronchodilators
- Supplemental oxygen
- Breath sounds
- Vital signs

Evaluation and Outcomes

The patient will:

- Have clear breath sounds
- Be without shortness of breath
- Identify "triggers"
- Understand pharmacologic therapy

Nursing Considerations

Patients should be instructed to receive yearly flu shots and the Pneumovax.

Patients can consider treatments for allergies and undergo allergy testing.

Patients should be instructed on proper use of inhalation medications.

49

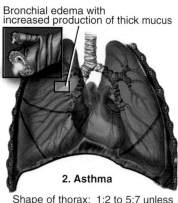

Bronchial edema with
increased production of thick mucus

2. Asthma

Shape of thorax: 1:2 to 5:7 unless
  chronic may have barrel chest
Tracheal position: midline
Percussion: hyperresonant
Adventitious sounds: wheezes

*Asthma is a condition that leads to
a narrowing of the airways, causing
hypoxia. There is also an increase
in the production of mucus. Patients
complain of shortness of breath and
wheezes are audible.*

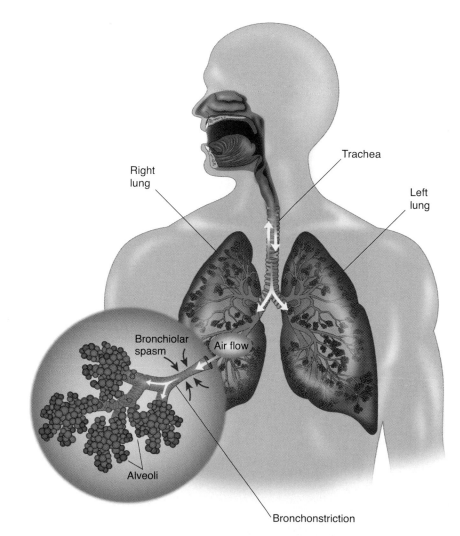

*The bronchoconstriction that occurs in asthmatics blocks the flow of oxygen to the
alveoli, causing extreme hypoxia. The mainstay of therapy is the use of bronchodilators to open up the airways.*

ATELECTASIS

Atelectasis is a collapse of the alveoli, affecting a part or an entire lung; it is caused by secretions, tumors, or postoperative complications.

Assessment

- Shortness of breath
- Decreased breath sounds over affected area
- Decreased oxygen levels
- Chest pain

Planning and Implementation

- Assess breath sounds
- Coughing and deep breathing exercises
- Supplemental oxygen
- Oxygen saturation levels

Evaluation and Outcomes

The patient will:

- Have a normal oxygen level
- Be without shortness of breath
- Have normal breath sounds
- Cough and deep breath

Nursing Considerations

- Atelectasis is a common postoperative complication making it imperative for the patient to cough and deep breathe and use the incentive spirometer after surgery.

- Encourage early ambulation after surgery to help prevent atelectasis.

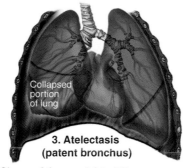

**3. Atelectasis
(patent bronchus)**

Shape of thorax: 1:2 to 5:7
Tracheal position: shifts to affected side
Percussion: dull
Adventitious sounds: crackles or wheezes

Atelectasis is a collapse of a portion of the alveoli even when the bronchi are intact. This is a common condition following surgery. Breath sounds are diminished over the portion of alveoli that are collapsed. Coughing and deep breathing exercises help prevent atelectasis.

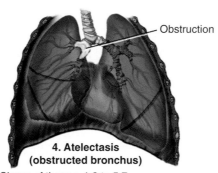

**4. Atelectasis
(obstructed bronchus)**

Shape of thorax: 1:2 to 5:7
Tracheal position: shifts to affected side
Percussion: dull
Adventitious sounds: absent

Another cause of atelectasis is occlusion of the bronchi from secretions. This occurs in patients with pneumonia. Breath sounds are absent or diminished over the affected area. Coughing and deep breathing exercises help prevent atelectasis.

BELL'S PALSY

Bell's palsy is a temporary unilateral facial paralysis resulting from damage to the 7th cranial nerve, and it is the most common cause of facial paralysis. The etiology of Bell's palsy is unknown, but may be viral or immunodeficiency.

Assessment

- Twitching
- Unilateral facial paralysis
- Excessive tearing
- Ptosis
- Drooling

Planning and Implementation

- Control secretions
- Eye protection
- Small, frequent meals with a soft diet
- Pain management

Evaluation and Outcomes

The patient will:

- Be free of pain
- Have return of facial movement
- Maintain adequate dietary intake
- Understand pharmacological treatment

Nursing Considerations

- Bell's palsy is more common in adults >40 years of age.

- Recovery is in 1-4 weeks with 70% achieving complete recovery.

- Teach the patient to keep the affected eye covered with an eye patch.

- Teach patient to apply warm moist heat over the affected area to help decrease the pain.

- Teach the patient to perform facial exercises three or four times a day to strengthen facial muscles. Exercises include whistling, grimacing, and blowing air out of the cheeks.

- Instruct patient that a soft diet may be needed to help decrease pain with eating.

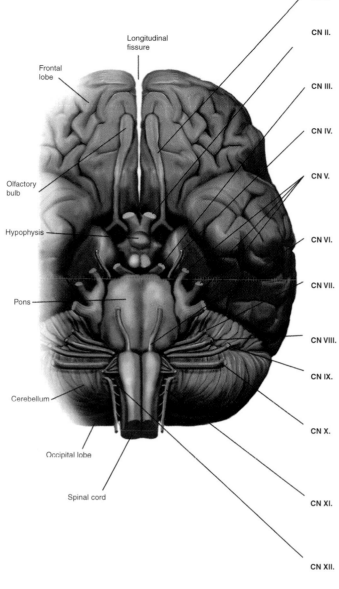

CN I.	Olfactory
	Function: Sense of smell (Sensory)
CN II.	Optic
	Function: Arises from retinas of the eyes and carries impulses associated with vision (Sensory)
CN III.	Oculomotor
	Function: Controls extrinsic eye muscles and regulates pupil size (Motor and Sensory)
CN IV.	Trochlear
	Function: Aids voluntary movements of eyeballs (Motor and Sensory)
CN V.	Trigeminal
	Function: Controls major sensory nerves of the face. Has 3 divisions: ophthalmic, maxillary, and mandibular (Motor and Sensory)
CN VI.	Abducens
	Function: Supplies the lateral rectus muscle of the eyes (Motor and Sensory)
CN VII.	Facial
	Function: Supplies the muscles of the face, scalp, taste buds, and lacrimal glands (Motor and Sensory)
CN VIII.	Vestibulocochlear
	Function: Supplies the ears (Sensory)
CN IX.	Glossopharyngeal
	Function: Supplies the tongue and pharynx, taste buds, and the carotid sinus (Motor and Sensory)
CN X.	Vagus
	Function: Runs close to common carotid arteries and internal jugular veins to the thorax and lower abdomen; has a broad parasympathetic distribution (Motor and Sensory)
CN XI.	Spinal Accessory
	Function: Supplies the trapezius and sternocleidomastoid muscles; responsible for proprioception (Motor and Sensory)
CN XII.	Hypoglossal
	Function: Supplies intrinsic and extrinsic muscles of tongue; involved in proprioception (Motor and Sensory)

The cranial with their respective functions. Bell's palsy affects cranial nerve VII, the facial nerve. This nerve is both motor and sensory supplying muscles of the face, scalp, taste buds, and lacrimal glands. There is loss of motor function of the facial muscles and pain from the sensory portion of the nerve.

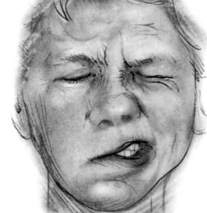

The patient with Bell's palsy usually is affected on one side of the face. Note the asymmetry of the facial expression. The pain occurs on the affected side of the face. The affected eye should be covered with an eye patch until the condition resolves, usually in 1-2 months.

BONE CANCER

Description/Definition

Bone cancer is caused by different types of primary tumors, including osteosarcomas, Ewing's sarcomas, chondrosarcomas, and fibrosarcomas. Osteosarcoma is the most common type of primary tumor, and is most often found in the distal femur, proximal tibia, and humerus. Bone cancer may also be a metastatic site from primary tumors of the prostate, breast, kidney, thyroid, and lungs.

Assessment

- Pain
- Swelling
- Low-grade fever
- Tender, palpable mass

Planning and Implementation

- Pain management
- Activities of daily living
- Maintain mobility
- Supportive care

Evaluation and Outcomes

The patient will:

- Understand medical therapy
- Maintain independence
- Perform activities of daily living
- Be pain-free

Nursing considerations

- Multiple myeloma is the most common primary bone tumor.

- Instruct the patient that treatment may include amputation of the affected limb.

- Monitor the patient with cancer for bone pain, since metastatic bone tumors are a complication.

- Nurses need to monitor the patient for an elevated level of serum calcium.

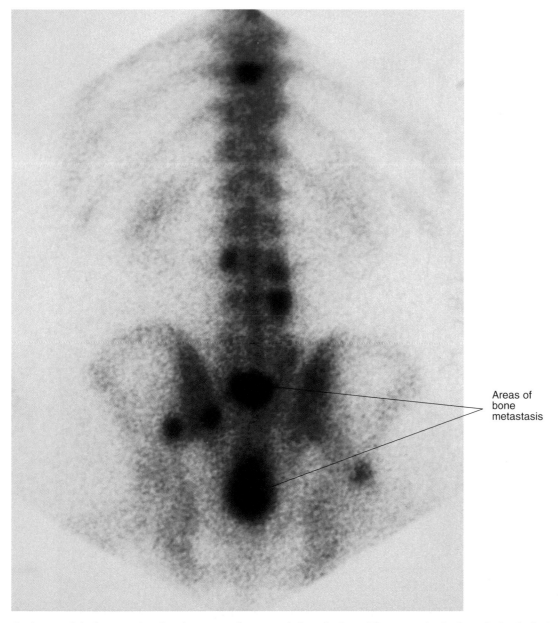

Areas of
bone
metastasis

An image of the lower spine showing areas of metastasis into the bone. The cancer in the bone is the dark circular areas. The patient would have complaints of lower back pain. (Courtesy of Viewing Medicine)

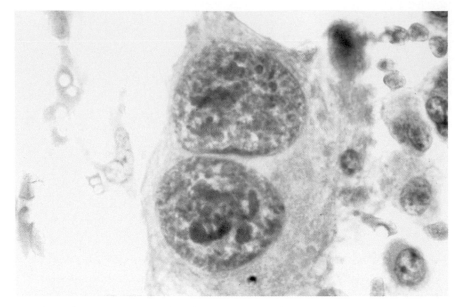

Histology of an osteosarcoma taken from an aspirate of a leg mass. (Courtesy of NCI)

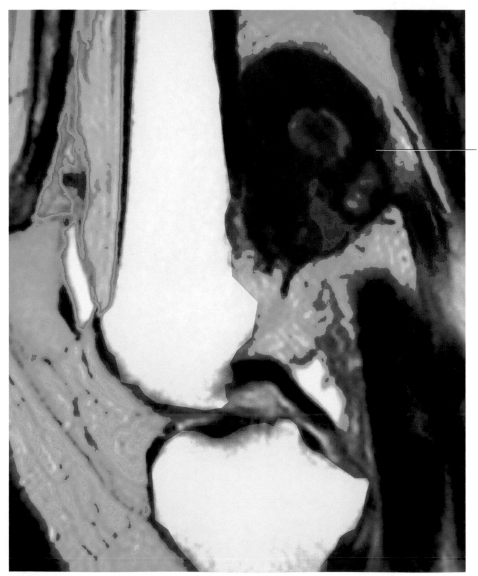

Bone tumor in red

An MRI scan of an osteosarcoma affecting the lower end of the fibia. The tumor is falsely colored in red. (Courtesy of Viewing Medicine)

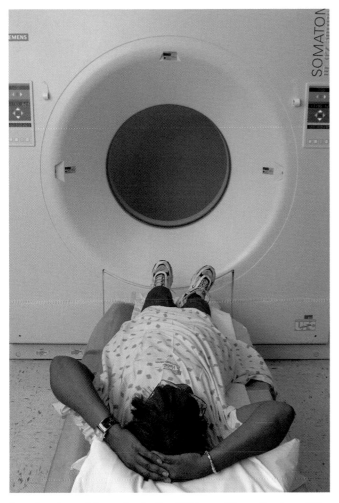

A patient in position to begin the CAT scan. The patient must lie flat and still during the time the scan is being done.

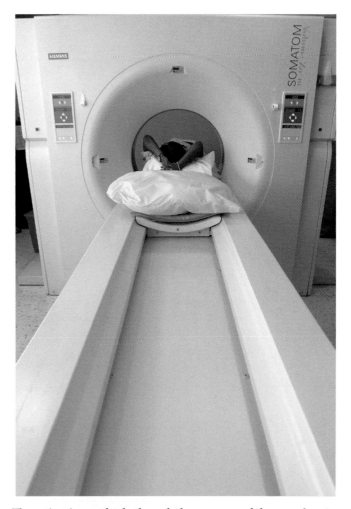

The patient is completely through the scanner and the procedure is complete. The process usually takes five to ten minutes to complete.

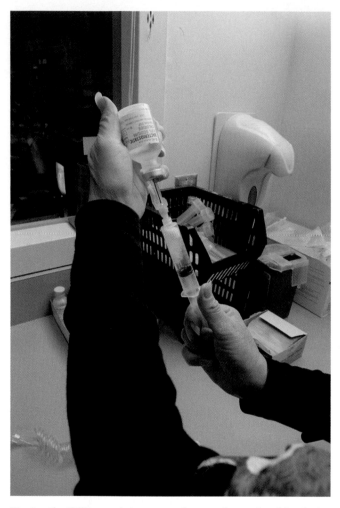

During the CAT scan, intravenous dye may be used and is administered by the technician in the radiology department. The patient should be checked for shellfish and iodine allergies prior to be given the contrast dye.

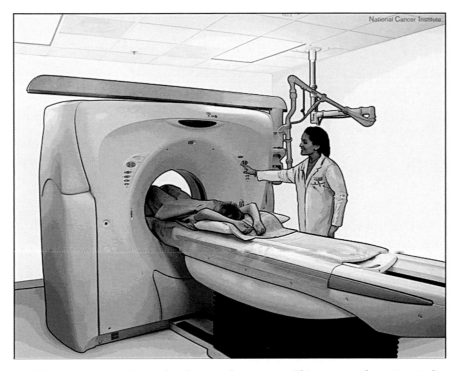

A CAT scan is commonly used to diagnose bone cancer. This requires the patient to lie still during the procedure. Patients may need pain medicine prior to the procedure because it may be uncomfortable for them to lie flat. Injection of intravenous contrast may be used to identify the areas of cancer. If contrast dye is to be used, patients need to be checked for allergies to shellfish or iodine. (Courtesy of NCI)

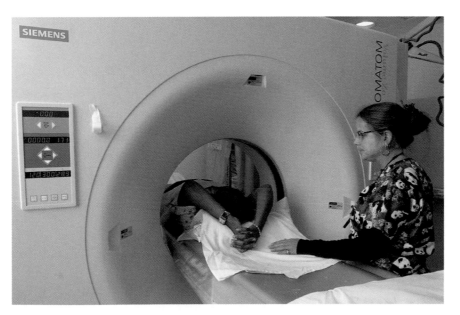

The patient slowly enters the scanning machine. The patient who is claustrophobic may require sedation for this procedure.

BREAST CANCER

Description/Definition

Breast cancer is the leading cause of death in women aged 35-54 years. The most common type is infiltrating ductal carcinoma, which originates in the epithelial cells lining the mammary ducts. Tumors invade lymph channels and carry tumor cells to the lymph nodes in the axilla. Sites of metastasis include bone, lungs, and brain. Breast cancer is the most common malignancy in women.

Assessment

- Lump in the breast
- Breast tenderness
- Discharge from the nipple/inversion of the nipple
- Family history, particularly on the mother's side

Planning and Implementation

- Location, size, and shape of mass
- Discharge from the nipple
- Family history (Maternal)
- Breast self-exam and routine mammograms

Evaluation and Outcomes

The patient will:

- Obtain routine mammograms
- Perform monthly self-breast exam
- Understand medical treatment
- Maintain body image

Nursing Considerations

- Nurses need to be aware that breast cancer does occur in men.

- Teach the patient to perform monthly self-breast exams at the same time of the menstrual cycle.

- Teach the patient to obtain yearly mammograms starting at age 40.

- If a mastectomy is performed, teach the patient to avoid deodorant, lotion, and ointments on the arm of the affected side.

- Instruct the patient that lymphedema (swelling) may occur on the extremity of the affected side, and blood pressure and venipunctures should be avoided on that arm.

- Nurses should provide information to patients on support groups available for patients with breast cancer.

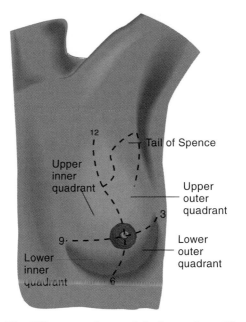

The different quadrants of the breast tissue. The Tail of Spence is located near the axilla, and patients must be taught to be sure to palpate this area when doing a self-breast exam.

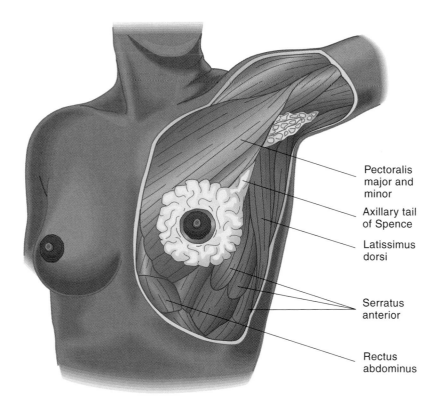

The major muscles of the breast. In a radical mastectomy, the muscles are removed along with all the breast tissue and lymph nodes. This is done to be sure that all cancerous cells are removed.

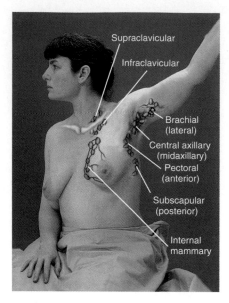

The lymphatic tissue associated with the breast. Cancer cells invade these lymph nodes and may be spread through these lymph nodes to other body tissues such as the lung or brain. This spreading is known as metastasis.

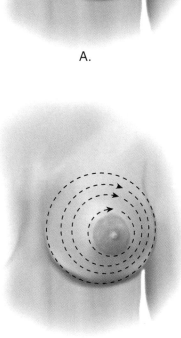

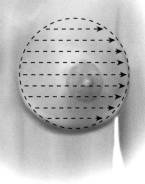

There are three different methods of palpation for a self-breast exam. These are the wedge, concentric circles, and parallel lines methods. In the wedge method, the patient divides the breast into six sections and starts at the outer edge and palpates inward to the nipple in each section or wedge. Using concentric circles, the breast is palpated starting at the outer edge and in a circular fashion palpates going inward to the nipple. Using parallel lines, the exam starts at the bottom of the breast and goes from the breast bone to the side of the body upward to the top of the breast.

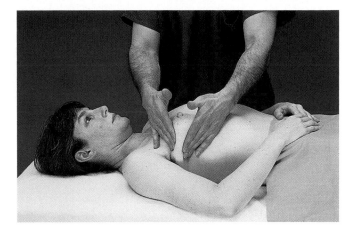

The nurse palpates the glandular tissue. Patients need to be taught to include palpation of this glandular tissue as well as the actual breast.

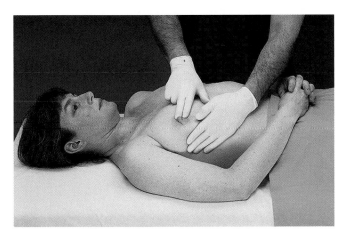

The nurse palpates the areola. The patient needs to be taught to palpate the areola in addition to the actual breast tissue when performing a self-breast exam.

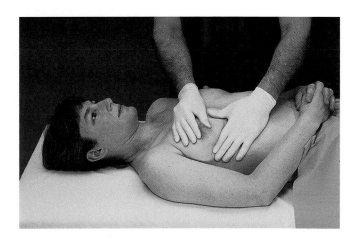

The last part of performing a breast exam is to squeeze the nipple to check for abnormal discharge.

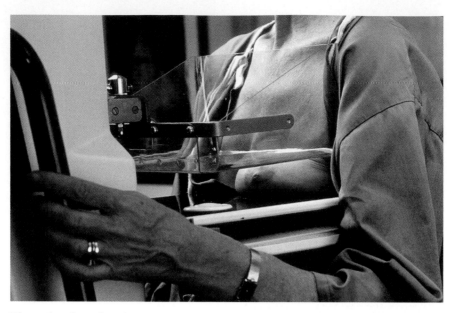

The patient is undergoing a mammogram. A mammogram is recommended as a screening for breast cancer. Yearly mammograms should begin at age 40. (Courtesy of NCI)

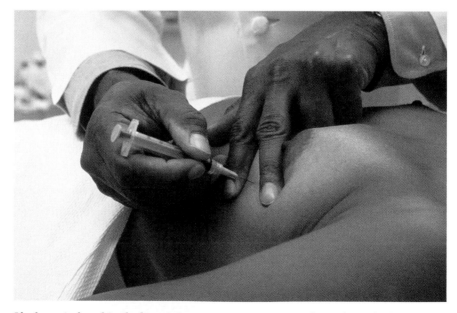

If a lump is found in the breast tissue a needle biopsy may be performed. The needle aspirates cells which are then examined for the presence of cancerous cells. The area is injected with an anesthetic prior to the insertion of the needle to perform the aspiration of cells. (Courtesy of NCI)

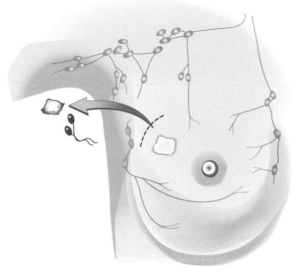

This illustrates removal of lymph nodes or a lymph node biopsy. These lymph nodes are then tested for the presence of cancerous cells. If cancerous cells are detected, further treatment is required. Treatment may include surgery, radiation, and/or chemotherapy depending upon how many of the lymph nodes were positive for the presence of cancer cells. (Courtesy of NCI)

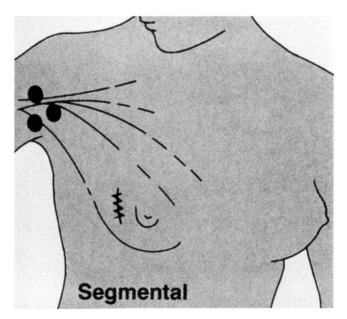

When the diagnosis of breast cancer is made, the patient may undergo a lumpectomy. In this procedure, only the lump in the breast is removed. A lumpectomy is considered when only a few lymph nodes were positive for the presence of cancer cells. (Courtesy of NCI)

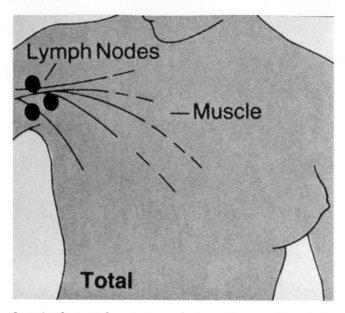

In a simple or total mastectomy, the breast tissue and the nipple are removed but the lymph nodes and muscle are left intact. The decision is individualized based upon the patient's history and surgeon's preference. (Courtesy of NCI)

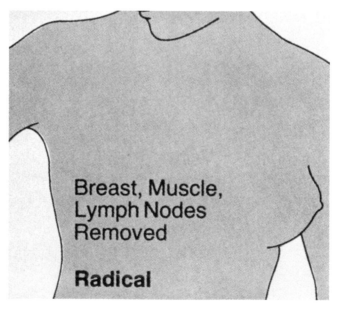

In a radical mastectomy the breast, nipple, muscle and lymph nodes are removed. Patients who have had lymph nodes removed are at risk for developing lymphedema in that extremity and should not have blood pressure, blood draws or IVs in that extremity. Lymphedema will always be present. (Courtesy of NCI)

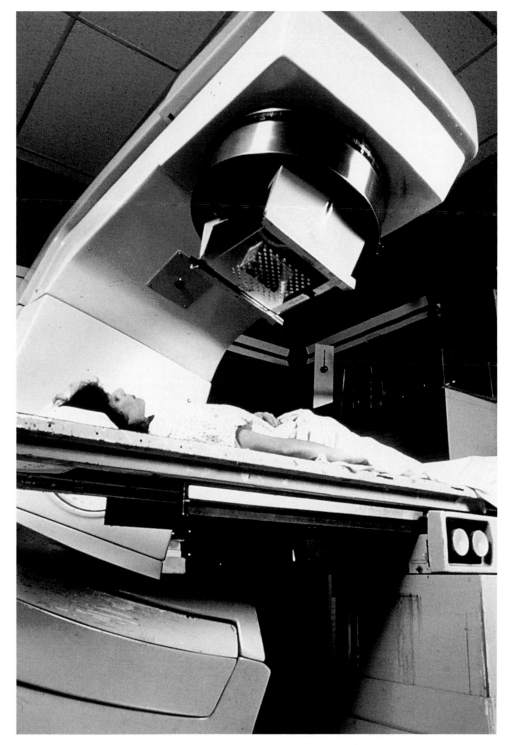

This patient is undergoing radiation therapy to treat breast cancer. The radiation may burn the skin, therefore, the nurse must assess the areas undergoing radiation for skin integrity and skin breakdown.

BREAST, FIBROCYSTIC DISEASE

Description/Definition

Fibrocystic disease, or cystic disease or dysplasia, is a benign condition in which there are one or more nodules that are palpable in the breast tissue, and which are usually associated with changes in hormonal levels. Fibrocystic changes typically occur during ovulation and prior to menses.

Assessment

- Lump in the breast
- Breast tenderness and fullness
- Swelling prior to menstrual cycle
- Discharge from the nipple

Planning and Implementation

- Breast self-exam
- Dietary history
- Pain management
- Use of vitamin therapy

Evaluation and Outcomes

The patient will:

- Verbalize relief of pain
- Perform monthly self-breast exams
- Identify dietary modification, e.g., limit caffeine intake, salt intake
- Understand hormonal therapy as prescribed

Nursing Considerations

- Teach patients to perform a self-breast exam during the same time each month of the menstrual cycle.

- Teach patients to avoid caffeine and limit salt intake, as this may cause the breasts to become more tender and painful.

- Instruct patients that fibrocystic breast disease often occurs in both breasts.

- Teach patients to wear a well-padded, supportive brassiere to give the breasts adequate support.

- Instruct patients that application of heat or cold may help alleviate the pain.

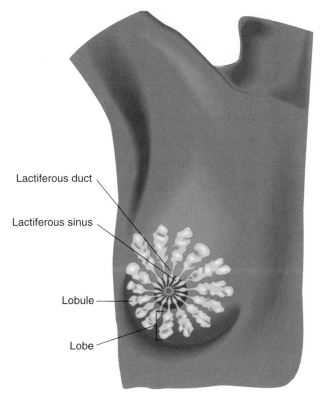

Lactiferous duct

Lactiferous sinus

Lobule

Lobe

The glandular tissue of the breast. Patients with fibrocystic breast disease feel lumps like marbles on self-breast exam.

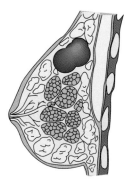

The cysts or lumps occur in the breast tissue and are painful to the patient.

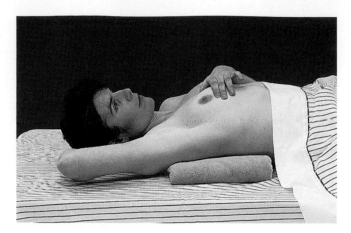

Self-breast exam can be done while lying in bed. Patients need to be taught to perform a self-breast exam at the same time each month.

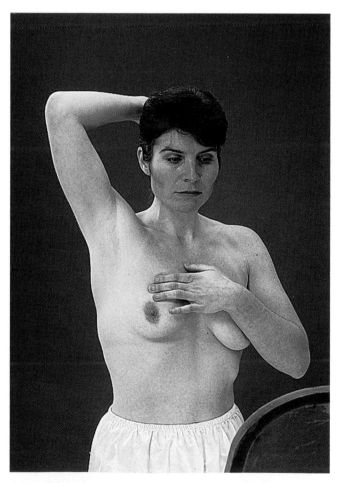

Self-breast exam can be done while standing. The breast is palpated in a circular fashion from the outer edge of the breast inward to the nipple.

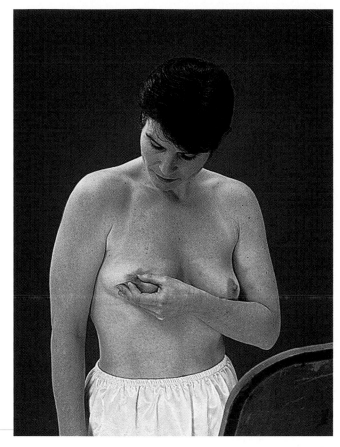

After palpation of the breast tissue, the nipple is palpated and then compressed to examine for discharge. Any discharge from the nipple is considered abnormal and should be reported to the physician.

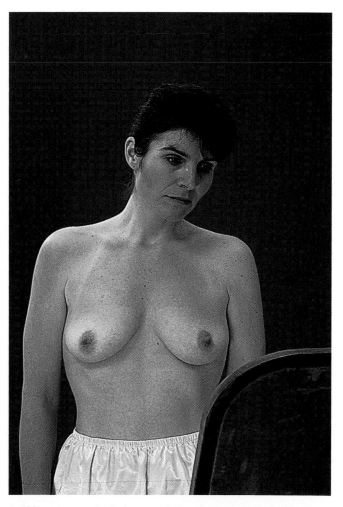

Self-breast exam includes examining the breasts with the arms at the side before a mirror. The breast is examined for abnormal lumps.

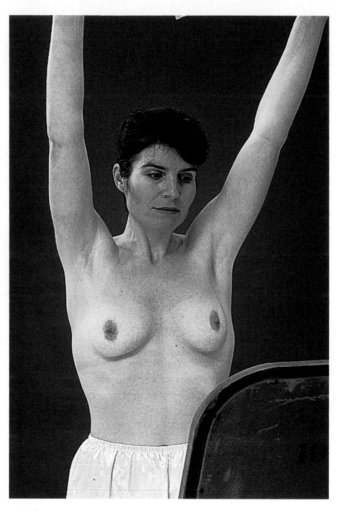

Self-breast exam includes standing before a mirror and raising the arms overhead to look for any abnormal lumps.

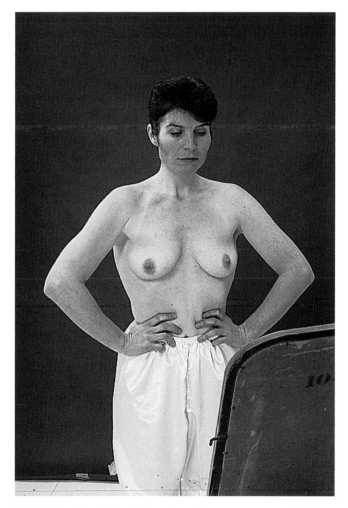

While standing in front of a mirror, the arms are pressed into the hips and the breast is examined for any abnormal lumps.

BUERGER'S DISEASE

Description/Definition

Buerger's disease is the acute inflammation and thrombosis of arteries and veins, typically affecting the hands and feet. It is also called thromboangitis obliterans.

Assessment

- Claudication
- Pain in the extremitites
- Paresthesia in the extremities
- Ulcerations

Planning and Implementation

- Circulation of the extremities
- Sensation and movement of extremities
- Pain
- Smoking history

Evaluation and Outcomes

The patient will:

- Verbalize need to stop smoking
- Be pain-free
- Maintain adequate sensation and function
- Maintain adequate skin integrity in extremities

Nursing Considerations

- Instruct patients to avoid tobacco, as patients who smoke are at a much higher risk for developing Buerger's disease.

- Teach patients to avoid extreme or prolonged exposure to cold.

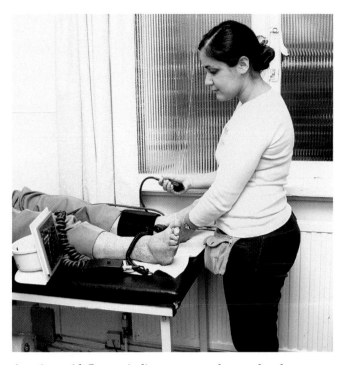

A patient with Buerger's disease may undergo a doppler pressure measurement. A blood pressure cuff is wrapped around the lower extremity and the blood pressure is checked. Because blood flow is diminished, the pressure may also be lowered compared to a blood pressure checked in the upper extremities. (Courtesy of Viewing Medicine)

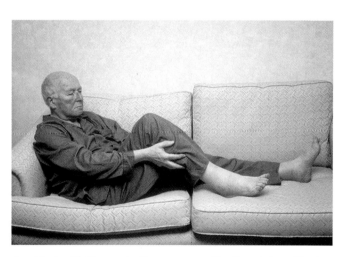

A patient with Buerger's disease may suffer from intermittent claudication or pain occurring in the lower leg. The pain in the lower leg is caused from inadequate blood flow to the muscles. The patient may feel this pain when walking, and it may go away when the activity is over. (Courtesy of Viewing Medicine)

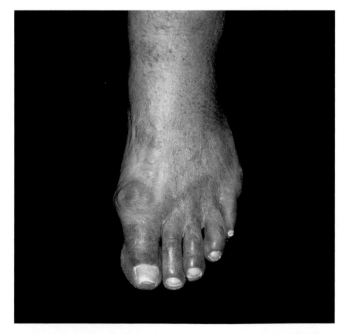

A ruby red or rubor color may be seen in the feet in a patient with Buerger's disease. Note the redness, especially over the toes. This discoloration is due to the poor arterial circulation. (Courtesy of Viewing Medicine)

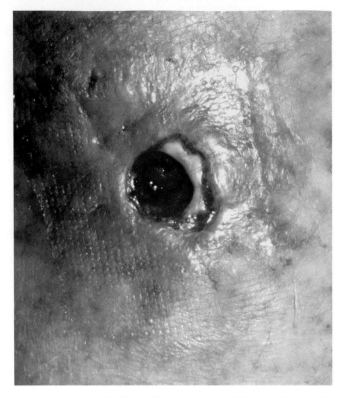

An ulceration on the lower leg as a result of decreased arterial blood flow. Because of the diminished blood flow, it is very difficult for these ulcers to heal and the ulcers are at a higher risk for infection. The treatment is a topical antibiotic and the wound is covered with a sterile dressing. (Courtesy of Viewing Medicine)

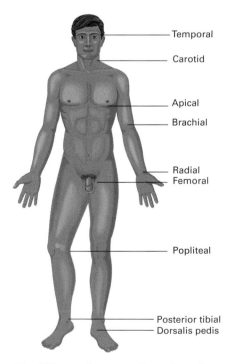

The different places to palpate the pulse. The nurse must assess the character and quality of pulses in the patient with Buerger's disease. The peripheral pulses may become diminished as the disease progresses.

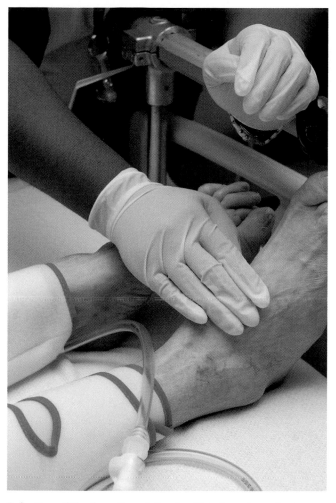

Palpation of the dorsalis pedal pulse. This is an important assessment in the patient with Buerger's disease because the arterial blood flow is diminished. A lack of a palpable pulse indicates poor blood flow, and will result in tissue ischemia and death. Patients will have severe pain as blood flow decreases.

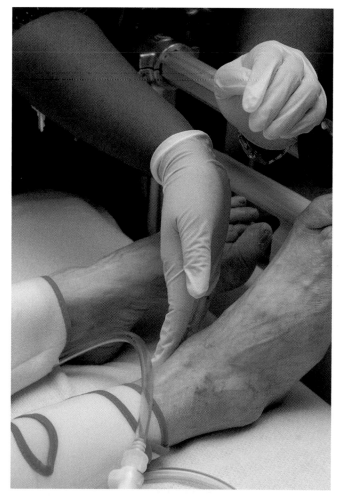

Palpation of the posterior tibial pulse. This is an important assessment in a patient with Buerger's disease, because the arterial blood flow is compromised. As blood flow decreases, patients experience severe pain in the extremity.

BURNS

Burns are an injury to the tissue caused from exposure to thermal, chemical, electrical of radioactive agents. Burns are classified by extent of tissue affected: superficial thickness extends through the epidermis, partial thickness extends into the dermis, and full thickness extends through the epidermis and dermis.

Assessment

- Percentage of skin affected
- Airway
- Vital signs, blood pressure
- Intravascular blood volume status
- Signs and symptoms of infection

Planning and Implementation

- Maintain adequate airway
- Maintain adequate blood volume
- Pain management
- Strict sterile technique for all procedures

Evaluation and Outcomes

The patient will:

- Be free of infection
- Have stable vital signs
- Be free of pain
- Maintain body image

Nursing Considerations

- Nurses need to be aware that skin in the elderly patient is thinner, therefore, burns tend to be more extensive in elderly patients.

- Nurses need to assess the patient with an electrical burn for the presence of rhabdomyolysis including assessing serum creatinine levels and elevated creatinine phosphokinase levels.

- Instruct patients that they may require several plastic surgery operations including the application of skin grafts following a severe burn injury.

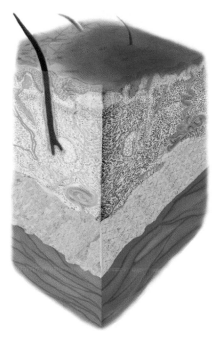

In first degree or superficial burns, the injury is to the epidermal layer of the skin. A sunburn is a superficial burn.

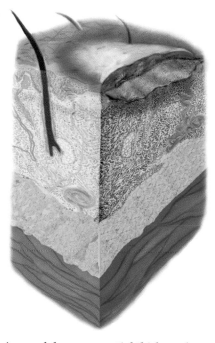

A second degree or partial thickness burn extends through the epidermis into the upper layers of the dermis. The skin is red and painful with blisters and swelling at the site. The nurse must monitor for signs of infection and volume loss.

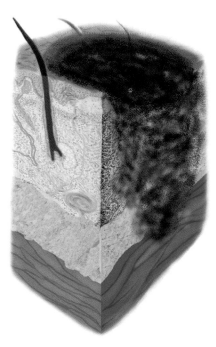

A third degree or full thickness burn extends through the epidermis, dermis, and into the subcutaneous tissue. The skin is dry, leathery, and charred in appearance. These burns usually require debridement and skin grafting. The nurse must assess for volume loss and monitor for signs of infection.

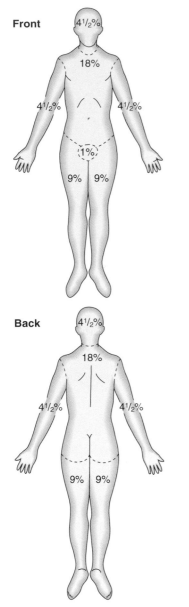

Front

4¹/₂%

18%

4¹/₂%   4¹/₂%

1%

9% 9%

Back

4¹/₂%

18%

4¹/₂%   4¹/₂%

9% 9%

The "Rule of Nines" is used to estimate the percentage of body surface
that is burned. Each section of the
body is given a percentage. The
areas that are burned are added
together and this is the percentage
of burned area. Percentages for
each section of the body are different for the adult, teen, and child, as
shown.

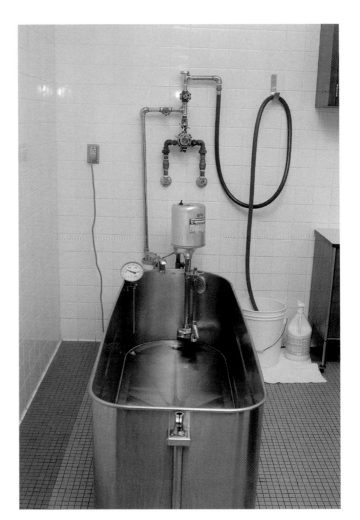

Whirlpool therapy is used to debride the burn wound. Patients
should be given pain medicine prior to whirlpool therapy.
Whirlpool therapy is used when dead tissue needs to be removed
from the burned area. Whirlpool therapy continues until the
dead tissue is completely removed.

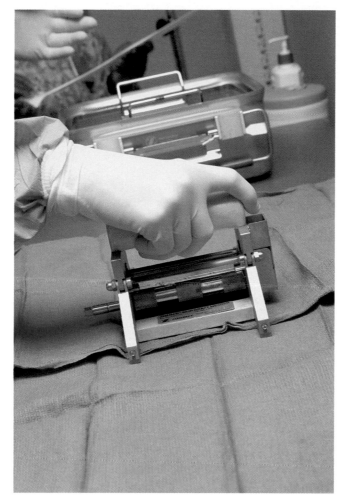

Skin grafting may be needed for treatment of burns. This equipment is used in the operating room to prepare for skin grafting. This piece of equipment is used to prepare the graft before it is placed on the patient.

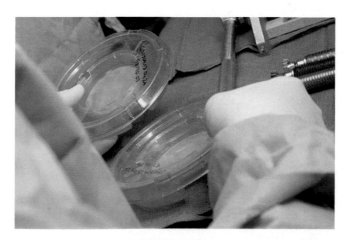

Pieces of skin graft that will be used to cover the burn wound.

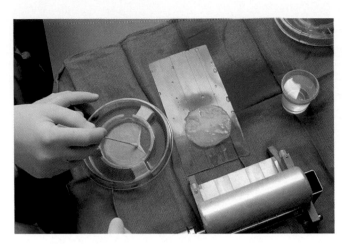

The pieces of grafting material being prepared for grafting.

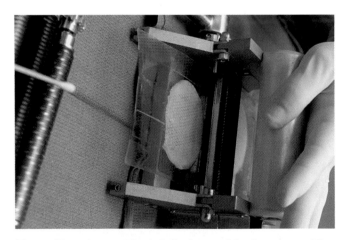

The grafting piece continues to be prepared by the surgeon. The equipment is used to smooth out the graft.

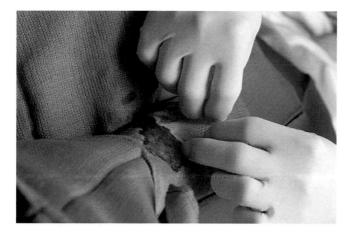

Application of the skin graft to the burn wound.

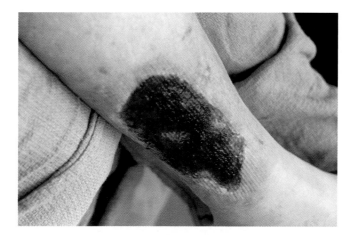

The skin graft on the wound. The graft is barely visible. The graft will adhere to the wound and provide a protective covering. Epithelial cells grow over the graft and the graft is incorporated into the patient's own skin.

CARDIAC ARRHYTHMIAS

Cardiac arrhythmias are caused by disturbances in the electrical conduction system in the heart. Arrhythmias may be caused by electrolyte imbalances or valvular dysfunction, and may be life-threatening. The most common arrhythmias are atrial fibrillation, ventricular tachycardia, and ventricular fibrillation.

Assessment

- Irregular pulse
- Chest pain
- Shortness of breath
- Lethargy
- Syncope

Planning and Implementation

- Administer oxygen
- Obtain 12-lead electrocardiogram
- Assess pulses
- Vital signs

Evaluation and Outcomes

- The patient will:
- Be free of chest pain and shortness of breath
- Return to a normal rhythm
- Have normal serum electrolyte values

Nursing Considerations

- Instruct patient on prescribed medications.

- Monitor serum potassium levels because low levels can be a cause of arrhythmias.

- Monitor serum magnesium levels since low levels may precipitate cardiac arrhythmias.

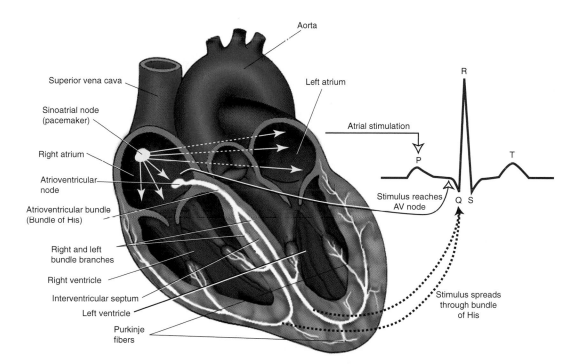

The cardiac conduction system. The sinoatrial node, located in the right atrium, is the pacemaker of the heart. The rhythm that originates from the sinoatrial node is called a sinus rhythm.

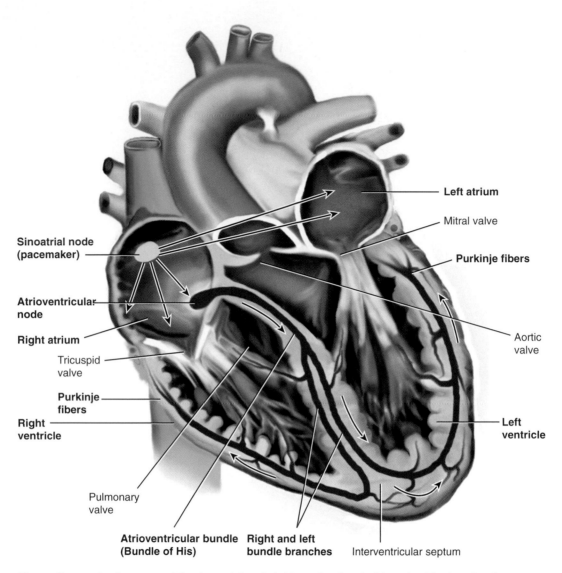

Sinoatrial node
(pacemaker)

Atrioventricular
node

Right atrium

Tricuspid
valve

Purkinje
fibers

Right
ventricle

Pulmonary
valve

Atrioventricular bundle **Right and left**
(Bundle of His) **bundle branches** Interventricular septum

Left atrium

Mitral valve

Purkinje fibers

Aortic
valve

Left
ventricle

The cardiac conduction system. The sinoatrial node initiates the electrical impulse. The impulse then is conducted through the atrium to the atrioventricular node, located in the lower portion of the right atrium above the tricuspid valve. The impulse is then conducted to the Bundle of His and then separates into the right and left bundle branches, which spread the impulse through the right and left ventricles, respectively. The terminal portion of the conduction system is at the Purkinje fibers located throughout each ventricle.

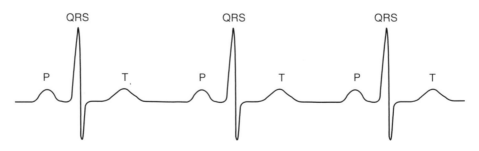

The electrical activity is represented on the electrocardiogram as a PQRST waveform. The P wave represents atrial electrical activity, the QRS and T waves represent ventricular electrical activity.

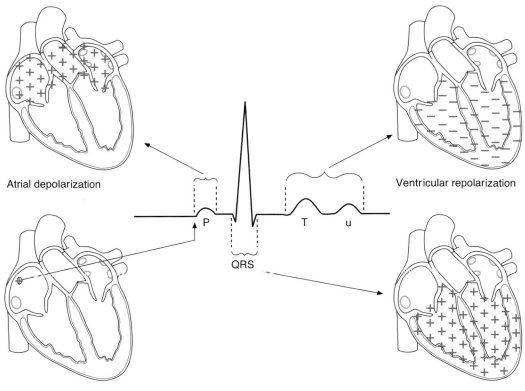

Atrial depolarization

Ventricular repolarization

Sinus node depolarization (no ECG deflection)

Ventricular depolarization

The correlation is shown between the electrical activity and the corresponding events in the heart.

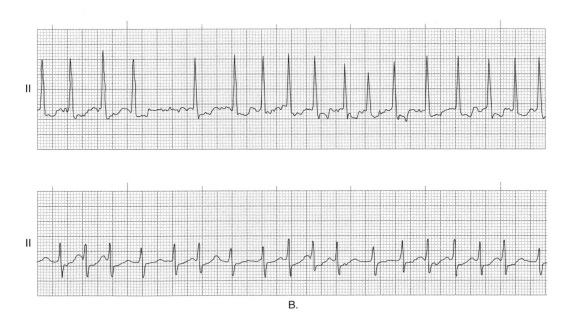

B.

This ECG represents atrial fibrillation, a common dysrhythmia. In this rhythm the atria quiver and do not contract. This leads to the stagnation of blood in the atria, which may lead to the possibility of clot formation.

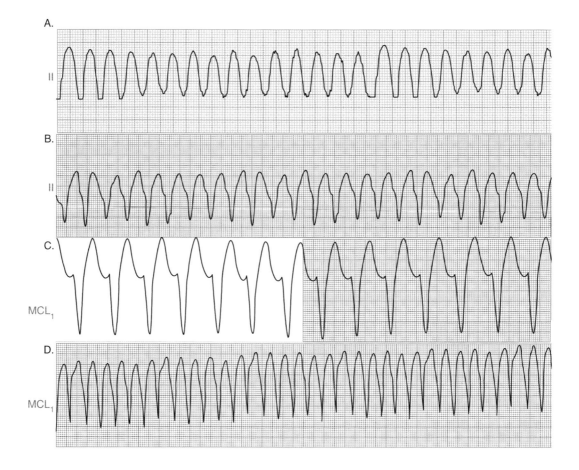

This ECG is ventricular tachycardia. This is a potentially life-threatening arrhythmia. The nurse needs to assess the patient by checking for responsiveness and assessing for breathing and a pulse.

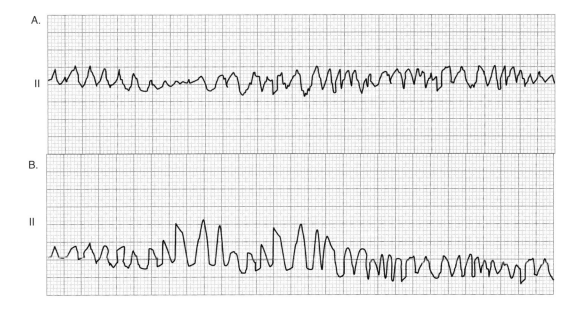

A.

II

B.

II

This ECG represents ventricular fibrillation. This is a life-threatening arrhythmia and leads to sudden death. The treatment is prompt defibrillation.

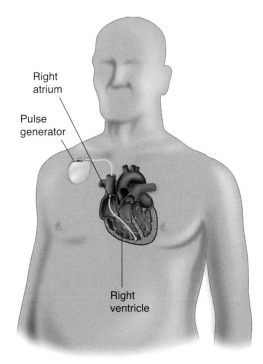

Right atrium

Pulse generator

Right ventricle

For patients who are susceptible to life-threatening dysrhythmias such as ventricular fibrillation, an internal cardioverter/defibrillator may be implanted. This device senses changes in the rhythm and delivers a shock to the heart.

CARPAL TUNNEL SYNDROME

Carpal tunnel syndrome is a neuropathy that occurs when there is a pressure on the median nerve at the point where it goes through the carpal tunnel of the wrist. It is associated with repetitive wrist motion.

Assessment

- Soreness of the wrist
- Tenderness of the wrist
- Weakness of the muscles of the thumb
- Numbness/tingling in the hand

Planning and Implementation

- Positive Tinel's sign (pain elicited by tapping over the medial nerve at the wrist)
- Positive Phalen's sign (pain and numbness when the wrist is flexed for a minute)
- Apply hand splints as ordered
- Administer non-steroidal medications as prescribed

Evaluation and Outcomes

The patient will:

- Maintain strength in the affected extremity
- Be free of pain
- Be able to perform activities of daily living
- Understand use of wrist splint

Nursing Considerations

- Patients may require modifications of occupational activities to relieve symptoms.

- Instruct patients that wearing a wrist splint at night may help decrease pain.

- Refer patients to their employee health department where they are employed; also refer them for potential Workers' Compensation.

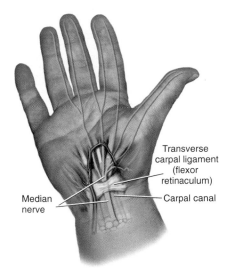

Transverse
carpal ligament
(flexor
retinaculum)

Median
nerve

Carpal canal

*The median nerve runs through the carpal
canal or tunnel located at the top of the
wrist.*

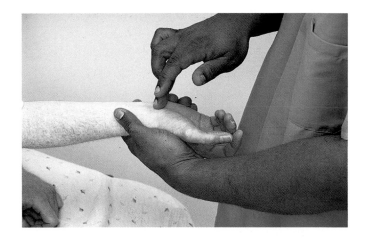

*Tinel's sign is used to assess for the presence of carpal tunnel
syndrome. To assess for this, the nurse taps over the medial nerve
at the wrist to elicit a pain response.*

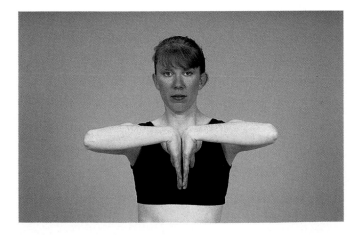

*Phalen's sign is also done to assess for carpal tunnel syndrome.
A positive Phalen's sign is pain and numbness when the wrist is
flexed for a full minute.*

CATARACT

A cataract is defined as an opacity of the lens of the eye. Cataracts result from the formation of protein clumps in the lens of the eye, and are characterized by a yellowish haze and visual disturbances.

Assessment

- Blurred vision
- Decrease in color vision
- Diplopia
- Presence of a white pupil

Planning and Implementation

- Teach patient to have routine eye exams
- Teach patient use of eye drops
- Treatment usually involves surgery
- Postoperative care teaching includes avoiding activities that increase intraocular pressure, including bending over, vomiting, coughing, sneezing, and lifting heavy objects.

Evaluation and Outcomes

The patient will:

- Understand postoperative care restrictions
- Be able to administer own eye drops
- Maintain safety
- Follow-up with routine eye exams

Nursing Considerations

- Instruct patients that cataracts form as part of the normal aging process, after traumatic eye injury, and may be a congenital defect in children.

- Instruct the diabetic patient that they may be more at risk for developing cataracts.

- Teach patients that their color perception may be altered.

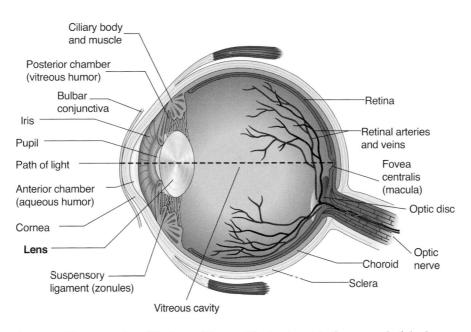

Ciliary body and muscle

Posterior chamber (vitreous humor)

Bulbar conjunctiva

Iris

Pupil

Path of light

Anterior chamber (aqueous humor)

Cornea

Lens

Suspensory ligament (zonules)

Vitreous cavity

Retina

Retinal arteries and veins

Fovea centralis (macula)

Optic disc

Optic nerve

Choroid

Sclera

A cataract is an opacity of the lens of the eye. The treatment is the removal of the lens with replacement of a new lens.

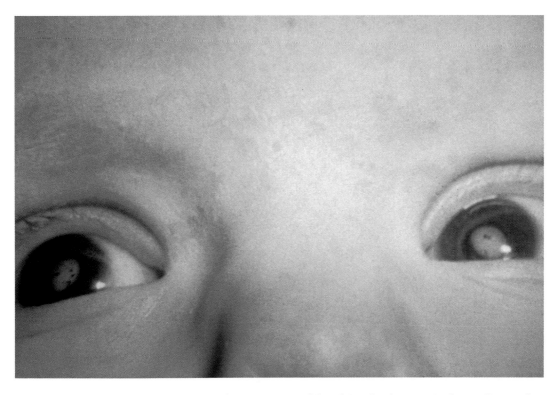

This patient has bilateral cataracts. Note the appearance of the white, cloudy areas in the pupil area of the eyes. The cataract is the white area. This patient would have cloudy vision with altered perception colors. (Courtesy of the CDC)

CELLULITIS

Cellulitis is an inflammation of the cellular or connective tissue, usually caused by Staphylococcus or Streptococcus bacteria. Other causes may be viral or fungal.

Assessment

- Recent history of skin trauma
- Redness and warmth over the affected area
- Edema of the area
- Pain and itching at the site

Planning and Implementation

- Assessment of the affected area
- Cleanse area with antibacterial soap
- Apply warm compresses
- Pain management
- Antibiotics, antifungals

Evaluation and Outcomes

The patient will:

- Be free of signs and symptoms of infection
- Be free of pain
- Understand and comply with treatment

Nursing Considerations

- Nurses should measure the circumference of the affected extremity in order to monitor the amount of swelling.

- Teach the patient to keep the affected area clean and dry and apply antibiotic ointment as ordered.

- Instruct patients that they may apply warm compresses to the affected area to assist with healing.

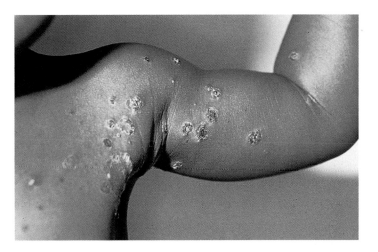

A patient with cellulitis on the face. Note the redness and swelling of the tissue. The area should be kept clean and dry to assist with healing. Antibiotic ointment may also be applied.

CEREBRAL HEMATOMAS, SUBDURAL AND EPIDURAL

Cerebral hematomas are located in the epidural or subdural spaces. Subdural hematomas, located beneath the dura, are typically venous and may be acute, subacute (occurring 6-20 days after injury) or chronic (slowly developing after minor trauma). Epidural hematomas, located above the dura, are from an arterial source, usually the middle meningeal artery.

Assessment

- Decreased level of consciousness
- Decreased heart rate and blood pressure
- Nausea and vomiting
- Decreased respirations

Planning and Implementation

- Neurologic assessment
- Vital signs
- Maintain airway
- Elevate head of bed
- Seizure precautions

Evaluation and Outcomes

The patient will:

- Maintain level of consciousness
- Maintain airway
- Maintain adequate vital signs
- Be free of seizures

Nursing Considerations

- Teach patients and families to immediately report to their physician signs and symptoms of increased intracranial pressure, such as a decreased level of consciousness, vomiting, and seizures.

- Any patients on blood thinners such as aspirin and Coumadin who has suffered a fall should be monitored for possible cerebral hematoma.

- A patients who has an epidural hematoma may experience a brief period of unconsciousness after the trauma but then become alert and oriented.

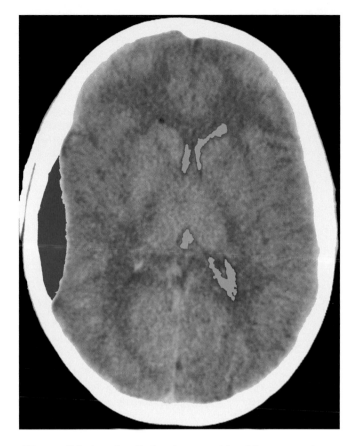

CT scan (falsely colored) showing an epidural hematoma (note the reddened area). The patient's neurological status should be assessed hourly.

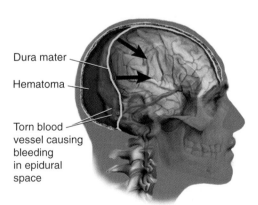

Dura mater

Hematoma

Torn blood vessel causing bleeding in epidural space

Epidural bleeds are also associated with skull fractures. Note the pressure the bleed puts on the brain tissue, causing displacement of the brain tissue. This shift leads to changes in the neurological status of the patient, such as a decrease in the level of consciousness, changes in vital signs, and changes in pupils.

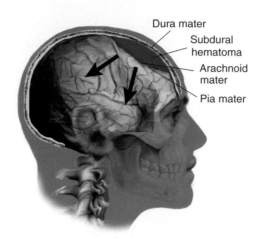

Dura mater
Subdural hematoma
Arachnoid mater
Pia mater

A subdural hematoma is located below the dura and is usually a result of a tear of veins under the dura mater. Subdural hematomas can develop rapidly or may accumulate slowly over a period of days, such as happens after a fall.

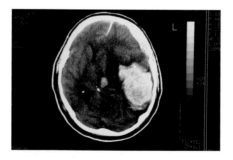

A CT scan reveals a subdural hematoma. It appears as the whitish area on the right side of the image.

CERVICAL CANCER

Cervical cancer is cancer of the cervix. Cervical cancer is classified as preinvasive, which is limited to the cervix, or invasive, which is found in the cervix and other pelvic structures. Cervical cancer is usually a squamous cell cancer.

Assessment

- Painless vaginal bleeding
- Abnormal vaginal discharge
- Weight loss
- Heavier or lighter than normal menses

Planning and Implementation

- Family history
- Monitor for postoperative complications
- Monitor for complications of radiation, chemotherapy
- Teaching on therapy

Evaluation and Outcomes

The patient will:

- Understand treatment options
- Be pain-free
- Have no complications from surgery, radiation, chemotherapy
- Maintain body image

Nursing Considerations

- Instruct patients that surgery alters the appearance of the vaginal opening and may result in scar tissue that causes painful intercourse and difficulties attaining orgasm.

- Discuss sexual concerns with the patient and significant other.

- Teach patients with daughters about the availability of the Human Papillovirus vaccine, which may decrease their daughter's risk of developing cervical cancer.

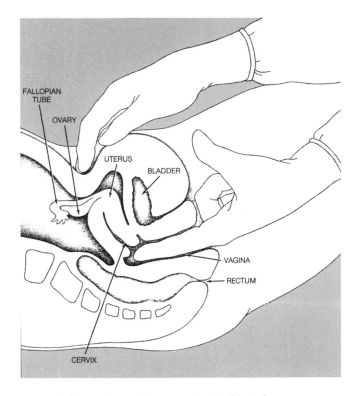

FALLOPIAN
TUBE

OVARY

UTERUS

BLADDER

VAGINA

RECTUM

CERVIX

A cervical exam is a routine screening to detect the presence of cervical cancer. Pressing down on the abdomen allows the examiner to palpate the cervix. (Courtesy of National Cancer Institute)

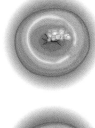

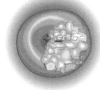

Cervical cancerous cells. The top picture shows the intial stages of the cancer, while the lower picture shows an advanced stage of the cancer.

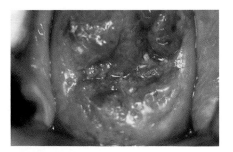

Cervical carcinoma in an advanced stage. The area may be painful and there may be a discharge from the cervix. (Courtesy of the CDC)

CHRONIC OBSTRUCTIVE PULMONARY DISEASE (COPD)

Chronic obstructive pulmonary disease (COPD) is a chronic lung disease which includes asthma, emphysema, and bronchitis, and is characterized by bronchoconstriction, mucus production, and dyspnea. Emphysema is the loss of lung elasticity and hyperinflation of the lungs. Bronchitis is inflammation of the bronchi.

AssessmentShortness of breath

- Chronic cough
- Use of accessory muscles
- Barrel chest

Planning and Implementation

- Administer oxygen
- Elevate head of bed
- Pulse oximetry
- Bronchodilators

Evaluation and Outcomes

The patient will:

- Be free of shortness of breath
- Oxygenate adequately on room air
- Maintain clear airway
- Perform activities of daily living
- Quit smoking

Nursing Considerations

- Monitor patients on high concentrations of oxygen, since high levels of oxygen may depress respiratory drive in COPD patients.

- Instruct patients that chocolate and milk may increase the thickness of secretions.

- Instruct the patient about smoking cessation programs/options.

- Instruct patients not to take over-the-counter cough suppressants.

- Instruct patients to receive yearly flu vaccinations and Pneumovax.

- Instruct patients on pursed lip breathing to help decrease their shortness of breath.

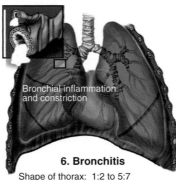

6. Bronchitis

Shape of thorax: 1:2 to 5:7
Tracheal position: midline
Percussion: resonant
Adventitious sounds: crackles or
    wheezes

Bronchitis is classified as a chronic obstructive pulmonary disease. In bronchitis there is inflammation and constriction of the airways, with an increase in mucus production. The nurse would hear rhonchi or wheezes on auscultation.

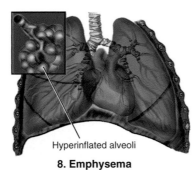

Hyperinflated alveoli

8. Emphysema

Shape of thorax: 1:1
Tracheal position: midline
Percussion: hyperresonant
Adventitious sounds: wheezes

Emphysema is classified as a chronic obstructive pulmonary disease. In emphysema there is destruction of the alveoli and the alveoli become hyperinflated. The breath sounds are diminished on auscultation and the lung fields are hyperresonant on percussion.

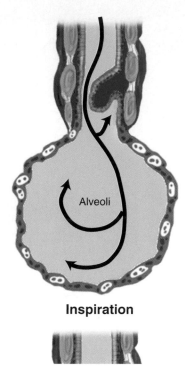

Inspiration

Air trapping commonly occurs in patients with COPD. During exhalation the airway closes, trapping the air in the alveoli and inhibiting gas exchange. This causes the patient to feel a shortness of breath. Pursued lip breathing is used to help prevent air trapping.

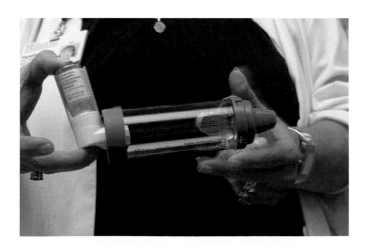

A patient with COPD is treated with inhalers. A spacer or plastic cylinder, as shown, is frequently used with the medication. The medication is inserted into one end of the spacer and the patient seals their lips around the mouthpiece. After the medication is dispensed, the patient is instructed to take a slow deep breath and hold in that breath up to ten seconds.

Early clubbing

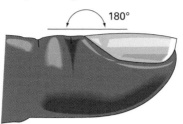

A finding in patients with COPD is clubbing of the nailbeds. This results from hypoxia over long periods of time.

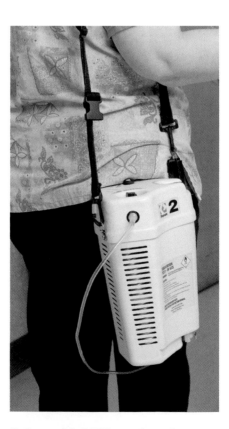

Patients with COPD may be on home oxygen therapy. The oxygen is portable and can by carried by a strap hanging from the shoulder.

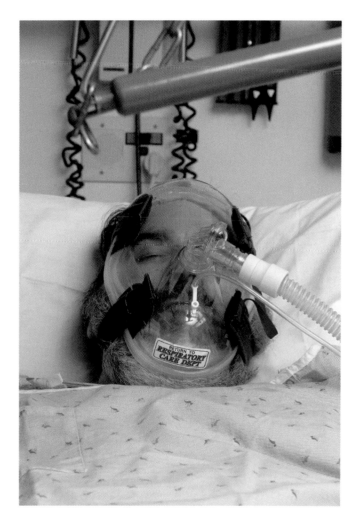

A BiPap mask may be used for COPD patients who are hypoxic. A positive pressure is applied to the airways, helping keep alveoli open and promoting gas exchange. This mask is very uncomfortable for patients. Patients may also have skin breakdown on the face from the pressure and weight of the mask.

CIRRHOSIS

Cirrhosis is a chronic liver disease that results in scarring and fibrosis of the liver and liver dysfunction. Causes include hepatitis C (postnecrotic), alcohol abuse (Laennec's), disorders of the biliary system (biliary), right-sided heart failure (cardiac), and medications such as Tylenol and cholesterol-reducing agents (statins).

Assessment

- Jaundice
- Generalized edema
- Ascites
- Decreased level of consciousness
- Bleeding

Planning and Implementation

- Neurological assessment
- Nutritional status
- Vital signs
- Fluid restriction

Evaluation and Outcomes

The patient will:

- Understand dietary modifications, e.g., sodium restrictions
- Have no bleeding
- Avoid alcohol use
- Have normal liver function tests

Nursing Considerations

- Teach patients that cirrhosis may cause amenorrhea in women.

- Teach patients to avoid alcohol.

- Instruct patients to increase their protein intake in their diet.

- Teach patients that cirrhosis may cause testicular atrophy, gynecomastia, and impotence in men.

- Teach patients to observe for signs of bleeding such as bruising, bleeding gums, and blood in the stool, since cirrhosis causes a decrease in the production of clotting factors.

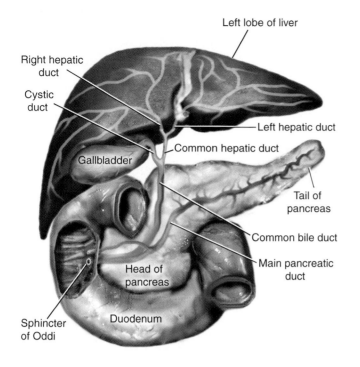

The liver, gall bladder, and pancreas. Destruction of the liver cells leads to cirrhosis.

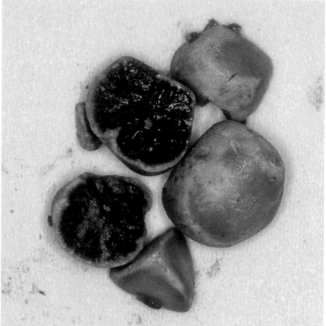

Gallstones seen in the gallbladder after surgical removal.

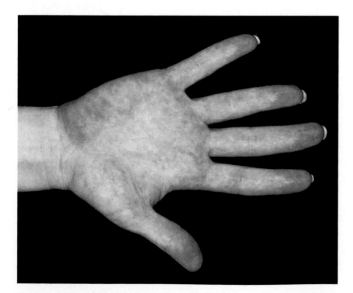

Palmar erythema or a redness in the palms seen in patients with cirrhosis.

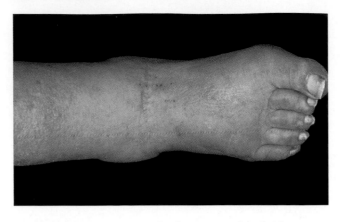

Patients with cirrhosis have fluid retention. This fluid reten-
tion leads to edema seen in the foot.

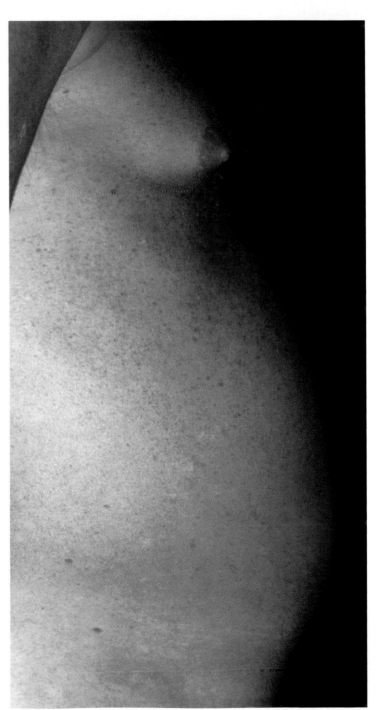

Fluid retention seen in cirrhosis leads to accumulation of fluid in the
abdomen or ascites.

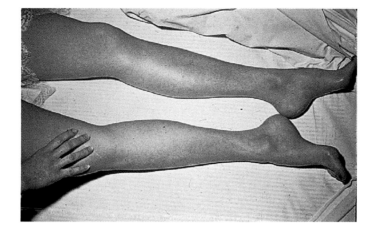

The patient with cirrhosis may also have jaundice or yellow-orange discoloration. Jaundice is seen on the skin and the sclera, and is caused by the accumulation of bilirubin in the blood.

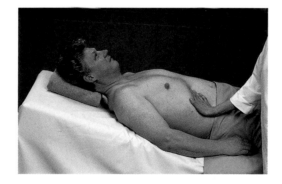

The nurse should assess the hepatojugular reflux in patients with cirrhosis. This is done due to the increased pressure in the portal vein. The patient is flat in bed and the nurse applies pressure on the right upper quadrant of the abdomen for 30-60 seconds. The nurse observes the neck for the presence of jugular venous distention, which is an abnormal finding indicating increased blood volume in the portal vein.

COLITIS, ULCERATIVE

Ulcerative colitis is a chronic inflammatory disease of the large intestine and rectum. It causes ulcers and irritation in the inner lining of the colon and rectum, with periods of exacerbation and remission. It is thought to be an autoimmune disease.

Assessment

- Bloody diarrhea
- Abdominal pain
- Fever
- Weight loss
- Tenesmus (pain and cramping)

Planning and Implementation

- History
- Vital signs
- Quantity, color, consistency of stools
- Accurate I and O
- May require surgical intervention

Evaluation and Outcomes

The patient will:

- Maintain adequate fluid intake
- Maintain stable vital signs
- Have no bloody diarrhea
- Understand medical therapy
- Maintain body image

Nursing Considerations

- Teach patients to avoid whole wheat grains, nuts, fresh fruits, and vegetables.

- Teach patients to avoid caffeine, pepper, and alcohol.

- Refer patients to local support groups.

- Monitor the perianal area for signs of skin breakdown and irritation from frequent loose stools.

- Teach patients to record the number, consistency, and amount of each stool.

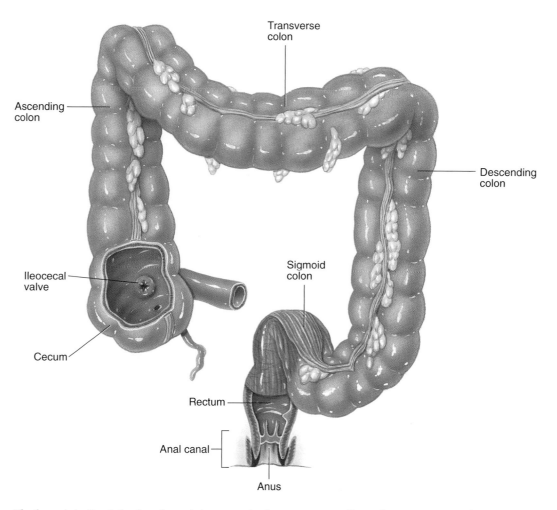

Transverse
colon

Ascending
colon

Descending
colon

Ileocecal
valve

Sigmoid
colon

Cecum

Rectum

Anal canal

Anus

The large intestine is broken down into segments: the cecum, ascending colon, transverse colon, descending colon and rectum. Ulcerative colitis can affect any area of the large intestine.

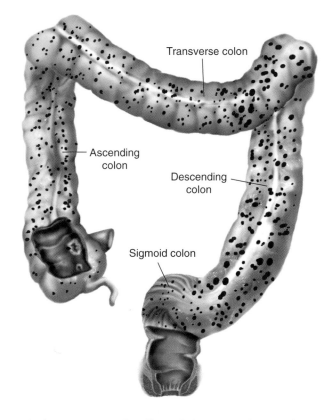

In the large intestine, the effects of ulcerative colitis can be seen throughout the colon leaving patchy areas that are inflamed leading to bleeding and the presence of blood in the stool. Patients may also complain os abdominal pain and cramping.

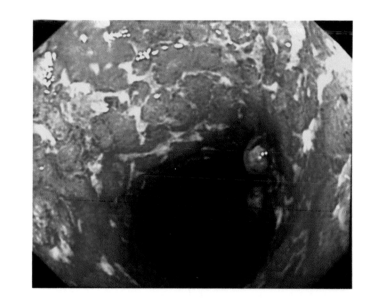

Ulcerative colitis seen through a colonoscope. Areas of ulceration and bleeding are seen, which is characteristic in ulcerative colitis. Polyps can also be seen in the image. This patient presented with frequent, loose stools and with blood present in the stools. (Courtesy of Viewing Medicine)

COLORECTAL CANCER

Colorectal cancer (CRC) is the presence of adenoma or adenocarcinoma tumors in the colon or rectum. Colorectal cancer results from the loss of key tumor suppression genes and activation of oncogenes that alter colonic mucosa cell division. Tumors occur in all areas of the colon.

Assessment

- Change in bowel patterns
- Presence of blood in the stool
- Weight loss
- Abdominal fullness

Planning and Implementation

- Normal bowel pattern
- Dietary history
- Hemetest stools
- Monitor complete blood count

Evaluation and Outcomes

The patient will:

- Understand treatment regimen
- Have normal bowel function
- Have no blood in the stool
- Be free of pain

Nursing Considerations

- Teach patients and families that risk factors for developing CRC include being older than 50, a diet high in animal protein intake, obesity, cigarette smoking; a history of adenomatous polyps, Crohn's disease, CRC or irritable bowel syndrome; and genetic disposition with a family history of CRC, familial adenomatous polyposis (FAP) or hereditary nonpolyposis colon cancer (HNPCC).

- Teach patients that treatment depends on the size and stage of CRC and may include surgery, chemotherapy, radiation, or palliative care.

- Refer patients to the enterostomal therapist if an ostomy will be needed.

- Teach patients and families that foods recommended for the prevention of colorectal cancer include fruits, vegetables, and whole grain products.

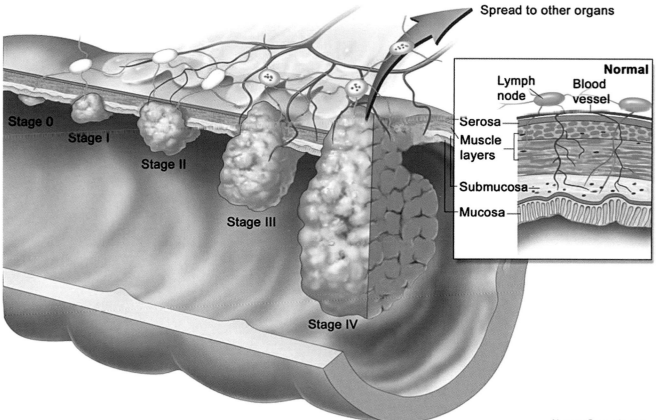

Spread to other organs

Stage 0

Stage I

Stage II

Stage III

Stage IV

Normal

Lymph node

Blood vessel

Serosa

Muscle layers

Submucosa

Mucosa

National Cancer Institute

The stages of colorectal cancer. In Stage 0, the disease has not grown beyond the lining of the colon or rectum. In Stage I, the cancer has grown through several layers of the colon but has not spread outside the colon itself. Standard treatment is a colon resection with no other treatment generally needed. In Stage II, the cancer has penetrated the wall of the colon and spread into nearby tissue. However, it has not yet reached the lymph nodes. Stage III is considered an advanced stage of colorectal cancer. The disease has spread to the lymph nodes, but not to other parts or organs in the body. For both colon and rectal cancer, sectional surgery is done first and is followed by chemotherapy and radiation therapy. In Stage IV, the disease has spread to distant organs such as the liver, lungs, and ovaries. When the cancer has reached this stage, surgery is generally aimed at relieving or preventing complications, as opposed to curing the patient of the disease. (Courtesy of NCI)

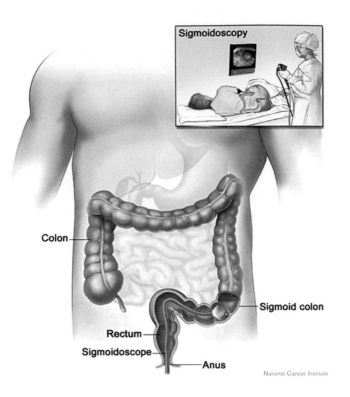

A colonoscopy or sigmoidoscopy is used as a screening tool for colon cancer. An initial routine screening is recommended for patients at age 50. Prior to the procedure the patient is given laxatives to cleanse the bowel. Conscious sedation is used during the procedure so the patient is responsive but may not remember having the procedure done. (Courtesy of NCI)

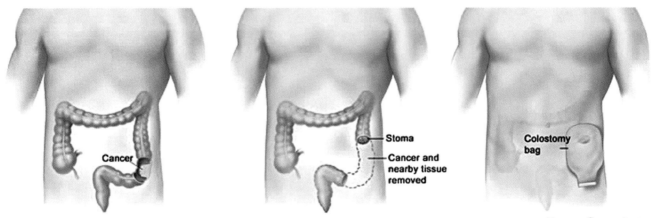

A treatment for colorectal cancer is removal of the segment of colon that is cancerous. After the colon segment is removed, an ostomy is created and patients wear an ostomy bag over the stoma. Fecal contents are excreted through the ostomy instead of continuing through the intestinal tract as normal. (Courtesy of NCI)

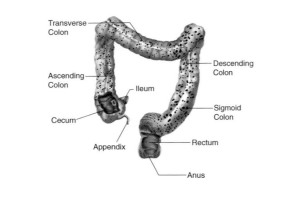

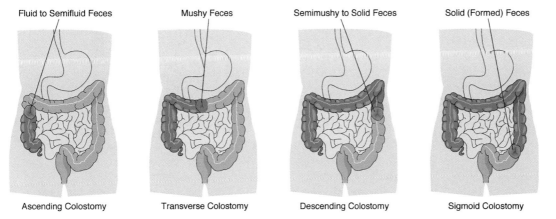

There are different sites of a colostomy. If the ascending colon is removed, the drainage from the ostomy will be semifluid. If the ostomy is in the transverse colon, there will be mushy fecal contents. If the ostomy is in the descending colon, the fecal drainage is semi-solid. If the ostomy is in the sigmoid colon, the fecal content is mainly solid.

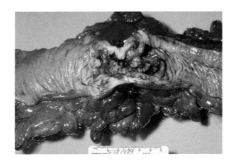

Cancerous mass in the colon as seen through a colonoscope. (Courtesy of the CDC)

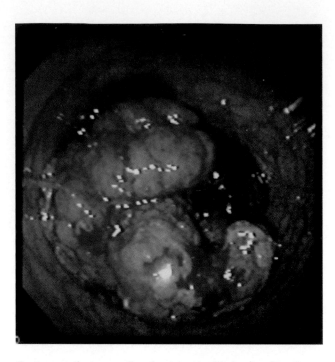

During a colonscopy, the physician is able to visualize the inside of the colon. This is what is seen if the patient has colon cancer. Note the reddened, bloody area on the growth within the colon.

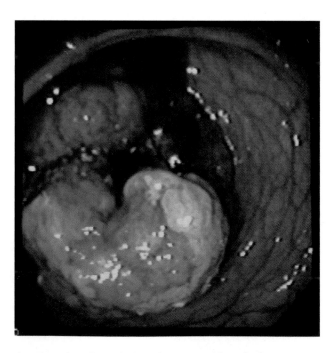

Another view through the colonoscope. Note the large cancerous mass within the colon.

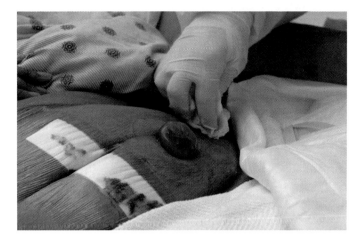

A stoma is created following the removal of a segment of the colon.

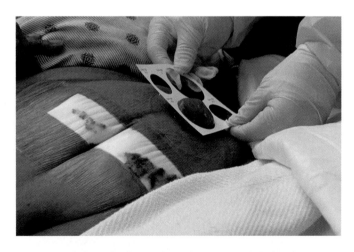

The stoma is measured in order to have a properly fitted ostomy bag.

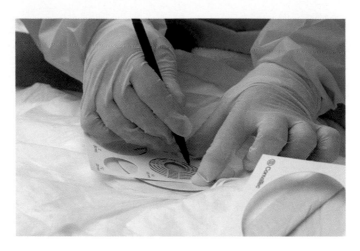

The ostomy bag is placed over the stoma and marked where it needs to be cut in order to assure a proper fit.

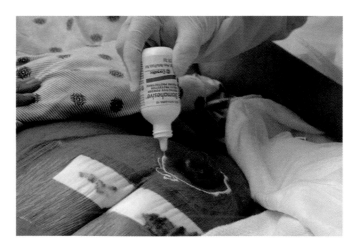

A special powder is placed around the stoma where the ostomy pouch will be placed. This powder helps protect the skin and prevent skin breakdown.

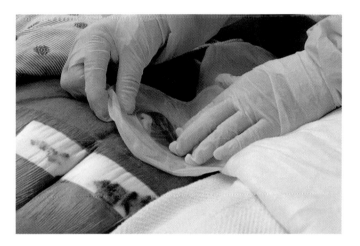

The ostomy bag is placed over the stoma. This needs to be replaced weekly or as needed. Patients are taught to care for their stoma prior to discharge from the hospital. This is usually done by a specially-trained enterostomal nurse.

CONJUNCTIVITIS

Conjunctivitis is the inflammation of the conjunctiva or thin membrane covering the white of the eye and the inner surface of the eyelid; it is caused by bacteria, viruses, or allergens. Infectious conjunctivitis is also called "pink eye."

Assessment

- Reddened eye
- Discharge, pus from the eye
- Itchy eye
- Watery eye
- Blurred vision

Planning and Implementation

- History
- Handwashing
- Administration of eye drops

Evaluation and Outcomes

The patient will:

- Be free of infection of the eye
- Avoid spread of bacteria to the other eye and to other people
- Appropriately apply eye drops
- Practice good handwashing

Nursing Considerations

- Teach patients infectious conjunctivitis is easily transmitted, and to use good handwashing techniques.

- Teach patients to refrain from using eye make up during infection.

- Teach patients that application of a warm compress to the eye may help decrease irritation and pain.

- Teach patients to not let others use their eyedrops.

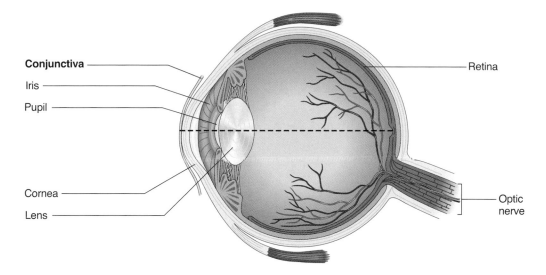

Conjunctiva

Iris

Pupil

Cornea

Lens

Retina

Optic nerve

The normal anatomy of the eye. The conjunctiva is the outer layer covering the eye and the inner surface of the eyelid. This layer becomes reddened with inflammation or infection. There may be discharge from the eye.

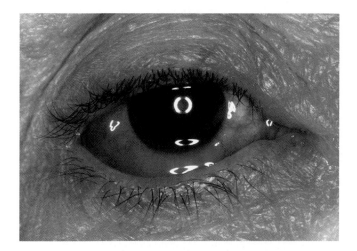

A patient with conjunctivitis, and the conjunctiva is extremely swollen. The eye is very painful. (Courtesy of Viewing Medicine)

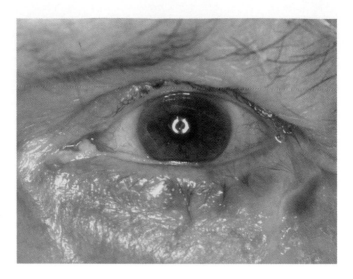

Conjunctivitis with infection. Pus is visible in the corner of the eye, and underneath the lower eyelid the pus is dried on the skin. (Courtesy of Viewing Medicine)

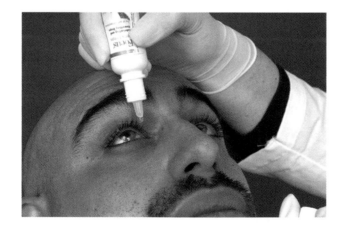

The application of eye drops. Patients with conjunctivitis may need antibiotic eye drops. In administration of eye drops, the medication is administered to the lower and inner surface of the eye. Be sure not to touch the tip of bottle of the medication on any surface, as this tip needs to be kept sterile.

CORNEAL DISORDERS

Corneal disorders encompass any disease or illness that affects the cornea, which is the transparent surface that covers the iris and is continuous with the conjunctival tissue. Corneal disorders include corneal abrasions, corneal burns, corneal ulcers, and corneal foreign bodies.

Assessment

- Eye redness
- Eye pain
- Eye itching
- Drainage from the eye

Planning and Implementation

- Assessment of the eye
- Visual acuity
- Clarity of vision
- Headaches

Evaluation and OutcomesThe patient will:

- Be free of redness, pain in the eye
- Maintain adequate visual acuity
- Be free of headaches

Nursing Considerations

- Teach patients that corneal tissue changes with age.

- Educate patients to prevent corneal abrasions through the use of protective eye wear.

- Instruct patients who wear contacts to not wear them beyond the recommended duration, in order to avoid corneal abrasions.

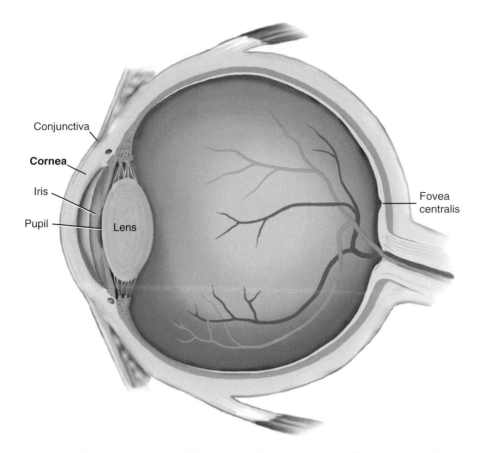

Conjunctiva

Cornea

Iris

Pupil

Lens

Fovea centralis

The normal anatomy of the eye. The cornea is the tissue covering the iris or colored part of the eye.

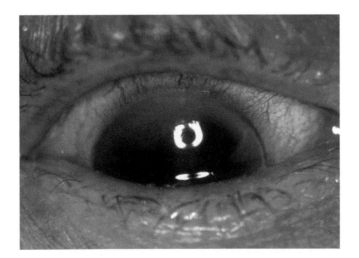

A corneal abrasion which has been stained green for better visualization. The patient needs to wear an eye patch to protect the eye. The abrasion will heal itself over time and no specific treatment is indicated. (Courtesy of Viewing Medicine)

CORONARY ARTERY DISEASE (CAD)

Coronary artery disease (CAD) is a narrowing or blockage of the blood vessels (coronary arteries) that supply blood and oxygen to the myocardium. It is caused by the buildup of fatty plaque (atherosclerosis) and the formation of clots within the lumen of the arteries.

Assessment

- Angina
- Shortness of breath
- Fatigue
- Diaphoresis

Planning and Implementation

- Vital signs
- Family history
- Risk factors
- Pain management

Evaluation and Outcomes

The patient will:

- Be free of angina
- Complete activities of daily living without symptoms
- Understand the need for a low fat diet
- Stop smoking
- Understand nitroglycerine administration

Nursing Considerations

- Teach women that their risk of CAD increases after menopause.

- Teach patients that if they experience chest pain, they should take their nitroglycerine. If there is no relief of chest pain in five minutes, they can take another dose. If there is still no relief of chest pain after three doses of nitroglycerine, they should call 911.

- Teach patients to check the expiration date of their nitroglycerine tablets or spray.

- Nurses must understand that women tend to describe their angina differently than do men and may complain of jaw pain and shoulder pain instead of the typical chest pain.

- Teach males patients that the use of phosphodiesterase inhibitors such as Viagra and Cialis may cause severe hypotension and cardiovascular collapse if taken within 24 hours of nitrate administration.

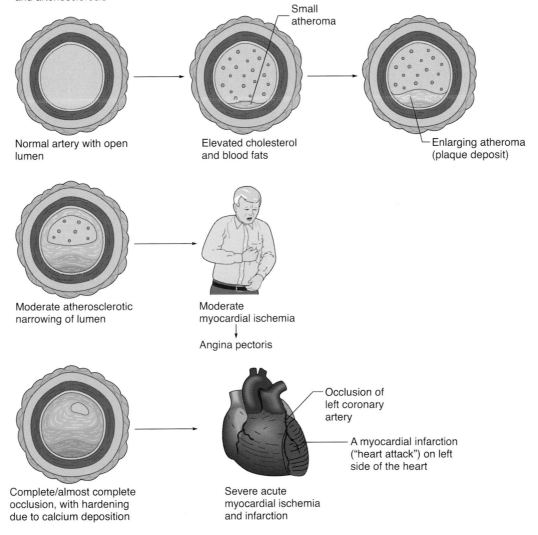

Cross sections through a coronary artery undergoing progressive atherosclerosis and arteriosclerosis

Small atheroma

Normal artery with open lumen

Elevated cholesterol and blood fats

Enlarging atheroma (plaque deposit)

Moderate atherosclerotic narrowing of lumen

Moderate myocardial ischemia

Angina pectoris

Complete/almost complete occlusion, with hardening due to calcium deposition

Severe acute myocardial ischemia and infarction

Occlusion of left coronary artery

A myocardial infarction ("heart attack") on left side of the heart

In coronary artery disease, cholesterol and fat build up within the lumen of the coronary artery. This is termed an atheroma. The atheroma gradually hardens and becomes calcified. The reduced lumen in the artery leads to a reduction in blood and oxygen flow to the myocardium causing angina and myocardial ischemia.

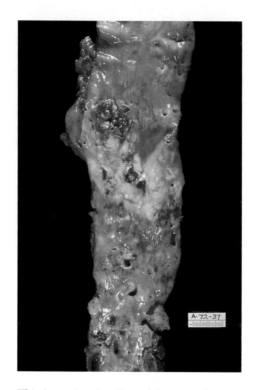

*This is a cut-out section of the aorta show-
ing the atherosclerosis process. The inside
of the aorta shows the fatty depositions on
the inner surface of the aorta. (Courtesy of
the CDC)*

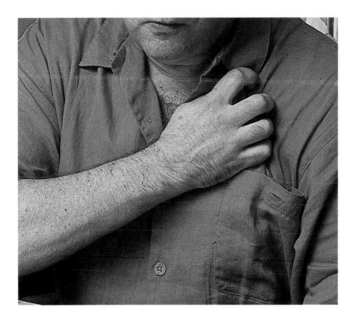

This the classic sign of a patient having chest pain or angina. Women may experience their pain in the jaw or in their shoulder, but may also experience this as a typical crushing feeling over the chest. The patient clutches or grabs at the chest area. The angina is caused by a reduction in blood and oxygen flow to the myocardium that results from fatty build-up in the lumen of the coronary arteries.

CROHN'S DISEASE

Crohn's disease, or regional enteritis, falls under the broad classification of inflammatory bowel disease and is a chronic, recurrent disease characterized by inflammation of any portion of the digestive tract with one-third of cases involving the small bowel. There are patchy areas along the GI tract that penetrate into the wall of the intestine.

Assessment

- Abdominal pain
- Diarrhea
- Weight loss
- Fatigue
- Fever

Planning and Implementation

- Nutritional supplements
- Vital signs
- Quantity, consistency, color of stools
- Skin integrity

Evaluation and Outcomes

The patient will:

- Maintain adequate nutritional status
- Maintain skin integrity
- Understand medical treatment

SpecialNursing Considerations

- Instruct patients that they will experience periods of exacerbation and remission.

- Teach patients that stress management techniques may help decrease periods of exacerbation.

- Monitor nutritional status, as patients may experience malabsorption from the disease in the small bowel.

- Instruct patients to have routine screening for colon cancer, since the incidence of colon cancer is higher in patients with Crohn's disease.

- Refer to community support groups.

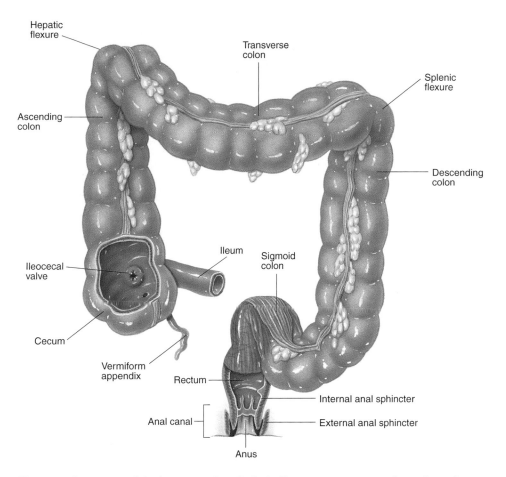

The normal anatomy of the large intestine. Crohn's disease can occur anywhere along the gastrointestinal tract.

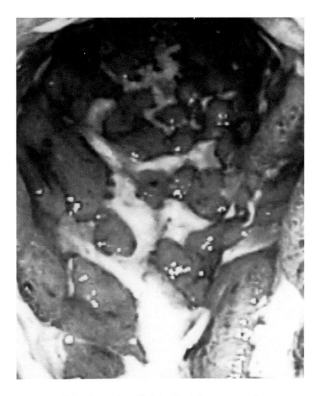

A view of the ileum (small intestine) from an endoscope, showing areas of bleeding and ulceration in a patient with Crohn's disease. The patient experiences abdominal pain and bleeding in the stool. (Courtesy of Viewing Medicine)

CUSHING'S SYNDROME

Cushing's syndrome is the oversecretion of cortisol from the adrenal cortex caused by a neoplasm or tumor, excessive secretion of ACTH from the pituitary, or increase exogenous intake of steroids.

Assessment

- Muscle weakness
- Hypertension
- Hirsutism
- Thinning of the skin
- Truncal obesity with thin extremities

Planning and Implementation

- Vital signs
- Monitor electrolyte values
- Signs of fluid overload
- Assist with activities

Evaluation and Outcomes

The patient will:

- Have normal vital signs
- Perform activities of daily living
- Maintain skin integrity
- Be free of infection

Nursing Considerations

- Teach patients to wear a MedicAlert bracelet.

- Instruct patients that tumors may need to be surgically removed

- Teach patients to monitor their blood sugar levels, as blood sugars rise with an increase in cortisol levels.

- Teach patients taking oral prednisone to monitor for side effects, including weight gain, gastric irritation, high blood sugars, and osteoporosis.

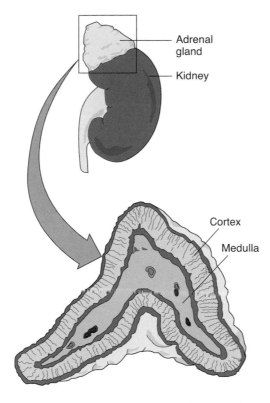

Adrenal
gland

Kidney

Cortex

Medulla

*Cushing's syndrome or Cushing's disease is the
oversecretion of hormones from the adrenal
gland. The adrenal gland is located on the top of
each kidney. The adrenal cortex, or outer layer of
the adrenal gland, oversecretes the hormones,
leading to Cushing's syndrome.*

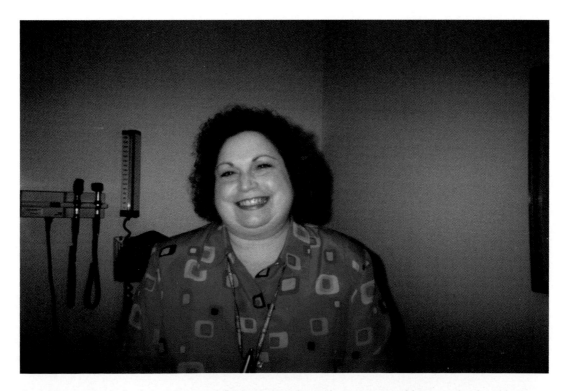

*Cushing's syndrome leads to sodium and fluid retention due to the increase in aldosterone levels. Aldosterone
causes the kidneys to increase reabsorption of sodium, which leads to an increase in water reabsorption,
causing swelling. This swelling is especially seen in the face. This is often referred to as "Moon Face."*

DEEP VEIN THROMBOSIS (DVT)

Deep vein thrombosis is the formation of a thrombus or clot in the venous system. Risk factors for developing DVT are based on Virchow's triad: trauma to the vessel, venous stasis, and hypercoagulability. DVTs usually occur in the deep veins of the lower extremities. Risk factors include immobility, estrogen use, pregnancy, and heart failure.

Assessment

- Pain in the affected area
- Swelling in the affected extremity
- Warmth over the site
- Redness over the site

Planning and Implementation

- Prevention is the key, ambulation
- Anticoagulation
- Sequential compression devices
- Elevation of the extremity

Evaluation and Outcome

The patient will:

- Be free of embolus/thrombosis
- Ambulate without difficulty
- Be free of bleeding if anticoagulated

Nursing Considerations

- Teach patients to avoid long periods of inactivity or sitting.

- Patients diagnosed with a DVT may require long-term Coumadin use and need to be taught to watch for signs of bleeding; they will also need to obtain lab tests to monitor prothrombin time (PT) and INR.

- Homans' sign frequently results in a false positive, so it is not routinely done.

- Prevention measures include early ambulation postoperatively, knee-high or thigh-high elastic stockings, and sequential compression devices.

- Medication prophylaxis includes low molecular weight heparin or a heparin infusion.

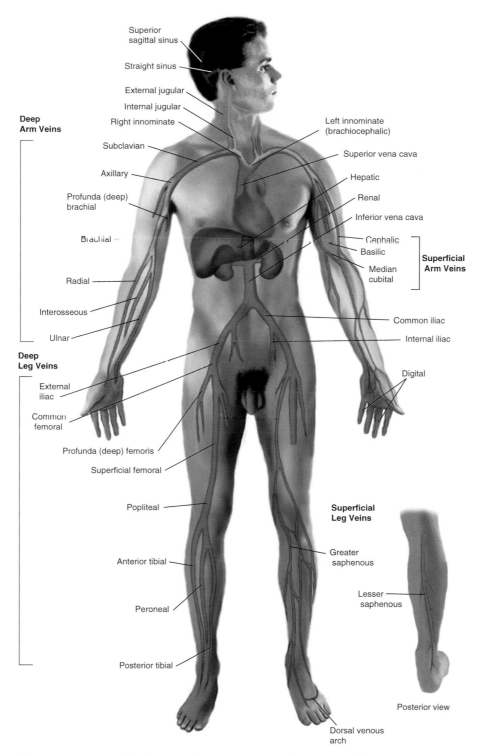

**Deep
Arm Veins**

Superior
sagittal sinus

Straight sinus

External jugular

Internal jugular

Right innominate

Subclavian

Axillary

Profunda (deep)
brachial

Brachial

Radial

Interosseous

Ulnar

**Deep
Leg Veins**

External
iliac

Common
femoral

Profunda (deep) femoris

Superficial femoral

Popliteal

Anterior tibial

Peroneal

Posterior tibial

Left innominate
(brachiocephalic)

Superior vena cava

Hepatic

Renal

Inferior vena cava

Cephalic

Basilic

Median
cubital

**Superficial
Arm Veins**

Common iliac

Internal iliac

Digital

**Superficial
Leg Veins**

Greater
saphenous

Lesser
saphenous

Posterior view

Dorsal venous
arch

The venous system of the body. A thrombus can occur in any part of the venous system, but most typically occur in the deep veins in the legs.

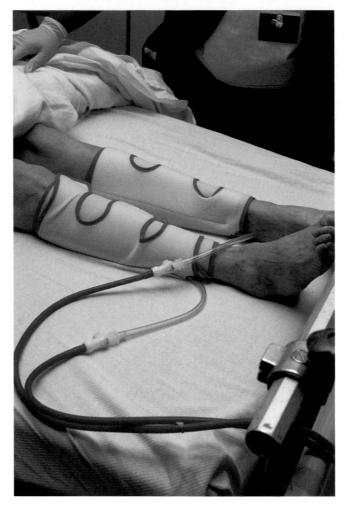

Compression stockings are used prophylactically to prevent deep vein thrombosis. These intermittently inflate and deflate, mimicking the action of the muscles on the venous system. Each time the stockings inflate they squeeze the veins in the legs, propelling blood forward and preventing venous stasis, which can result in clot formation.

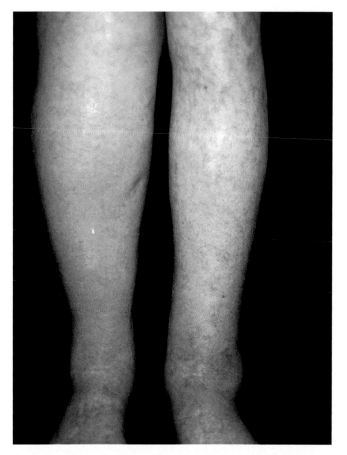

A patient with a DVT in the right leg. Notice how the right leg is reddened and swollen compared to the left leg. If a DVT occurs, the nurse should not massage the affected leg as this may cause the clot to dislodge and travel to the lungs or the brain. (Courtesy of Viewing Medicine)

DIABETES INSIPIDUS

Diabetes insipidus results from insufficient antidiuretic hormone (ADH), occurring due to posterior pituitary disturbances (central diabetes insipidus) or a lack of sensitivity of circulating ADH from the nephrons in the kidney (nephrogenic diabetes insipidus).

Assessment

- Polydipsia
- Polyuria
- Level of consciousness
- Hypovolemia (tachycardia, hypotension, dry mucous membranes, weight loss)
- Visual disturbances

Planning and Implementation

- Vital signs
- Intake and Output
- Monitor serum electrolyte values
- Intravenous fluid replacement

Evaluation and Outcomes

The patient will:

- Have normal vital signs
- Have normal urinary output
- Have normal serum electrolyte values
- Maintain level of consciousness

Nursing Considerations

▬ Diabetes insipidus may result from head trauma, craniotomy, or brain tumors.

▬ Antidiuretic hormone replacement (vasopressin, desmopressin or DDAVP) is given either intravenously or as a nasal spray due to lack of absorption if given orally.

▬ Intake and output need to monitored hourly.

▬ The urine specific gravity should be measured at least once daily.

▬ Patients with chronic diabetes insipidus should wear a Medic Alert bracelet.

▬ Patients taking lithium should be monitored for signs and symptoms of diabetes insipidus, as this is a potential side effect of this medication.

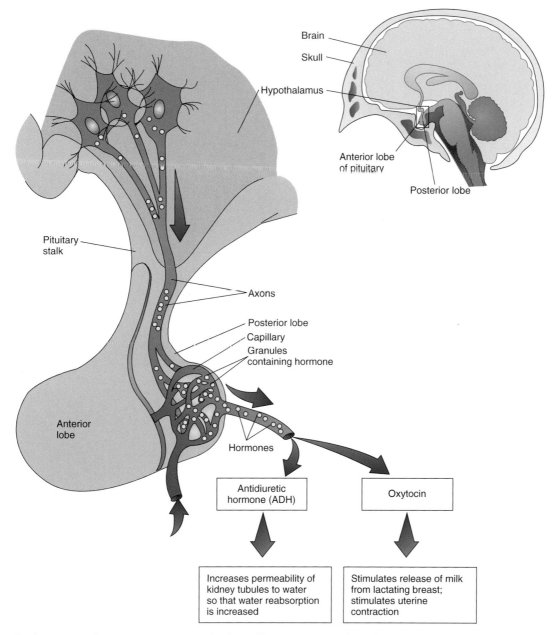

Brain

Skull

Hypothalamus

Anterior lobe
of pituitary

Posterior lobe

Pituitary
stalk

Axons

Posterior lobe
Capillary
Granules
containing hormone

Anterior
lobe

Hormones

Antidiuretic
hormone (ADH)

Oxytocin

Increases permeability of
kidney tubules to water
so that water reabsorption
is increased

Stimulates release of milk
from lactating breast;
stimulates uterine
contraction

Diabetes insipidus may occur as a result of insufficient secretion of antidiuretic hormone, which is secreted from the posterior pituitary.

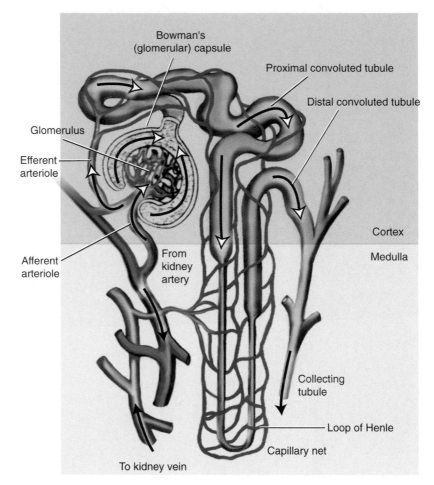

Antidiuretic hormone produces effects in the nephron of the kidney, and an insufficient amount of this antidiuretic hormone can lead to the loss of high volumes of urine.

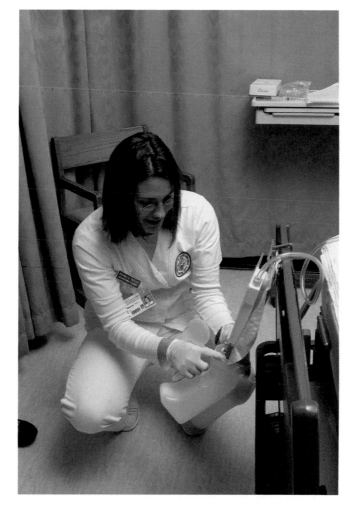

The nurse needs to closely monitor the urine output of patients suspected of having or being at risk for developing diabetes insipidus.

DIABETES MELLITUS (DM)

Diabetes mellitus refers to a group of chronic disorders of metabolism that are characterized by hyperglycemia (high blood glucose) and disturbances in the metabolism of carbohydrates, fats, and proteins as a result of a lack of insulin (Type I diabetes) or insulin deficiency or resistance (Type 2 diabetes).

Assessment

- Polyuria
- Polydipsia
- Polyphagia
- Weight loss

Planning and Implementation

- Monitor blood glucose values
- Monitor for signs of hyperglycemia including Kussmaul's respirations, acidodis, fruity odor to breath
- Monitor electrolyte values
- Fluid replacement
- Teaching

Evaluation and Outcomes

The patient will:

- Identify signs and symptoms of hypo/hyperglycemia
- Perform daily blood glucose checks
- Correctly administer insulin
- Identify appropriate dietary choices

Nursing Considerations

- African-American, Hispanic American, Native American, Asian Americans, and Pacific Islanders are at higher risk for developing DM.

- 20% of patients 65 and older have DM.

- Diabetes affects 16 million patients, and obesity is the number one modifiable risk factor.

- Older adults with diabetes are at a higher risk for the development of dehydration as a result of hyperglycemia.

- Compared to Caucasians, minority groups have a higher risk for the development of complications of diabetes.

- Diabetes associated with pregnancy is termed gestational diabetes mellitus.

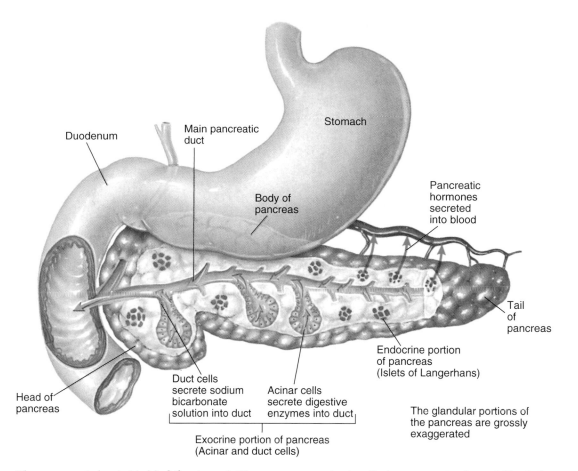

Duodenum

Main pancreatic duct

Stomach

Body of pancreas

Pancreatic hormones secreted into blood

Tail of pancreas

Endocrine portion of pancreas (Islets of Langerhans)

Duct cells secrete sodium bicarbonate solution into duct

Acinar cells secrete digestive enzymes into duct

The glandular portions of the pancreas are grossly exaggerated

Head of pancreas

Exocrine portion of pancreas (Acinar and duct cells)

The pancreas is located behind the stomach. The pancreas secretes insulin in response to elevated blood glucose levels. A lack of insulin results in diabetes mellitus.

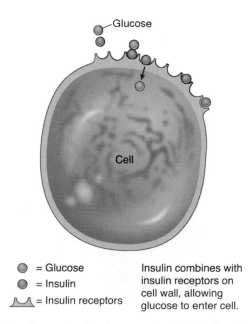

Glucose

Cell

● = Glucose
● = Insulin
⏝⏝ = Insulin receptors

Insulin combines with insulin receptors on cell wall, allowing glucose to enter cell.

Insulin carries the glucose molecule into the cell by binding to insulin receptors on the cell wall. Once insulin is inside the cell, the cell uses it for energy.

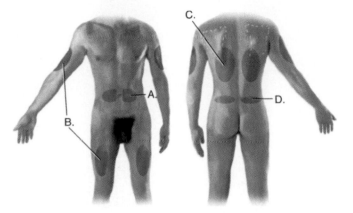

Insulin is administered subcutaneously. There are several areas or sites available for subcutaneous injections. These include the abdomen, lateral and anterior aspects of the upper arm and thigh, and scapular area on the back. Patients should be taught to rotate the sites of injection, since injection of insulin into the same site repeatedly causes lipodystrophy and the insulin may not be absorbed into the body.

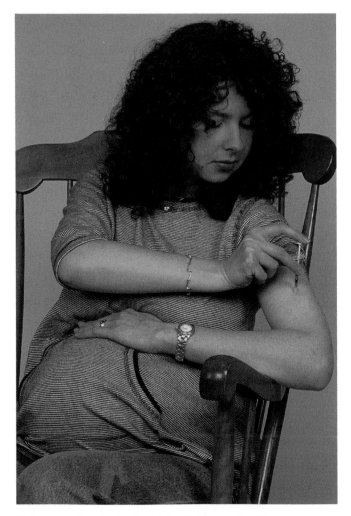

Patients are taught to administer their own insulin.

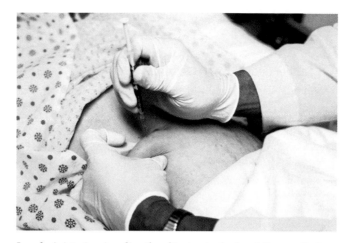

In administering insulin, the skin is pinched and the needle is inserted at a 90 degree angle.

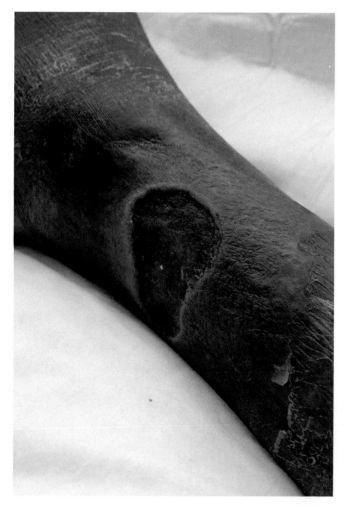

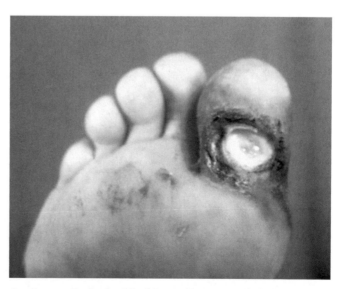

A venous ulcer seen on the lower leg. The patient with diabetes mellitus is at risk for developing venous ulcers. These ulcers may not be felt by the patient and easily become infected. Patients should be taught to inspect their feet daily to check for open areas.

An ulcer on the back of the big toe. Patients with diabetes mellitus must be taught good foot care, including visual inspections of their feet daily and wearing properly fitted shoes. Diabetics are slow to heal, so this ulcer may take a long time to heal and may become easily infected. Treatment includes daily dressing changes.

DIVERTICULITIS

Diverticulitis is the inflammation of diverticula or saclike outpouches of the mucosa of the bowel, from the retention of undigested foods. Diverticulitis is closely associated with a diet low in fiber and high in refined foods, decreased activity levels, and constipation.

Assessment

- Left lower quadrant pain
- Fever
- Nausea and vomiting
- Abdominal distention
- Blood in the stool

Planning and Implementation

- Assess bowel pattern
- Hemetest stools
- NPO or clear liquids during acute phase
- Pain management

Evaluation and Outcomes

The patient will:

- Have normal vital signs
- Be free of infection
- Ingest diet high in fiber, fruits and vegetables, and avoid foods with seeds

Nursing Considerations

- Antibiotics are used during the acute phase.

- Alcohol should be avoided, since it is an irritant to the bowel.

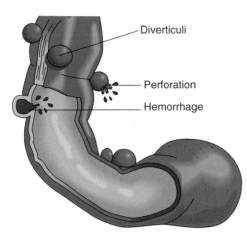

Diverticuli are outpouchings in the wall of the large intestine. Treatment at this stage includes a high fiber diet and avoiding foods with seeds. There can be bleeding from the diverticuli, causing bloody stool or melena. Patients notice their stools are dark and tarry in color. Eventually the diverticuli can perforate, causing internal bleeding. At this point the patient has severe abdominal pain and the abdomen is rigid and tender to the touch.

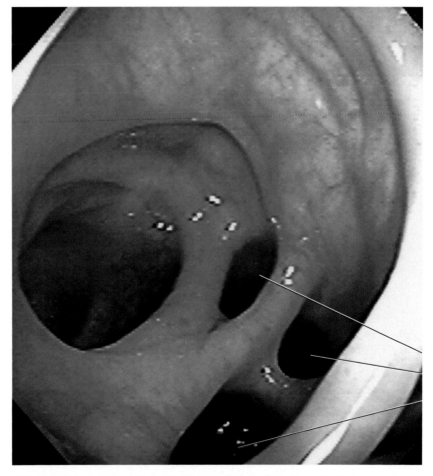

Diverticuli as seen through a colonoscopy. The diverticuli are the holes or outpouchings in the lower part of the picture. No bleeding is apparent, so the patient is taught to increase the fiber intake in their diet. Yearly colonoscopies are recommended. (Courtesy of Viewing Medicine)

EMBOLISM

An embolism is an obstruction or occlusion of a blood vessel by an embolus, which is an abnormal particle circulating in the blood comprised of either a clot, fat, or air. The embolism typically occurs in the brain (cerebral embolism) or the lungs (pulmonary embolus), leading to symptoms.

Assessment

- Altered level of consciousness
- Shortness of breath
- Chest pain
- Diminished breath sounds

Planning and Implementation

- Vital signs
- Lung sounds
- Administer oxygen
- Assess for presence of deep vein thrombosis

Evaluation and Outcomes

The patient will:

- Maintain level of consciousness
- Oxygenate adequately on room air
- Have stable vital signs
- Be free of signs and symptoms of a deep vein thrombosis

Nursing Considerations

- Patients at high risk for a deep vein thrombosis should be monitored for signs of an embolism.

- An embolism may travel to the lungs (pulmonary embolism) or the brain (cerebral embolism), so nurses must monitor for these potential complications.

- Prevention of thrombus formation through early postoperative ambulation, elastic stockings, sequential compression devices, and anticoagulation is critical to prevent embolism.

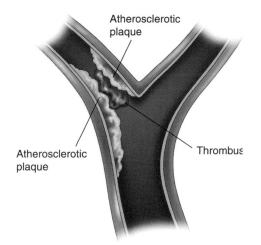

An embolism results when a thrombus is formed and dislodges and moves within the blood vessel. Thrombi are formed from the aggregation of platelets, usually around areas of plaque within the blood vessel.

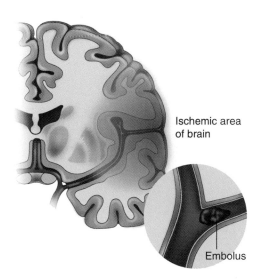

The embolus can lodge in a vessel and occlude blood flow distally, resulting in ischemia (lack of blood and oxygen) and necrosis (tissue death). If the embolus is in a cerebral vessel, the patient may suffer an embolic stroke. Symptoms of an embolic stroke include weakness, facial drooping, slurred speech, and visual disturbances. Treatment of an embolic stroke includes anticoagulation.

ENDOCARDITIS, BACTERIAL

Bacterial endocarditis is an inflammation of the endocardium or inner layer of the heart, including the heart valves. Vegetative lesions form on the valves, altering their normal function. Treatment is a surgical replacement of the affected valve. Bacterial endocarditis is also referred to as infective endocarditis.

Assessment

- Fever, chills
- Murmurs
- Shortness of breath
- Splinter hemorrhages in the nailbeds

Planning and Implementation

- Vital signs
- Administer antibiotics
- Treat hyperthermia
- Prepare patient for surgery

Evaluation and Outcomes

The patient will:

- Have stable vital signs
- Be free of signs of infection
- Maintain cardiac function
- Understand need for valve replacement

Nursing Considerations

- Bacterial endocarditis occurs primarily in patients with a history of intravenous drug abuse, previous valve replacement, or mitral valve prolapse.

- Patients with mitral valve prolapse need to take prophylactic antibiotics prior to any dental work.

- Patients will be on long-term antibiotic therapy.

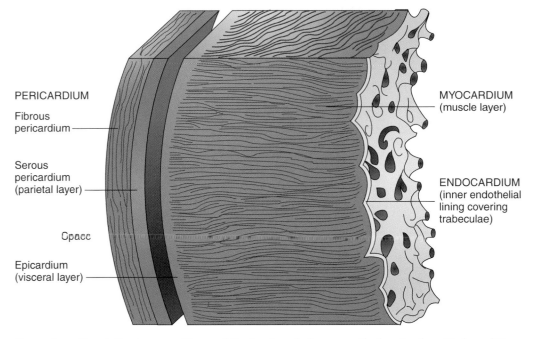

PERICARDIUM

Fibrous
pericardium

Serous
pericardium
(parietal layer)

Space

Epicardium
(visceral layer)

MYOCARDIUM
(muscle layer)

ENDOCARDIUM
(inner endothelial
lining covering
trabeculae)

The endocardium is the innermost layer of the heart, and also covers the heart valves. Endocarditis affects the valves of the heart.

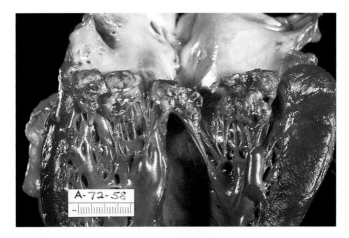

Bacterial endocarditis will attack the valves of the heart. This results in vegetation or growths that form on the valves.

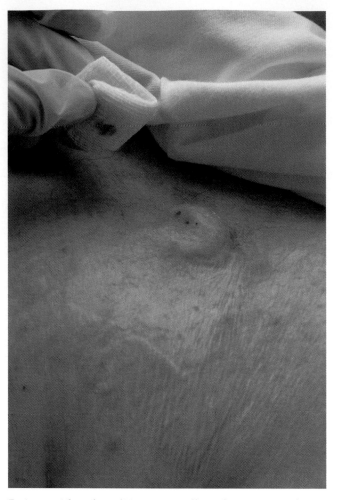

Patients with endocarditis are typically on long-term antibiotics. This may require placement of a central venous access port as seen here in the upper chest area. The port is surgically placed and is left in place for long-term antibiotic therapy. The port is accessed by a needle directly through the skin.

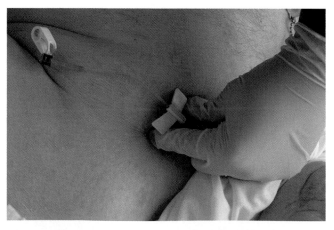

The central venous port is accessed with a butterfly needle inserted directly through the skin. The antibiotic is infused through this catheter directly into the access port into the central venous system.

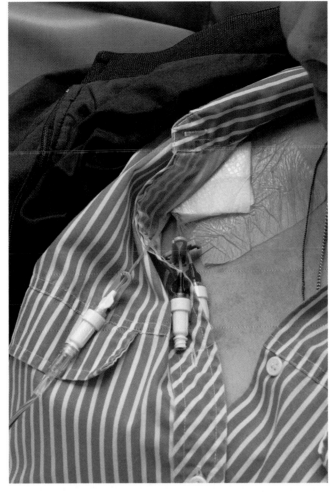

Another example of a central venous catheter into the subclavian vein. It may be used for short-term antibiotic administration. This catheter has three lumens that may be used for administration of three different medications at the same time. This catheter may not be used for as an extended length of time as those catheters that are surgically implanted.

ESOPHAGEAL VARICES

Esophageal varices are extreme dilations of the veins in the mucosa of the esophagus as a result of portal hypertension, usually secondary to cirrhosis. Portal hypertension is high blood pressure in the portal vein, which is the major vein coming from the liver. Varices typically occur in the lower segment of the esophagus.

Assessment

- Bloody emesis
- Hypotension and tachycardia
- Dark, tarry stools
- Low urinary output

Planning and Implementation

- Vital signs
- Amount/character of emesis
- Administer blood products
- Monitor complete blood count

Evaluation and Outcomes

The patient will:

- Have stable vital signs
- Be free of bleeding
- Understand medical/surgical therapy

Nursing Considerations

- Nurses need to instruct patients to eliminate alcohol ingestion.

- Patients should be taught to avoid constipation by using stool softeners and increasing water and fiber intake.

- Patients need to be instructed to seek medical help immediately if vomiting blood or if having dark, tarry stools.

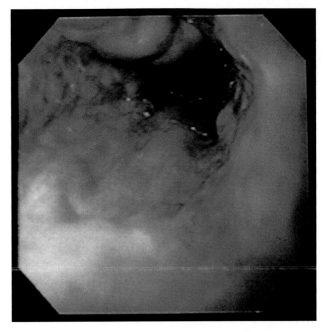

The esophageal varices are visualized through the endo-scope. Note the dilation seen in the upper part of the esoph-agus, which is the engorgement of blood in the venous sys-tem of the esophagus from the high venous pressure in the portal vein. Patients may experience abdominal pain, heart-burn, nausea, and vomiting.

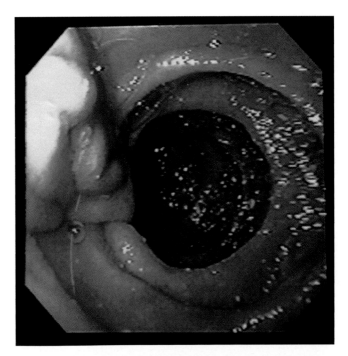

A view of esophageal varices through an endoscope. The dila-tion of the esophageal venous system is seen in the left side of the picture. Through the endoscope, metal bands may be placed around the varices, preventing the varices from rupturing and bleeding.

FLAIL CHEST

Flail chest is rib cage instability resulting from multiple broken ribs. The instability causes hypoxia and inadequate ventilation. It is usually caused by severe trauma.

Assessment

- Paradoxical movement over affected area (chest wall goes in with inspiration and out with expiration)
- Dyspnea
- Hypotension
- Chest pain
- Tachycardia and tachypnea
- Decreased pulse oximetry

Planning and Implementation

- High Fowler's position if the patient is not hypotensive
- Administer oxygen
- Anticipate intubation and mechanical ventilation
- Treat pain and anxiety
- Patient may have surgical stabilization of the fractures

Evaluation and Outcomes

The patient will:

- Oxygenate adequately on room air
- Have equal, symmetrical chest expansion
- Be free of shortness of breath

Nursing Considerations

- Flail chest is typically associated with high-speed motor vehicle accidents.

- Patients need to be taught to splint their chest when breathing to decrease pain.

- Patients need to perform coughing and deep breathing exercises or use the incentive spirometer hourly to prevent pneumonia.

- Nursing care is focused on pain relief, since breathing is extremely painful.

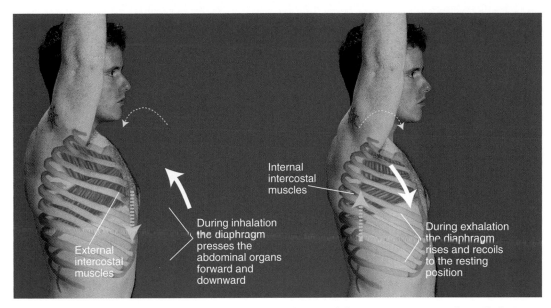

In normal respiration the chest expands downward, and outward during inspiration, and recoils during expiration.

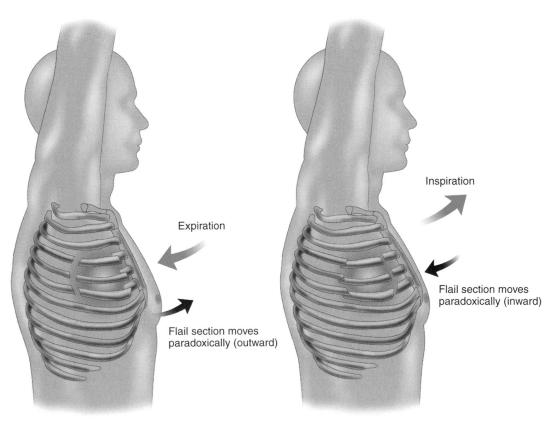

In flail chest there is paradoxical movement of the chest during respiration. The chest wall moves inward during inspiration and outward during expiration. Flail chest is seen in patients with rib fractures. This is a very painful condition and patients require frequent pain medication to maximize breathing effort and prevent pneumonia.

FRACTURES

A fracture is any break or disruption in the continuity of a bone.

Assessment

- Pulse, color, temperature, distal to fracture
- Deformity
- Numbness
- Pain
- Hypotension, tachycardia (shock)

Planning and Implementation

- Cover open wounds
- Splint fracture
- Frequent vital signs
- Treat pain
- Elevate extremity
- Monitor neurovascular status (pain, pallor, pulse, paresthesia, paralysis)

Evaluation and Outcomes

The patient will:

- Be free of pain
- Maintain adequate circulation and sensation distal to the fracture
- Be free of infection
- Be able to complete activities of daily living

Nursing Considerations

- Hip fractures occur most often in older women, due to osteoporosis.

- Older adults are more at risk for problems associated with skin or skeletal traction due to inadequate circulation and sensation, therefore the nurse must frequently assess pulses and sensation distal to the fracture.

- Fat emboli are a common complication of fractures and result from the release of fat globules from yellow bone marrow into the bloodstream. Patients may experience shortness of breath, chest pain, low oxygen saturations, cyanosis, and tachycardia due to a fat embolus.

- Osteomyelitis, infection of the bone, is most commonly seen in open fractures.

- If a cast is applied, teach the patient to notify the doctor if the cast becomes tight or there is numbness, tingling, or pain distal to the cast.

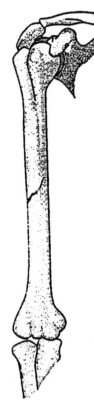

Greenstick
(incomplete)

A greenstick fracture is an incomplete fracture, not going through the entire bone. One side of the bone is broken while the other side is bent. This type of fracture typically occurs in children because of the pliable nature of their bones. The fracture usually heals in one week.

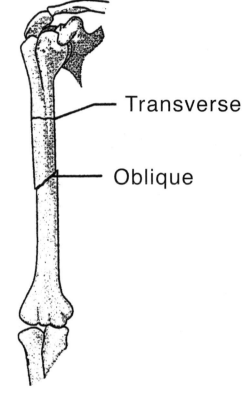

Transverse

Oblique

Closed
(simple, complete)

In a closed or simple fracture, the bone does not break through the skin. There is little to no damage to surrounding soft tissue. The treatment is application of a plaster cast after the ends of the bone have been aligned.

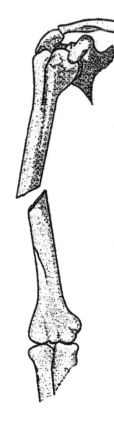

Open
(compound)

In an open or compound fracture, the bone comes through the skin. Because there is a break in the skin, the patient is at a greater risk for infection with this type of fracture. Patients need to go to surgery to have the area thoroughly cleaned before the fracture is set.

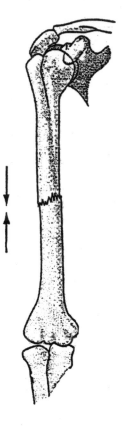

Impacted

In an impacted fracture, the portion of bone that is fractured is wedged into the portion of the bone that is not broken. The fracture is stable unless the fragments are pulled apart.

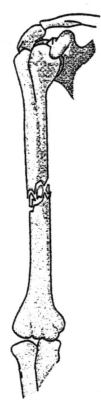

Comminuted

In a comminuted fracture, the bone breaks into pieces. The fracture is produced from a very high force or normal force in a very fragile bone. Treatment includes placement of external or internal fixators to stabilize the bone. These fractures take a longer time to heal.

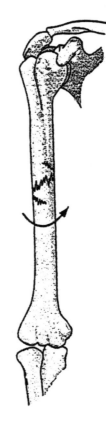

Spiral

A spiral fracture is a fracture in which the bone has been twisted apart. These fractures are very unstable, therefore there may never be union of the bone pieces. Treatment includes surgical placement of rods and screws to realign the bone.

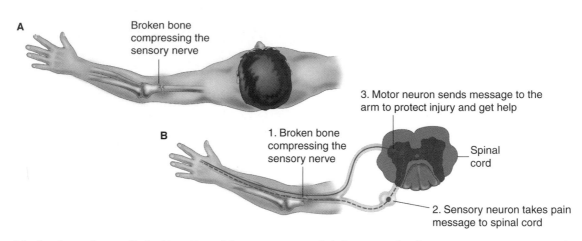

A broken bone also results in disruption of the sensory nerve. It is important for the nurse to assess sensory and motor function distal to the site of the fracture.

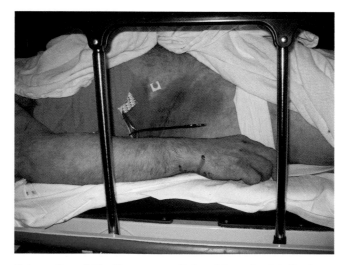

Retroperitoneal bleeding may result from hip and pelvic fractures.

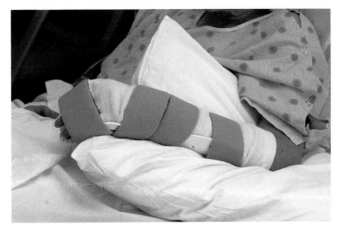

A splint may be used to stabilize a fracture. A splints is used as a temporary means to stabilize a fracture until medical care is available.

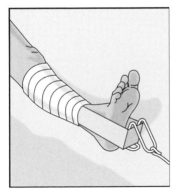

Skin traction is used to stabilize a fracture. The extremity is wrapped and weights are applied distal to the fracture. Skin traction is used for dislocated joints or simple fractures, and helps decrease muscle spasms associated with a fracture. Weights of only 5-10 pounds are used.

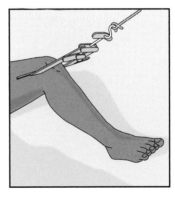

Skeletal traction is used to stabilize a fracture and involves the insertion of a pin through the bone. Skeletal traction is used for fractures of long bones. Weights are attached to the pins and hung over the edge of the bed. The nurse needs to be sure the weights are hanging freely and not leaning up against the bed frame.

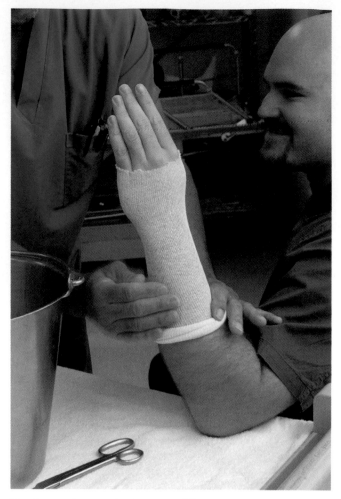

The fractured extremity is prepared for casting. First a knit stocking is placed over the extremity.

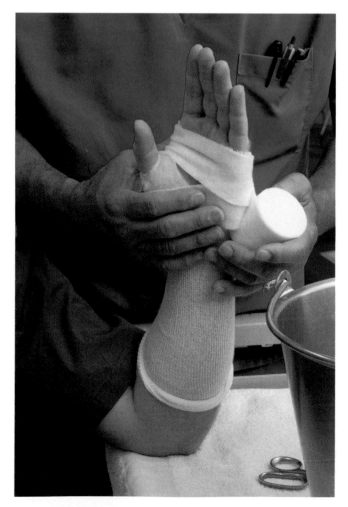

After application of the knit stocking, the arm is wrapped with a dry bandage.

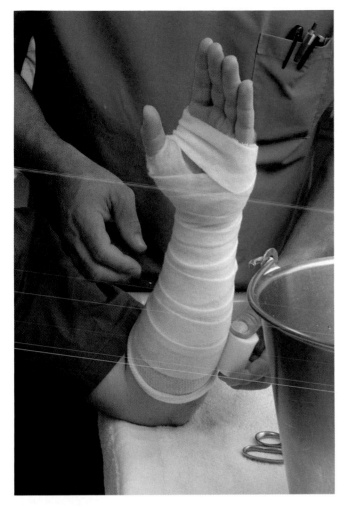

The application of the dry bandage is completed.

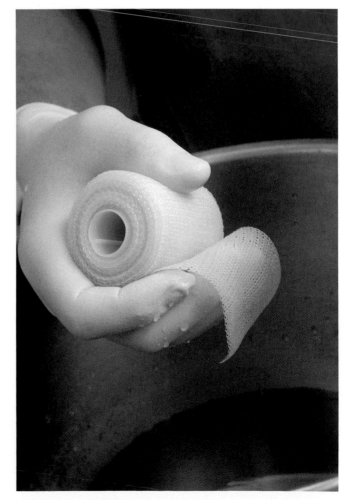

The plaster bandage is soaked is water.

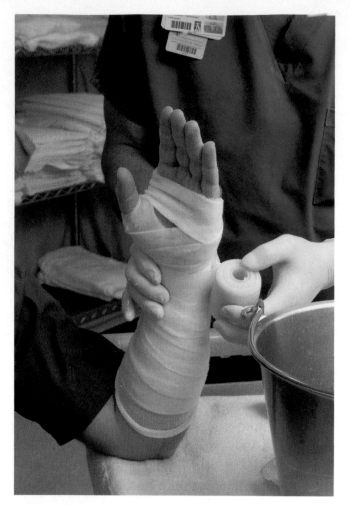

The soaked plaster bandage is then wrapped on the arm.

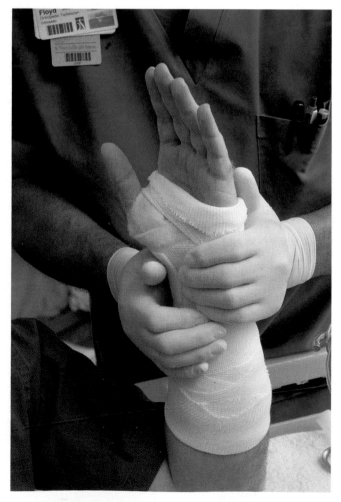

The bandage is smoothed out to an even surface.

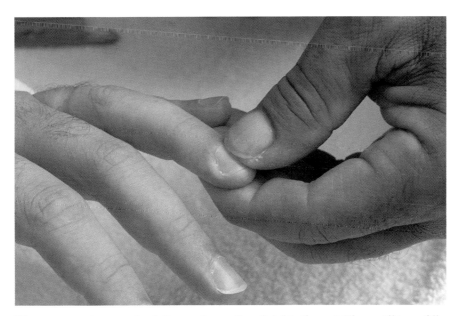

The nurse must assess circulation and sensation distal to the cast. The capillary refill is being checked to assess circulation and the nail is pinched also to assess feeling or sensation. The assessment of circulation and sensation is most important the first 24-48 hours after the cast is applied, since swelling is most often to occur during this period.

GASTRITIS

Gastritis is the inflammation of the stomach lining and may be acute or chronic. Causes include infection (*Helicobacter pylori*), nonsteroidal anti-inflammatory drugs, alcohol, smoking, and radiation. If untreated, gastritis can lead to ulcer formation. Treatment of gastritis can prevent ulcer formation.

Assessment

- Epigastric pain, guarding, distention
- Poor appetite
- Nausea and vomiting
- Signs of ulcer hemorrhage: melena (blood in the feces), hematemesis (vomiting blood), and hemorrhagic shock (low BP, tachycardia)
- Signs of ulcer perforation: melena, hematemesis, hemorrhagic shock, and a rigid, intensely painful abdomen

Planning and Implementation

- Treat nausea and vomiting
- Administer antacids, H2 receptor antagonists, and proton pump inhibitors
- If H pylori present, anticipate administering antibiotics (bismuth subsalicylate, metronidazole, and tetracycline)
- Monitor stools for melena
- Monitor for hematemesis
- Offer small, frequent meals

Evaluation and Outcomes

The patient will:

- Be free of gastric pain
- Maintain adequate nutritional intake
- Avoid precipitating factors
- Understand pharmacologic treatment

Nursing Considerations

- Precipitating factors include alcohol, non-steroidal anti-inflammatory medications, spicy foods, nicotine, and caffeine.

- Teach patients taking nonsteroidal anti-inflammatory drugs to report any abdominal pain or bloody emesis or stools.

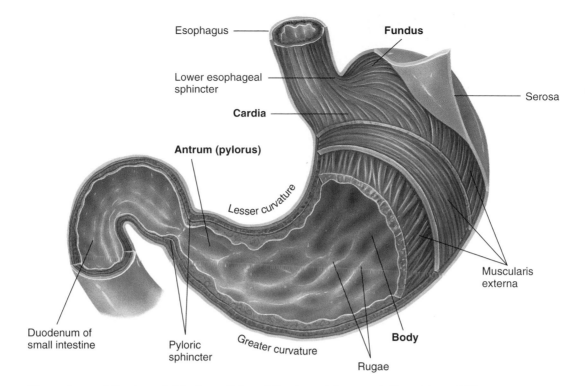

The anatomy of the stomach. The inner lining of the stomach becomes inflamed in gastritis.

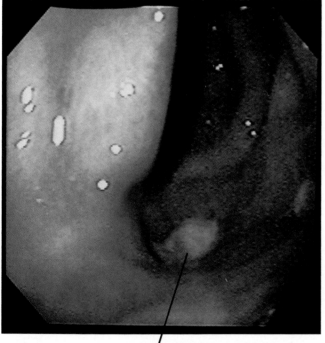

Gastric Ulceration

This endoscopic picture shows a gastric ulcer. The ulceration is the patchy whitish discoloration seen through the endoscope. Treatment at this stage includes medications to decrease acid production in the stomach.

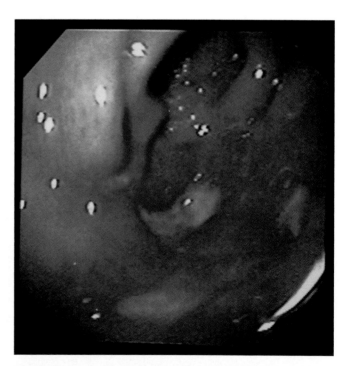

The presence of a stomach ulcer—the whitish patchy area seen on an endoscopy. Gastric ulcers can result from chronic gastritis. Patients may experience stomach pain, indigestion and heartburn or dyspepsia.

GASTROENTERITIS

Gastroenteritis is the inflammation of the mucous membranes of the stomach and intestines, resulting in an increased frequency and water content of stools and vomiting. It may be viral or bacterial in origin.

Assessment

- History of onset of diarrhea, vomiting
- Vital signs
- Signs and symptoms of dehydration
- Character, quality, amount of stools

Planning and Implementation

- Intravenous fluid replacement
- Daily weights
- Intake and Output
- Clear liquids

Evaluation and Outcomes

The patient will:

- Be free of diarrhea and vomiting
- Maintain weight
- Maintain adequate fluid intake
- Maintain skin integrity

Nursing Considerations

- Elderly patients develop dehydration more quickly

- Teach patients not to share eating utensils, glasses, and dishes.

- Teach patients to wash hands after each bowel movement to minimize risk of disease transmission

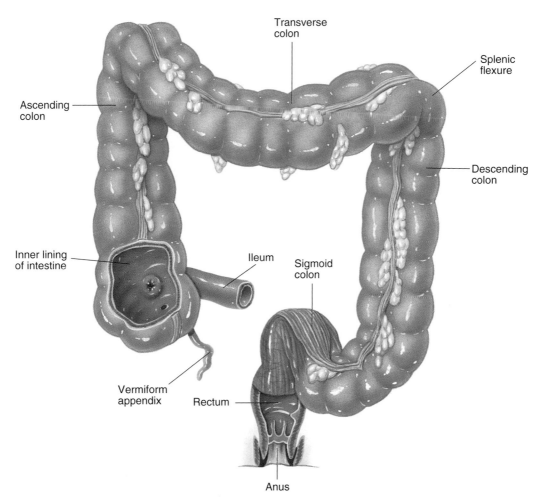

The normal anatomy of the large intestine. Gastroenteritis is the inflammation of the inner lining of the gastrointestinal tract, resulting in vomiting and watery diarrhea. With the presence of inflammation the large intestine is unable to absorb water, thus leading to the watery diarrhea seen in gastroenteritis.

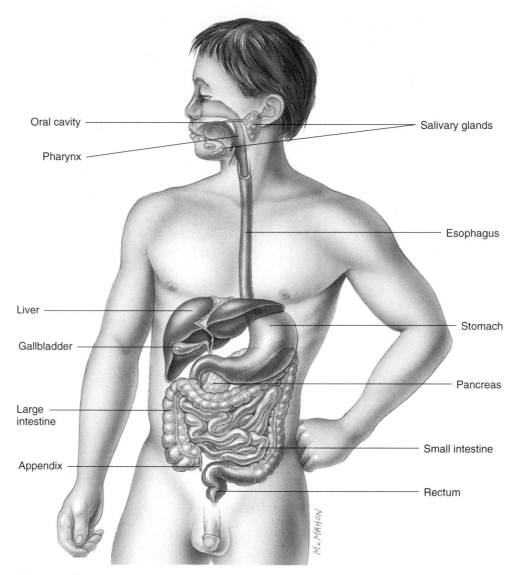

The normal anatomy of the gastrointestinal tract. Gastroenteritis can occur anywhere along the gastrointestinal system.

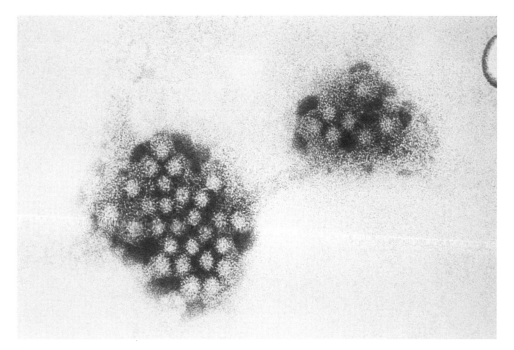

An electron microscope picture of the Norovirus. The Norovirus is a type of food poisoning caused by eating foods or drinking liquids that are contaminated with the virus. Symptoms last 1-2 days.

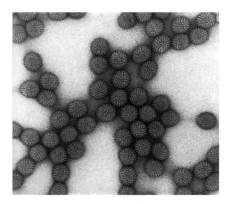

An electron microscope view of the rotavirus. The rotavirus is a common cause of gastroenteritis. Patients are infected through ingestion of contaminated food or water or contact with contaminated surfaces. This virus commonly causes diarrhea in children.

GASTROESOPHAGEAL REFLUX DISEASE (GERD)

Gastroesophageal reflux disease (GERD) refers to the backing up of gastric contents into the esophagus, causing irritation of the esophageal mucosal and eliciting an inflammatory response. The esophagus may become inflamed (esophagitis) and ulcerations may develop in the esophagus if left untreated.

Assessment

- Pyrosis (heartburn, low sternal or epigastric pain) especially after a large meal or with bending forward
- Esophagitis
- Pharyngitis
- Hoarseness
- Water brash (excess saliva stimulated by acid reflux)

Planning and Implementation

- Eat 4 to 6 small meals per day
- Upright position while eating and for one hour after meals
- Avoid hot and cold beverages
- Avoid alcohol, caffeine, and tobacco
- Avoid eating before bedtime
- Administer antacids, H2 blockers, and proton pump inhibitors as ordered

Evaluation and Outcomes

The patient will:

- Be free of dyspepsia
- Understand pharmacologic treatment
- Avoid irritants such as fatty foods, alcohol, caffeine, and nicotine

Nursing Considerations

- Weight reduction may help decrease symptoms in the obese patient.

- Teach patients to elevate head of bed by 8 to 12 inches to prevent reflux at night.

- Teach patients to avoid wearing clothing that is tight around the waistline.

- Teach patients to eat frequent small meals and avoid eating two to three hours before sleeping.

- Teach patients to sit upright for one hour after meals.

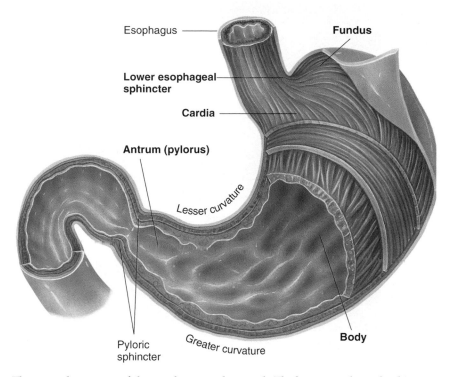

The normal anatomy of the esophagus and stomach. The lower esophageal sphincter stops stomach contents from backing up into the esophagus. In gastroesophageal reflux disease, the esophageal sphincter fails and the acid from the stomach backs up into the esophagus.

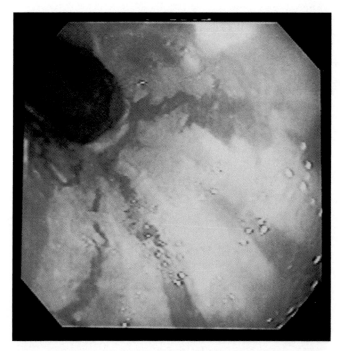

An endoscopic image of esophagitis. Esophagitis is a common finding in patients with gastroesophageal reflux disease. The whitish areas seen are the result of reflux of stomach acids seen in GERD.

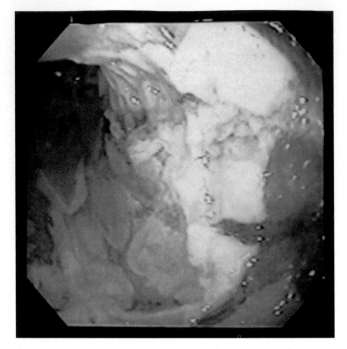

An image of severe esophagitis as seen through an endoscope. Instead of pink tissue, the lining is white in color.

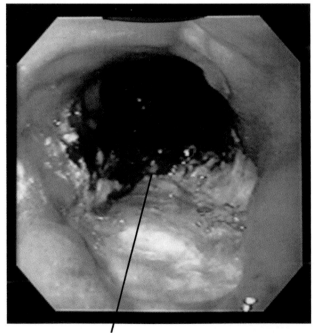

Bleeding From Ulceratior

An esophageal ulcer seen through an endoscope. The patchy white area is the ulceration and fresh blood is seen at the top of the whitish area.

Active Bleeding

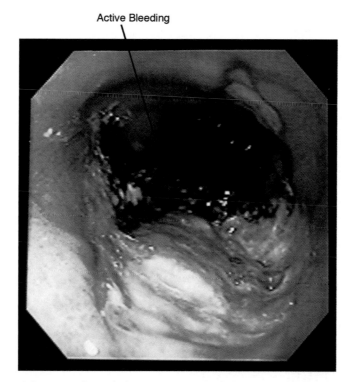

A large esophageal ulceration. Note the blood seen at the base of the white ulceration. The patient would present with bloody emesis and would require an immediate endoscopy to cauterize the bleeding area.

GENETIC DISORDERS, AMYOTROPHIC LATERAL SCLEROSIS

Amyotrophic lateral sclerosis (ALS) is a neurological disorder that causes the upper and lower motor neurons to degenerate and die. The loss of neuron function causes the muscles to gradually weaken and atrophy. There is no known cure for ALS.

Assessment

- Sensation in the upper and lower extremities.
- Muscle strength in the upper and lower extremities
- Dysphagia
- Fatigue while talking

Planning and Implementation

- Prevent complications of immobility
- Provide for comfort
- Provide for rest periods
- Emotional support for patient and family

Evaluation and Outcomes

The patient will:

- Be free of complications of immobility
- Understand the progression of the disease
- Maintain a support system

Nursing Considerations

- ALS is also called Lou Gehrig's disease, named after a famous baseball player who was diagnosed with this disease.

- Men are affected more than women.

- ALS most commonly affects people between the ages of 40 and 60 years.

- About 5 to 10 percent of all ALS cases are inherited.

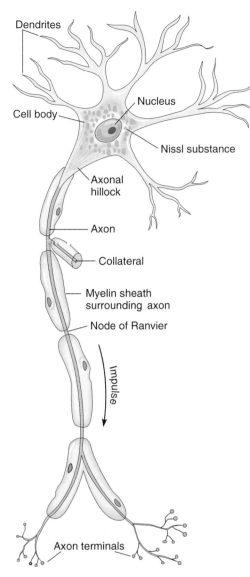

The normal neuron. In ALS the motor neurons degenerate and die, leading to muscle weakness and paralysis.

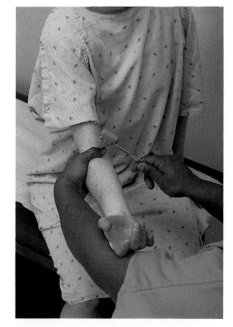

The nurse should assess the reflexes in the upper arms in patients with ALS. The biceps tendon reflex is shown in this picture. As the disease progresses the reflexes become weaker to absent.

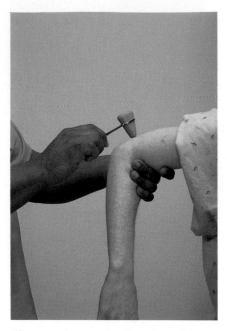

The nurse is assessing the triceps deep tendon reflex. The reflex becomes weak to absent as ALS progresses.

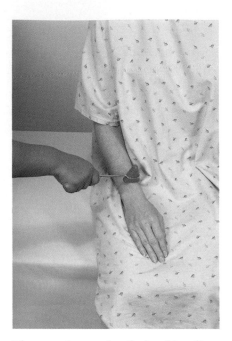

The nurse is assessing the brachioradialis deep tendon reflex.

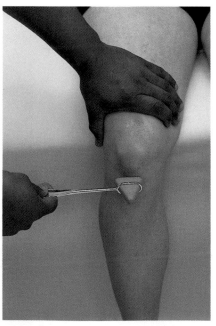

The nurse should assess the reflexes in the lower extremities in patients with ALS. The nurse is assessing the patellar reflex. As the disease progresses the reflexes become weaker to absent.

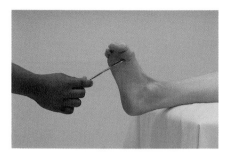

The nurse is assessing the Babinski reflex.

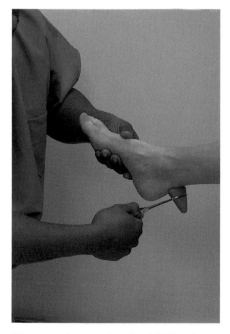

The nurse is assessing the Achilles deep tendon reflex. As ALS progresses the reflexes become weaker and eventually absent.

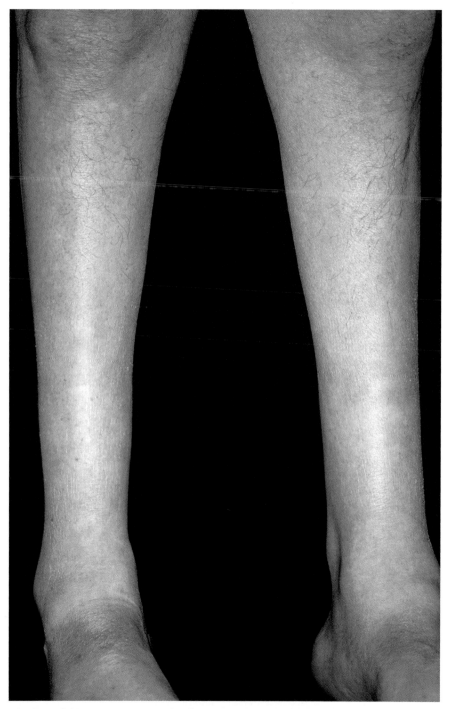

The legs of this patient are atrophied, meaning the muscle tissue has decreased in size. This is due to the progressive loss of neuromuscular function seen in ALS.

GENETIC DISORDERS, CYSTIC FIBROSIS

Cystic fibrosis (CF) is a genetic disease of the mucus and sweat glands. CF is caused by a defective gene that directs the body's epithelial cells to produce a defective form of a protein called CFTR (or Cystic Fibrosis Transmembrane Conductance Regulator) found in cells that line the lungs, digestive tract, sweat glands, and genitourinary system. The mucus becomes thick, sticky, and hard to move, so the lungs become infected and the pancreas can't secrete enzymes needed for absorption of nutrients.

Assessment

- Malnourished
- Thick pulmonary secretions
- Bulky, foul-smelling stools
- Stomach pain and discomfort

Planning and Implementation

- Coughing and deep breathing
- Provide adequate nutrition
- Maintain hydration status
- Chest percussion and postural drainage

Evaluation and Outcomes

The patient will:

- Be free of pulmonary infections
- Maintain adequate nutritional status
- Be free of pain

Nursing Considerations

- 40% of patients with cystic fibrosis are over the age of 18.

- The average life span for those who live to adulthood is approximately 35 years.

- The patient inherits two defective genes, one from each parent.

- CF is more common in Caucasians, especially those of Northern or Central European descent.

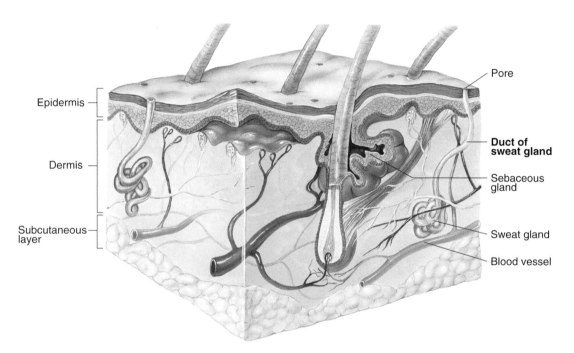

Epidermis

Dermis

Subcutaneous layer

Pore

Duct of sweat gland

Sebaceous gland

Sweat gland

Blood vessel

Normal anatomy of the skin. Cystic fibrosis affects the sweat and mucus glands located in the skin and throughout the body. The mucus becomes very thick in the lungs and pancreas, altering organ function.

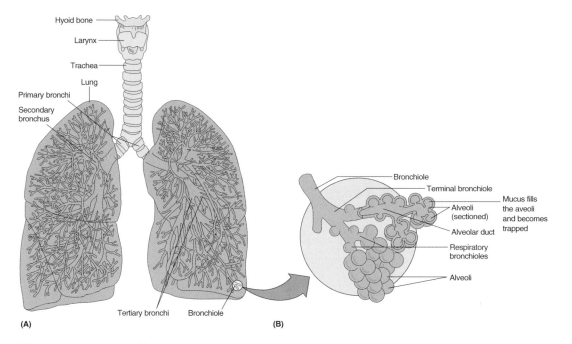

Hyoid bone
Larynx
Trachea
Lung
Primary bronchi
Secondary bronchus
Tertiary bronchi
Bronchiole

(A)

Bronchiole
Terminal bronchiole
Mucus fills the aveoli and becomes trapped
Alveoli (sectioned)
Alveolar duct
Respiratory bronchioles
Alveoli

(B)

The patient with cystic fibrosis has alveoli that become plugged with thick mucus, leading to the development of frequent respiratory infections.

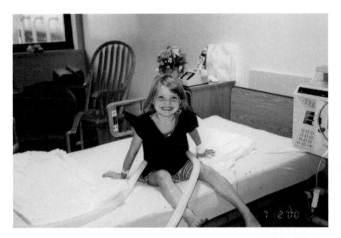

A ThAIRapy vest is used for patients with cystic fibrosis. The purpose of the vest is to provide chest physiotherapy to break up the thick secretions in the alveoli, so the patient can expectorate the thick mucus.

GENETIC DISORDERS, MARFAN'S SYNDROME

Marfan's syndrome is a genetically inherited connective tissue disease that causes deformations and defects in the ocular, skeletal, and cardiovascular systems. Marfan's syndrome is caused by mutations in the gene fibrillin-1. Fibrillin-1 plays an important role as the "scaffolding" for elastic tissue in the body. Disruption of scaffolding (by mutations in fibrillin-1) results in changes in elastic tissues, particularly in the aorta, eye, and skin. Mutations in fibrillin-1 also cause overgrowth of the long bones of the body, resulting in the tall stature and long limbs seen in Marfan patients.

Assessment

- Skeletal structure
- Assess spinal deformities.
- Cardiac auscultation
- Supraventricular arrhythmias

Planning and Implementation

- Assess heart sounds
- Monitor electrocardiogram
- Routine eye examinations

Evaluation and Outcomes

The patient will:

- Maintain normal cardiac function
- Be able to perform activities of daily living
- Maintain adequate vision

Nursing Considerations

- Marfan's syndrome is inherited as an autosomal dominant trait.

- Marfan's syndrome appears in 4-6 of every 100,000 people.

- There is 50% incidence of transmittance to offspring, with no sex-linked characteristics.

- Those diagnosed with Marfan's need to be on prophylactic antibiotics prior to dental procedures, because of an increased risk of endocarditis.

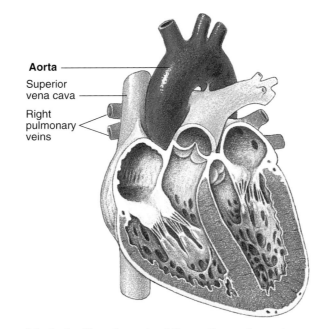

Aorta
Superior
vena cava
Right
pulmonary
veins

Marfan's affects the aorta of the cardiovascular system.
The aorta may tear easier, leading to rupture and death.

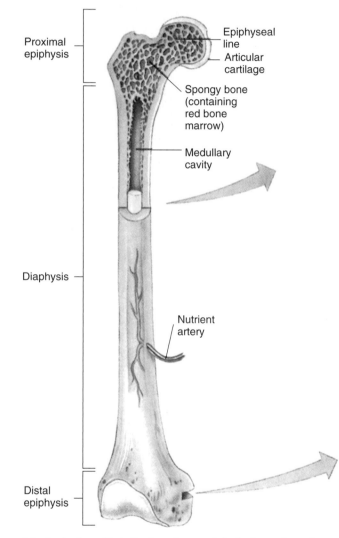

Proximal
epiphysis

Epiphyseal
line

Articular
cartilage

Spongy bone
(containing
red bone
marrow)

Medullary
cavity

Diaphysis

Nutrient
artery

Distal
epiphysis

*Marfan's also affects the long bones of the body, such as the
humerus and femur. The result of Marfan's is overgrowth of the
long bones. Patients with Marfan's are tall with long limbs.*

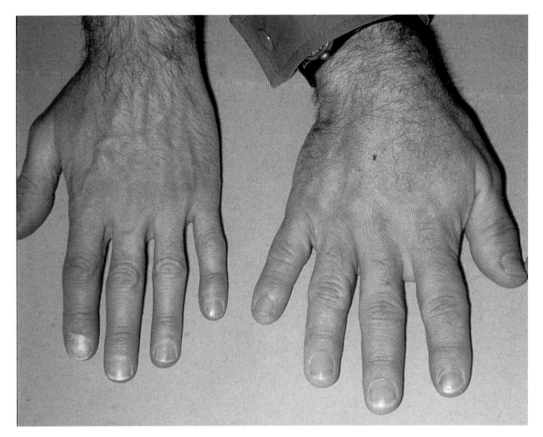

The hand on the right depicts an enlarged hand seen in a person with Marfan's. Notice how large the hand is compared to the hand on the left from a person who does not have Marfan's. (Courtesy of Viewing Medicine)

GENETIC DISORDERS, POLYCYSTIC KIDNEY

Polycystic kidney disease (PKD) is a genetic disorder characterized by the growth of numerous cysts in the glomeruli and tubules of the kidney. The cysts slowly replace the kidney tissue, leading to renal failure. Autosomal dominant PKD is the most common inherited form.

Assessment

- Protruding and distended abdomen
- Abdominal pain
- Hematuria or cloudy urine
- Flank pain
- Hypertension

Planning and Implementation

- Assess amount, character, and quantity of urine
- Palpate for enlarged kidney
- Monitor blood pressure
- Monitor for edema

Evaluation and Outcomes

The patient will:

- Maintain adequate kidney function
- Maintain normal blood pressure
- Be free of pain
- Be able to perform activities of daily living

Nursing Considerations

- Patients with polycystic kidney disease suffer from frequent urinary tract infections and should inform their doctor immediately if they have pain or burning with urination.

- Patients should be instructed to treat the pain associated with this disease with over-the-counter analgesics, such as Tylenol.

- Patients should be taught to check their blood pressure monthly, since polycystic kidney disease may result in hypertension.

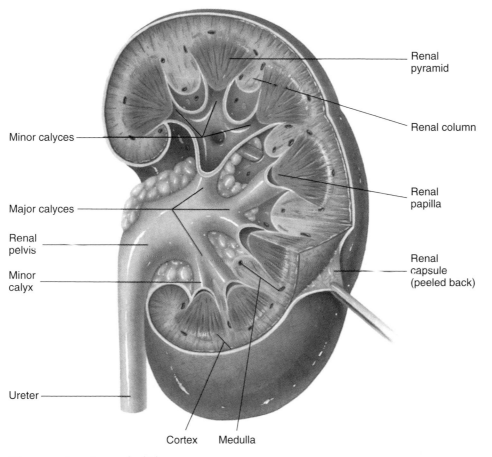

Renal
pyramid

Renal column

Renal
papilla

Minor calyces

Major calyces

Renal
pelvis

Minor
calyx

Renal
capsule
(peeled back)

Ureter

Cortex   Medulla

The normal anatomy of a kidney.

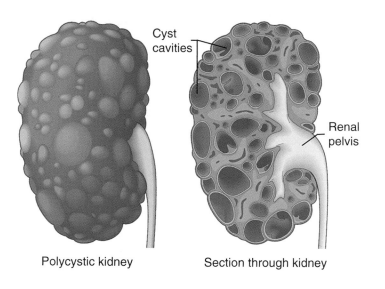

Polycystic kidney   Section through kidney

In polycystic kidney disease there are multiple cysts located throughout the kidney.

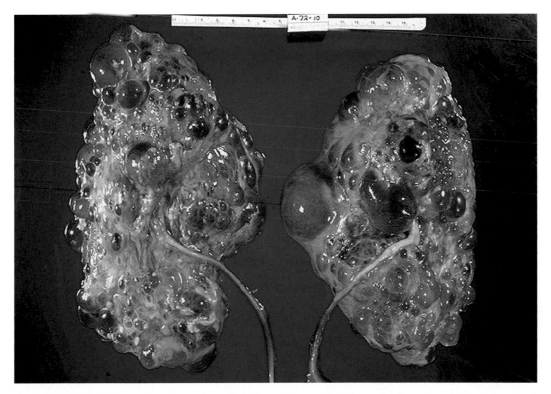

Pathology of the kidneys showing polycystic kidney disease. Note the multiple cysts or blebs throughout the kidneys.

GENITAL HERPES

Genital herpes is a sexually transmitted disease caused by the herpes simplex virus.

Assessment

- Vesicles or blisters in or on the genitals (penis, scrotum, vulva, vagina, cervix) and/or perianal area
- Fever
- Tingling sensation in the skin
- Headache

Planning and Implementation

- Assess genital area and note presence of blisters
- Vital signs
- History of sexual contacts
- Pain management

Evaluation and Outcomes

The patient will:

- Understand genital herpes is a sexually transmitted disease
- Prevent further spread of the disease
- Understand pharmacologic treatment
- Maintain body image

Nursing Considerations

- The incubation period is 2 to 20 days, with an average of one week.

- Teach patients to wear gloves while applying ointments.

- Genital-to-oral transmission can occur.

- Teach patients to avoid sexual contact when lesions are present and use condoms during all sexual activity.

- Educate patients about available support groups.

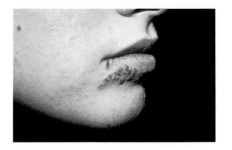

The herpes simplex virus. (Courtesy of Robert A. Silverman, M.D., clinical Associate Professor, Department of Pediatrics, Georgetown University)

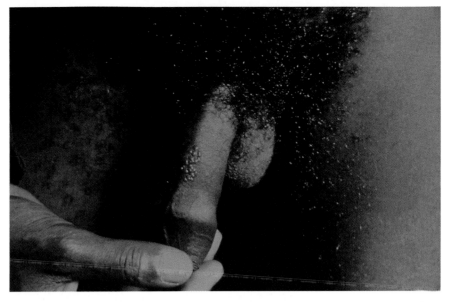

Herpes simplex virus of the penis. The lesions are painful and may cause pain and burning with urination. Treatment is with antiviral drugs. (Courtesy of the CDC)

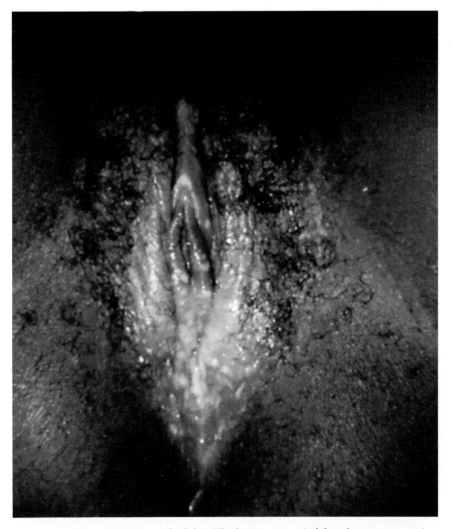

Herpes simplex virus seen on the labia. The lesions are painful and may cause pain and burning with urination. The presence of genital herpes increases a womeanís risk of cervical cancer. Treatment includes antiviral drugs. (Courtesy of the CDC)

GENITAL WARTS

Genital warts or venereal warts are a sign of Human Papillomavirus, a sexually transmitted disease causing warts or bumps in the genital areas of men and women.

Assessment

- Soft, moist skin colored bumps in the genital area
- Itching, burning in genital area
- Discomfort, pain or bleeding during intercourse

Planning and Implementation

- Inspection of genital area
- Handwashing
- Teaching on transmission

Evaluation and Outcomes

The patient will:

- Understand the warts are sexually transmitted
- Maintain good hygiene practices
- Use a condom during sexual intercourse

Nursing Considerations

- Genital warts can lead to cancer of the cervix in women and cancer of the penis in men.

- There is a long incubation period.

- Warts can be removed but the virus remains.

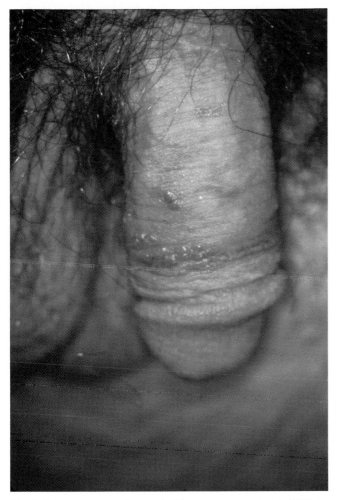

Genital warts seen on the penis. The warts are not painful but may cause itching. Drainage from the warts may also occur. Warts may occur on the urethra, penis, scrotum, and rectal area in men. Warts may be removed by cryotherapy or laser therapy. (Courtesy of the CDC)

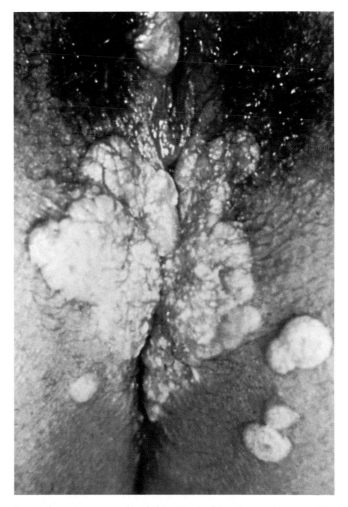

Genital warts seen on the labia. Genital warts may be caused by the Human Papillomavirus and may increase a woman's risk of developing cervical cancer. A vaccine against this virus is now available. (Courtesy of the CDC)

GOITER

A goiter is an enlargement of the thyroid gland. A simple goiter occurs when the thyroid gland is unable to produce enough thyroid hormone to meet the body's needs.

Assessment

- Enlarged neck
- Difficulty swallowing
- Painful swallowing
- Stridor

Planning and Implementation

- Assess airway
- Assess swallowing
- Neck vein distention

Evaluation and Outcomes

The patient will:

- Maintain an adequate airway
- Maintain ability to swallow

Nursing Considerations

- The use of ionized table salt prevents endemic goiter.

- Goiter occurs more commonly in females.

- There is a familial history with the presence of a goiter.

- Goiter is more common after the age of 40.

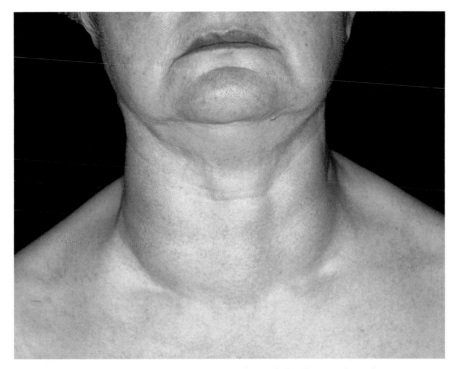

A goiter seen in a patient with an overactive thyroid gland. Note the enlargement in the neck. The thyroid gland is grossly enlarged and results in the mass seen in the neck. The nurse needs to monitor the patient for an adequate airway and the ability to swallow. (Courtesy of Viewing Medicine)

GONORRHEA

Gonorrhea is a sexually transmitted disease caused by the gram-negative bacteria, Neisseria gonorrhoeae, and is transmitted by sexual contact and during childbirth through an infected birth canal.

Assessment

- Dysuria
- Penile discharge in men; vaginal discharge in women
- Anal itching and burning
- Pharyngitis

Planning and Implementation

- Sexual history
- Number of sexual contacts
- History of sexually transmitted diseases
- Presence of symptoms

Evaluation and Outcomes

The patient will:

- Report the need for treatment to all sexual contacts
- Adhere to treatment regimen
- Verbalize the need to practice safe sex

Nursing Considerations

- Initial symptoms occur 3 to 10 days after sexual contact with an infected individual.

- Gonorrhea is the most reported communicable disease in the United States.

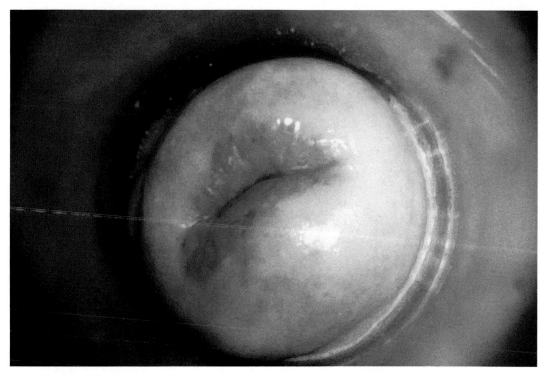

Neisseria gonorrhea infection of the cervix as seen through a colposcopy. The patient may be asymptomatic. (Courtesy of the CDC)

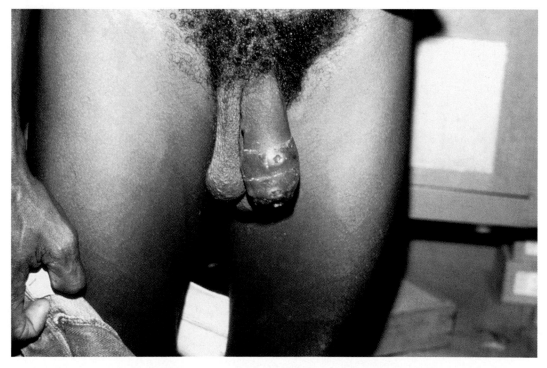

Penile infection caused from Neisseria gonorrhea. Symptoms include painful urination, penile discharge, and anal itching and irritation. Treatment includes antibiotics. (Courtesy of the CDC)

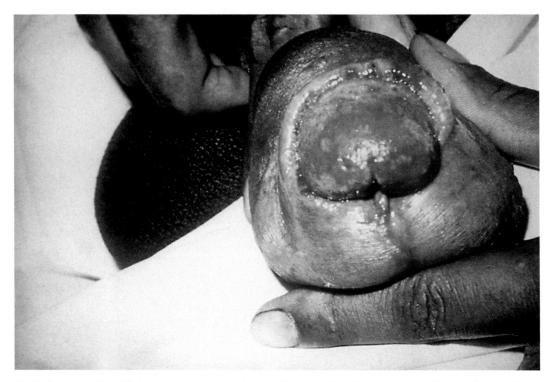

Penile infection from Neisseria gonorrhea with paraphimosis. Paraphimosis causes the foreskin to adhere to the glans penis and cannot be retracted. This is very painful. (Courtesy of the CDC)

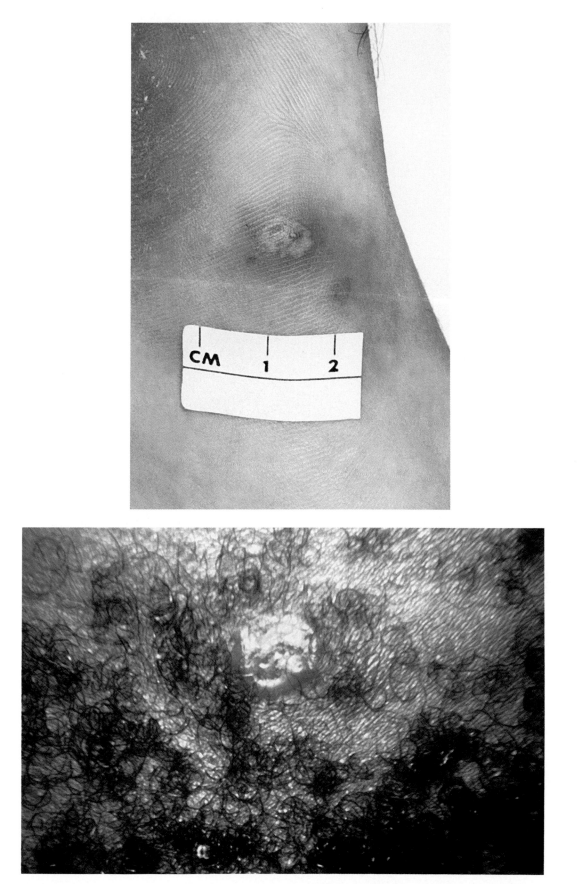

Skin infections caused by Neisseria gonorrhea. Treatment includes antibiotics. (Courtesy of the CDC)

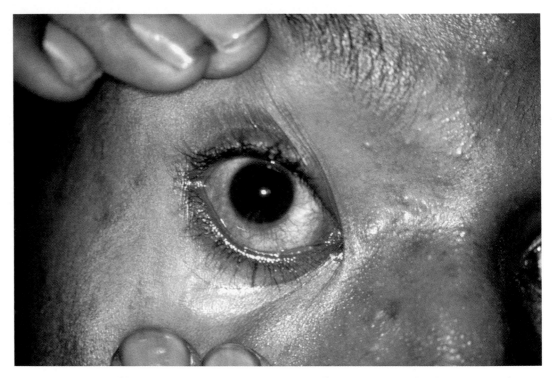

Conjunctivitis caused by Neisseria gonorrhea bacteria. The infection may spread to the eye by touching the eye. Symptoms include red, watery eyes, with drainage from the eyes. Treatment is with antibiotics. (Courtesy of the CDC)

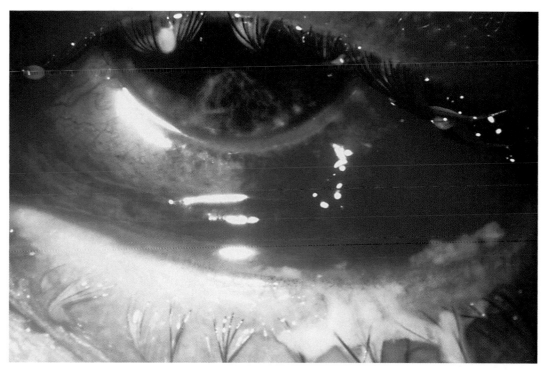

Severe conjunctivitis caused from Neisseria gonorrhea. This resulted in partial blindness for the patient. (Courtesy of the CDC)

GOUT

Gout is a metabolic disorder with a hereditary tendency causing hyperuricemia (excessive uric acid), producing nodules or tophi consisting of uric acid. The tophi may be found in the joints and cause an acute foreign body reaction, such as swelling and fever.

Assessment

- Pain
- Swelling
- Decreased ROM to affected joint
- Affected joints commonly include ears, hands, feet

Planning and Implementation

- Bedrest (1st 24 hours)
- Heat
- Ice
- Elevation of extremity
- Low purine diet
- Administer NSAIDs as ordered

Evaluation and Outcomes

The patient will:

- Be free of pain
- Be able to perform activities of daily living

Nursing Considerations

- Avoid foods high in purine including alcohol, organ meats, anchovies, sardines, herring, mussels, codfish, scallops, trout, haddock, bacon, turkey, veal, and venison.

- Nonsteroidal anti-inflammatory drugs can be used to treat the pain.

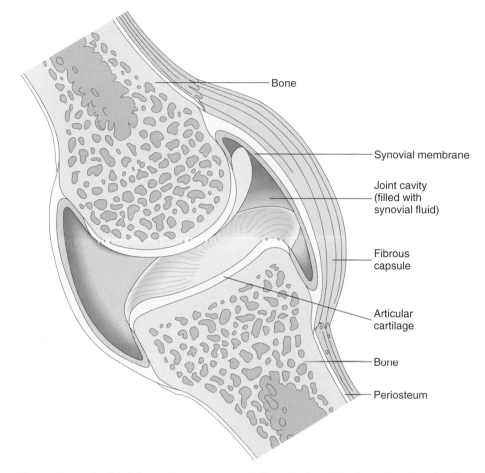

Bone

Synovial membrane

Joint cavity (filled with synovial fluid)

Fibrous capsule

Articular cartilage

Bone

Periosteum

The anatomy of a joint. In gout, excess accumulation of uric acid leads to deposits of nod-ules within the joints. These nodules cause pain in the joints, especially the distal phlanx or "great toe".

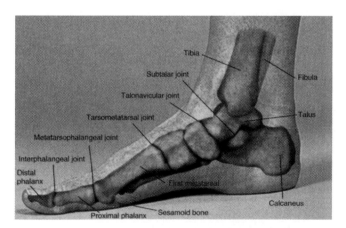

The hallmark symptom of gout is pain in the great toe.

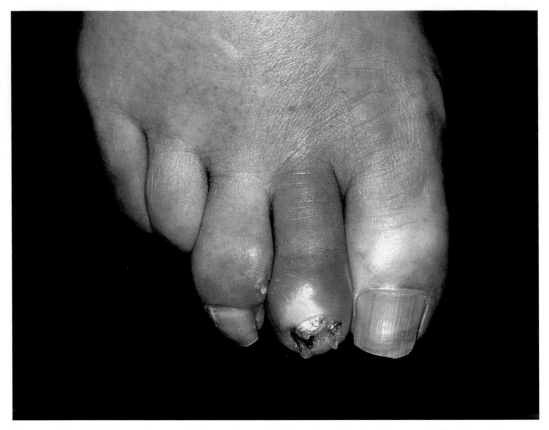

The second and third toes have tophi formations, which are deposits of sodium urate. Tophi usually are found in the joint of the foot and are painful. The tophus on the second toe is white and creamy in color and very reddened. The third toe is also reddened and swollen. Patients should keep the affected foot elevated to help decrease swelling. (Courtesy of Viewing Medicine)

GRAVES' DISEASE

Graves' disease or a toxic diffuse goiter is the most common cause of hyperthyroidism.

Assessment

- Tachycardia, hypertension, tachypnea
- Goiter
- Fever
- Agitation, nervousness, anxiety

Planning and Implementation

- Vital signs
- Electrocardiogram
- Gastrointestinal symptoms
- Airway

Evaluation and Outcomes

The patient will:

- Maintain adequate airway
- Have stable vital signs
- Have normal thyroid function
- Have a normal cardiac rhythm

Nursing Considerations

- Treatment for hyperthyroidism includes pharmacological and surgical intervention.

- Hyperthyroidism is more common in women.

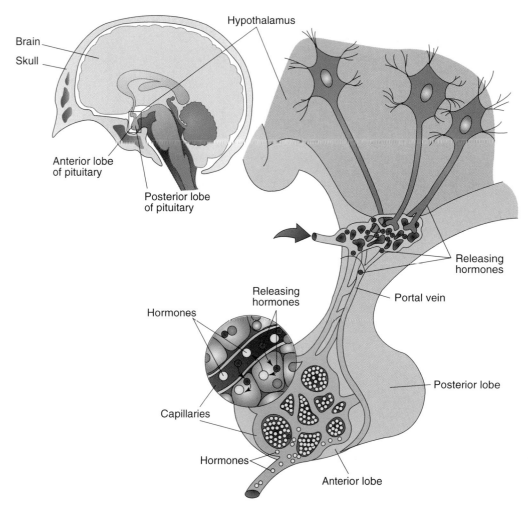

Brain

Skull

Hypothalamus

Anterior lobe
of pituitary

Posterior lobe
of pituitary

Releasing
hormones

Releasing
hormones

Hormones

Portal vein

Capillaries

Posterior lobe

Hormones

Anterior lobe

Graves' disease is the excess of thyroid hormone in the body. The thyroid gland is stimulated to release thyroid hormone by thyroid stimulating hormone released from the anterior lobe of the hypothalamus.

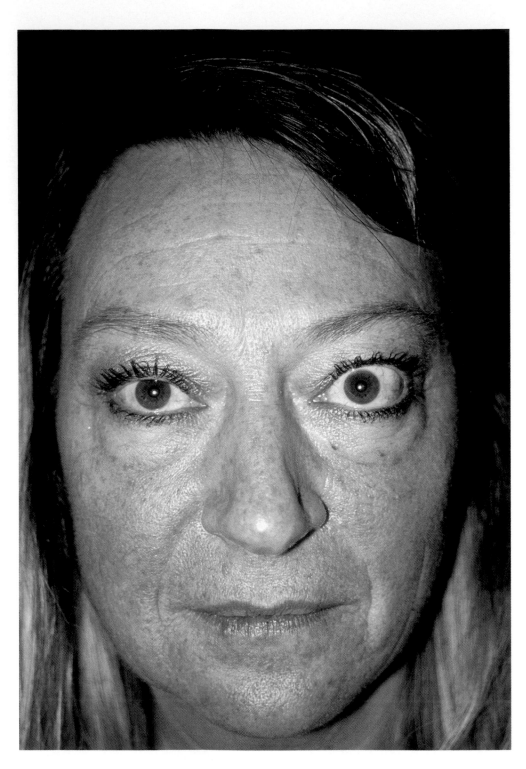

Exopthalamus, or bulging eyes, seen in a patient with Grave's disease. The patient should be instructed to use lubricant eye drops to prevent dryness of the eyes.

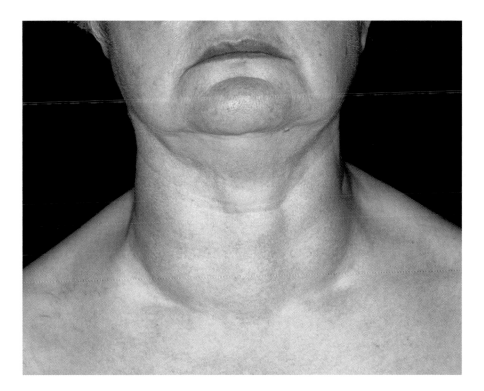

An excess of thyroid hormone production as seen in Grave's disease leads to the enlargement of the thyroid gland, also called a goiter.

GYNECOMASTIA

Gynecomastia is the enlargement of the breast tissue in males caused by the proliferation of the glandular tissue.

Assessment

- Enlarged breasts
- Increased serum estrogen levels
- Decreased serum testosterone levels

Planning and Implementation

- Medications
- Assess enlargement of breast tissue
- Medical history

Evaluation and Outcomes

The patient will:

- Maintain adequate body image
- Understand treatment possibilities.

Nursing Considerations

- Nurses should conduct a thorough history of medication use in patients with gynecomastia, since one of the causes of gynecomastia includes drugs such as anti-ulcer drugs, chemotherapy agents, and some antibiotics.

- Nurses should inform the patient that one potential treatment for gynecomastia is surgical reduction.

- Nurses need to teach patients with gynecomastia that breast tenderness can be reduced with analgesics and the application of cold compresses.

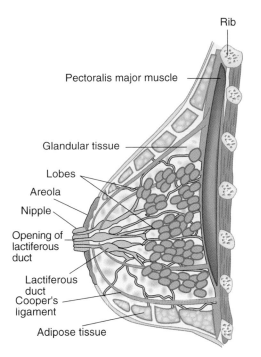

Gynecomastia is the enlargement of breast tissue
seen in males.

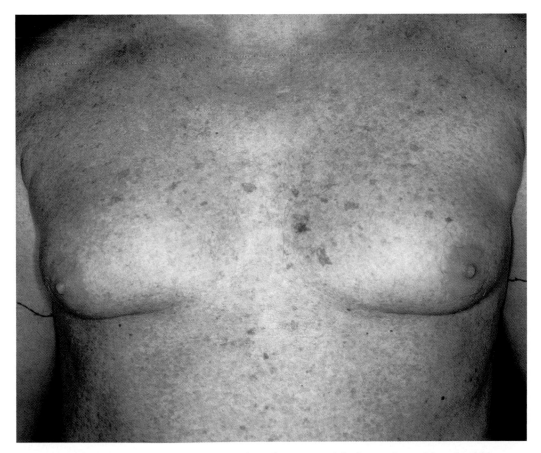

*Gynecomastia seen in a male patient. Notice the enlargement of the breast tissue. Men should be
assessed for a potential disturbance in body image related to the increase in size of the breast tissue.
(Courtesy of Viewing Medicine)*

HEMOPHILIA

Hemophilia is a group of hereditary diseases that result in a deficiency of clotting factors. Depletion of factors VIII, IX, and X collectively makes up approximately 95% of the bleeding disorders. The lack of clotting factor puts patients with hemophilia at higher risk for bleeding.

Assessment

- Joint or muscle pain
- Bruising
- Hemarthrosis (bleeding into joints)—weight bearing joints most commonly affected
- Hemorrhage (may be fatal after trauma or surgery)
- Oxygenation status

Planning and Implementation

- Frequent vital signs (signs of shock—hypotension and tachycardia)
- Anticipate blood and factor replacement
- Observe for hemorrhage, especially at surgical site
- Monitor clotting factors
- Monitor patient for hypersensitivity reactions to factor replacement (chest tightness, uticaria, hypotension)

Evaluation and Outcomes

The patient will:

- Have stable vital signs
- Be free of bleeding
- Wear MedicAlert bracelet

Nursing Considerations

- Refer patients for genetic counseling. Hemophilia A affects 1 in 10,000 males and is an X-linked recessive disorder transmitted from mother to sons and Hemophilia B affects 1 in 40,000 males and is an X-linked recessive disorder transmitted from mother to sons.

- Teach patients to watch closely for signs of bleeding including bruising, bloody gums, and blood in the stools.

- Teach patients to wear a MedicAlert bracelet.

- Teach patients to avoid medications that inhibit blood clotting such as aspirin and ibuprofen.

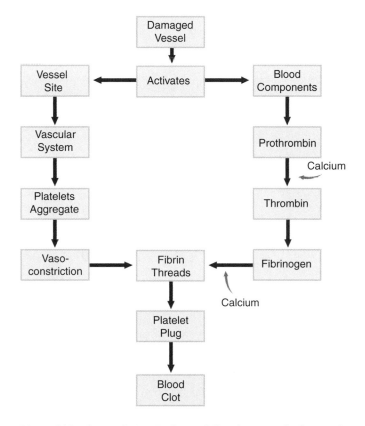

Normal blood coagulation. In hemophilia, there is a depletion of clotting factors, leading to abnormal clotting and bleeding.

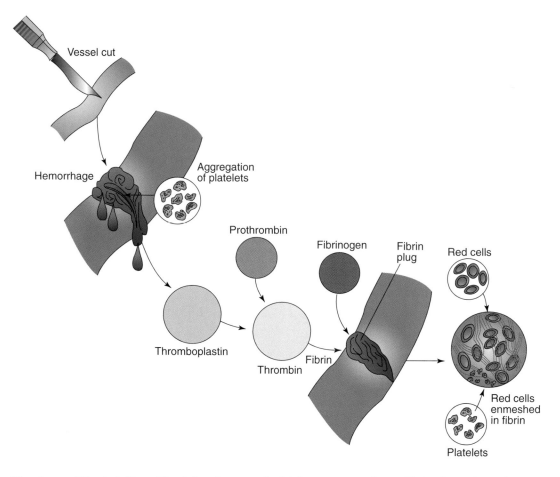

The stages of blood clotting. After injury to a vessel, platelets aggregate then a fibrin plug is formed to seal the vessel. In hemophilia, a deficiency in clotting factors leads to the inability of the body to produce a fibrin plug.

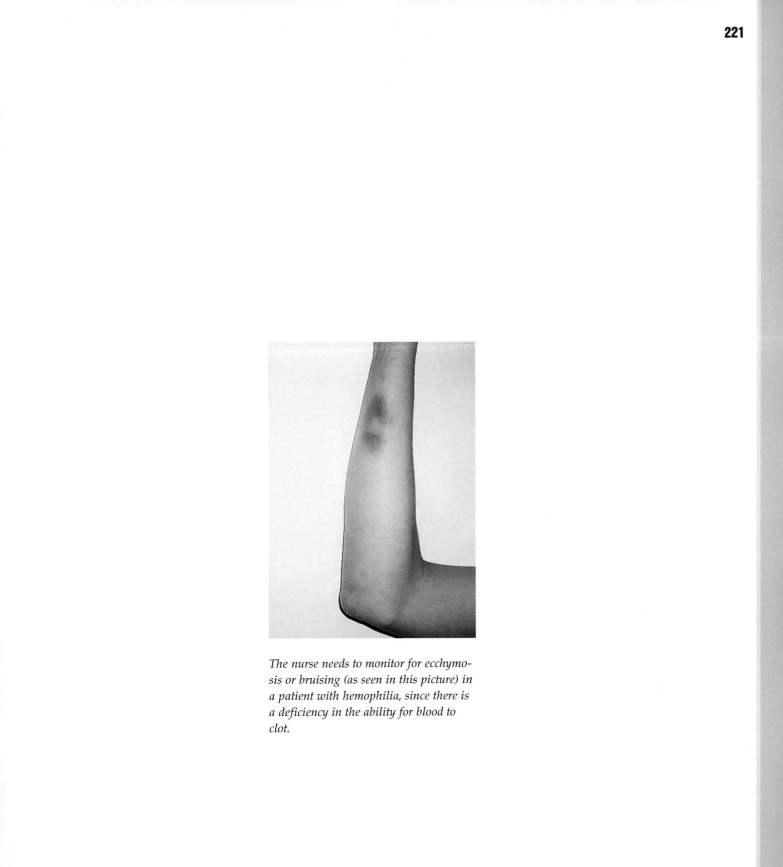

The nurse needs to monitor for ecchymosis or bruising (as seen in this picture) in a patient with hemophilia, since there is a deficiency in the ability for blood to clot.

HEMORRHOIDS

Hemorrhoids are swollen or dilated veins in the anal or rectal region. Internal hemorrhoids are located above the anal sphincter and external hemorrhoids are located outside of the anal sphincter.

Assessment

- Bleeding
- Pain
- Itching
- Burning

Planning and Implementation

- Inspection of anal area
- Assess for bleeding
- Provide therapy for relief of pain and burning
- High fiber diet and fluids to promote regular bowel movements

Evaluation and Outcomes

The patient will:

- Be free of symptoms
- Verbalize need for high fiber diet and adequate fluid intake
- Verbalize understanding of therapies to relieve symptoms
- Understand need for possible surgical intervention

Nursing Considerations

- Instruct women of childbearing age that hemorrhoids may occur during pregnancy.

- Teach patients to increase their fiber intake to promote regular bowel pattern to reduce risk of developing hemorrhoids.

- Teach the patient that stool softeners may also help decrease pain with hemorrhoids.

- Teach patients that over-the-counter medications are helpful to decrease the pain and itching associated

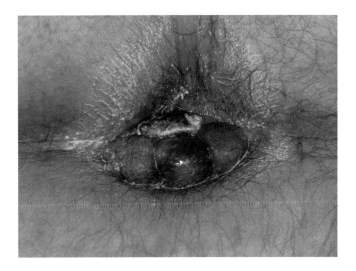

The hemorrhoids are visible on the outer aspects of the anus.
The patient feels burning, itching, and pain in the area.
(Courtesy of Viewing Medicine)

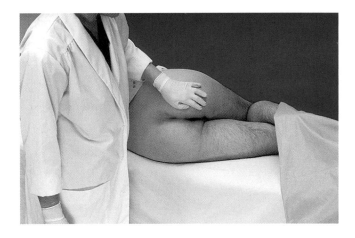

The patient should be placed in a lateral recumbent position in
order for the nurse to assess for the presence of hemorrhoids.

HODGKIN'S LYMPHOMA

Hodgkin's Lymphoma is a lymphatic cancer that develops in a lymph node or chains of lymph nodes. Affected lymph nodes in Hodgkin's lymphoma contain Reed-Sternberg cells. Hodgkin's disease is labeled in stages I through IV. Stage I involves one lymph node region. Stage II involves two or more lymph node regions on the same side of the diaphragm. Stage III involves lymph nodes on both sides of the diaphragm. Stage IV involves other organs besides the lymph system. The earlier it is diagnosed, the better the prognosis.

Assessment

- Lymph node enlargement, painless or painful
- Fever, weight loss
- Night sweats
- Generalized malaise

Planning and Implementation

- Meticulous skin care
- Monitor for infection
- Promote adequate nutritional intake
- Promote rest periods to combat fatigue
- Anticipate administering blood products, granulocyte colony-stimulating factor, and epogen products

Evaluation and Outcomes

The patient will:

- Verbalize understanding of treatment of chemotherapy and radiation
- Be free of infection, bleeding, and anemia
- Maintain skin integrity

Nursing Considerations

- Teach male patients that treatment may result in sterility.

- While undergoing therapy, teach patients to monitor body temperature and avoid crowded areas to reduce risk of infection.

- Teach patients to watch for skin breakdown and avoid using harsh soaps at the site where radiation is administered.

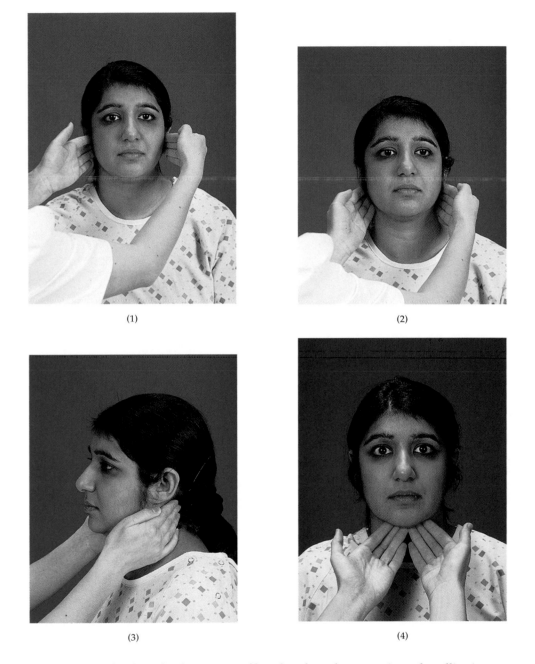

(1)

(2)

(3)

(4)

The nurse should palpate for the presence of lymph node tenderness, pain, and swelling in a patient with Hodgkin's lymphoma. These pictures illustrate the sequence and appropriate places of palpation.

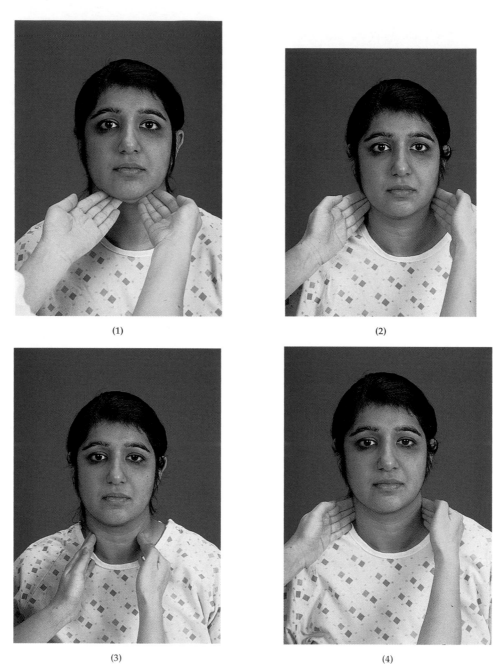

(1)

(2)

(3)

(4)

The nurse should palpate for the presence of lymph node tenderness, pain, and swelling in a patient with Hodgkin's lymphoma. These pictures illustrate the sequence and appropriate places of palpation.

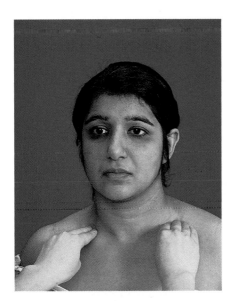

The nurse should palpate for the presence of lymph node tenderness, pain, and swelling in a patient with Hodgkin's lymphoma. This picture illustrates the sequence and appropriate places of palpation.

HYPERLIPIDEMIA

Hyperlipidemia is the elevation of lipids in blood including cholesterol and triglycerides. The increase in lipid levels causes formation of plaque in the interior of the blood vessels narrowing the lumen and restricting blood flow.

Assessment

- Dietary intake
- Family history
- Activity levels
- Lipid panel

Planning and Implementation

- Assess for risk factors
- Assess dietary intake
- Monitor lipid panel
- Administer medications to reduce lipid levels (niacin, statins)

Evaluation and Outcomes

The patient will:

- Verbalize need to reduce dietary intake of fat
- Understand pharmacologic treatment
- Verbalize need to monitor lipid levels on a routine basis

Nursing Considerations

- Teach patients to avoid foods high in fats such as organ meats, cream, butter, and fast foods.

- Instruct patients that increasing exercise may help decrease lipid levels in the blood.

- Teach patients on statins (lipid-lowering medications) to report right upper quadrant abdominal pain, pale yellow urine, or clay-colored stools as this may indicate liver dysfunction, which is a side effect of these medications.

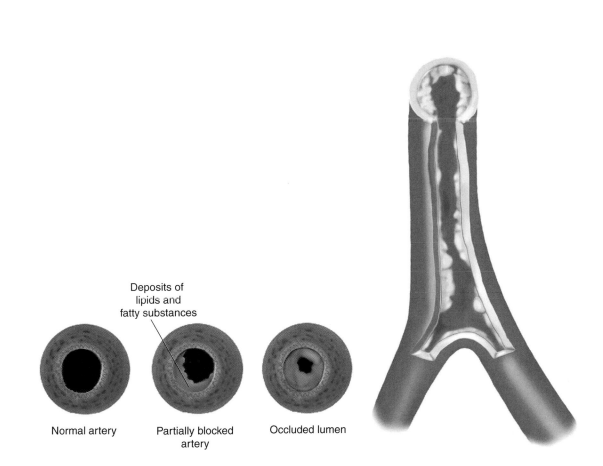

Deposits of
lipids and
fatty substances

Normal artery

Partially blocked
artery

Occluded lumen

A. A cross section of the artery. The buildup of fat within the vessel is the result of hyperlipidemia. B. The buildup of fatty substances within the inner lumen of the arteries can lead to total occlusion of the artery and ischemia.

HYPERTHYROIDISM

Hyperthyroidism is the continuous secretion of thyroid hormones resulting in elevated triiodothyronine (T3) and thyroxine (T4) hormone and low thyroid-stimulating hormone (TSH) levels. Thyrotoxic crisis is a life-threatening complication of hyperthyroidism.

Assessment

- Enlarged thyroid
- Tachycardia, palpitations
- Fatigue
- Heat intolerance
- Weight loss
- Exopthalmos

Planning and Implementation

- Monitor oxygenation status
- Monitor for cardiac arrhythmias
- Ensure adequate fluid and nutritional intake
- Provide eye care (artificial tears, shielding at night)
- Monitor for hypothyroidism after therapy
- Monitor for thyrotoxic crisis or thyroid storm (brought on by infection, stress, pregnancy)

Evaluation and Outcomes

The patient will:

- Have stable vital signs
- Maintain a regular cardiac rhythm
- Maintain adequate nutritional intake
- Verbalize understanding of treatment

Nursing Considerations

- Teach patients with exopthalmos to use artificial tears and elevate the head of bed at night to relieve eye soreness.

- Teach patients receiving antithyroid therapy the signs and symptoms of hypothyroidism, such as slow heart rate, fatigue, constipation, weight gain.

- Patients receiving radioactive iodine therapy need discharge instructions to sleep alone; avoid close contact with children; practice personal hygiene; wash towels and clothes daily; and avoid preparing food with bare hands.

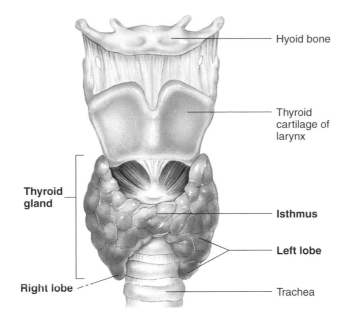

The normal anatomy of the thyroid gland. The thyroid gland is a butterfly-shaped organ located on the anterior part of the trachea. The isthmus connects the right and left lobes of the thyroid gland.

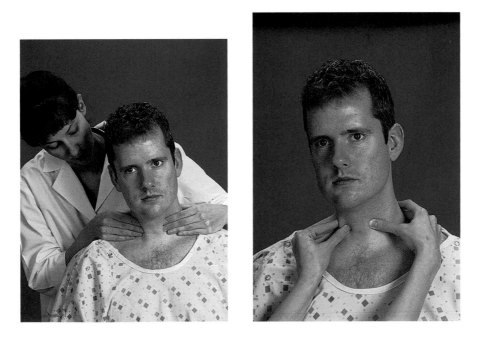

On assessment, the nurse needs to palpate for enlargement of the thyroid gland. This can be done using a posterior or anterior approach. In hyperthyroidism, the thyroid gland will be enlarged.

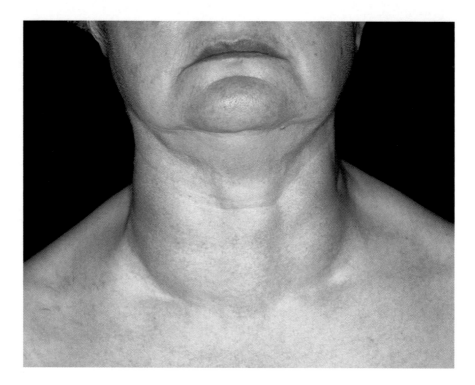

A goiter or enlarged thyroid is present in hyperthyroidism due to the overactivity of the thyroid gland. The patient needs to be assessed for an adequate airway and any difficulty with swallowing, as the enlarged thyroid gland may compress the trachea and esophagus. (Courtesy of Viewing Medicine)

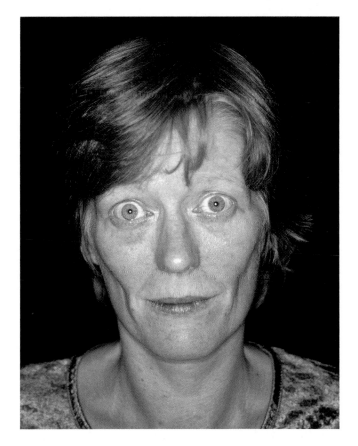

In hyperthyroidism, an assessment finding is exopthalmos or bulging of the eyes and patients may appear to "stare" with the eyes. The eyes become dry and painful. Artificial tears may be used to lubricate the eyes. (Courtesy of Viewing Medicine)

HYPOPITUITARISM

Hypopituitarism is caused by the inability of the pituitary gland to synthesize and secrete hormones. Deficiencies in adrenocorticotropic hormone (ACTH) lead to vascular collapse, and deficiencies in thyroid-stimulating hormone (TSH) lead to suppression of heart rate and respirations.

Assessment

- Fatigue
- Weakness
- Sensitivity to cold
- Infertility
- Hypotension

Planning and Implementation

- Anticipate surgical removal if tumor present
- Anticipate administering supplemental hormones (thyroid, sex, and growth)
- Monitor blood pressure
- Discuss infertility concerns

Evaluation and Outcomes

The patient will:

- Have stable vital signs
- Verbalize need for lifelong replacement of deficient hormones
- Wear MedicAlert bracelet
- Maintain body image

Nursing Considerations

- Teach patients they will be on lifelong hormone replacement.

- Instruct female patients that hormone replacement therapy (human chorionic gonadotropin) will be needed for reproduction.

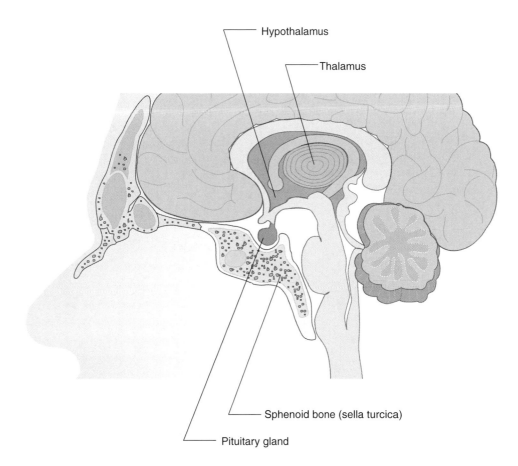

Hypothalamus

Thalamus

Sphenoid bone (sella turcica)

Pituitary gland

Normal anatomy of the brain showing the location of the pituitary gland.

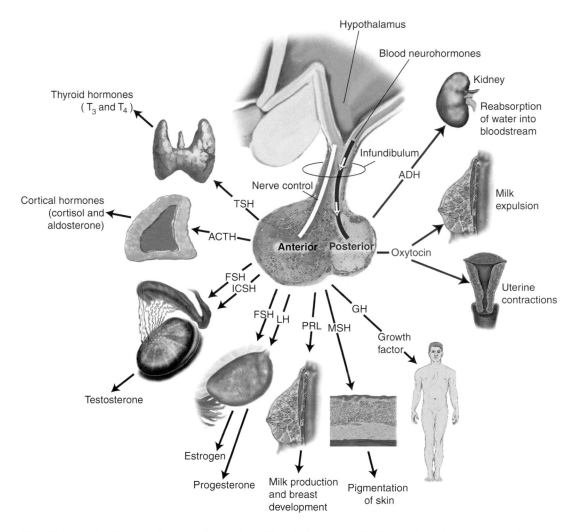

The pituitary gland and its hormonal secretions. The pituitary gland is divided into the anterior and posterior lobes. Pituitary hormones are responsible for growth (secretion of growth hormone), metabolism (secretion of thyroid hormone), development of sexual characteristics (secretion of estrogen and testosterone), glucose metabolism (secretion of cortisol), and blood volume (secretion of aldosterone).

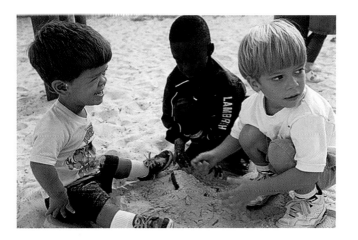

Hypopituitarism results in a decreased secretion of growth hormone, resulting in dwarfism in children. This can be treated with administration of human growth hormone until the normal period of growth ends, usually in the end of the teenage years.

HYPOTHYROIDISM

Hypothyroidism is the clinical state where there is deficient production of thyroid hormone by the thyroid gland. Symptoms of the condition may range from general malaise to myxedema coma when heart rate and respirations are too slow to sustain life.

Assessment

- Fatigue
- Weight gain
- Dry skin
- Cold intolerance
- Bradycardia
- Constipation
- Confusion

Planning and Implementation

- Provide frequent rest periods
- Monitor vital signs
- Provide warm environment
- Encourage fluid intake
- Monitor and treat constipation
- Administer medications (levothyroxine (T4) is the drug of choice, liothyronine (T3) may be administered as well)

Evaluation and Outcomes

The patient will:

- Have stable vital signs
- Maintain adequate oxygenation status
- Understand need for lifelong pharmacologic therapy
- Maintain adequate nutritional intake

Nursing Considerations

- Women and the elderly are more commonly affected with hypothyroidism.

- Teach patients that thyroid replacement therapy will be lifelong.

- Teach patients to take the thyroid medication in the morning on an empty stomach to maximize absorption.

- Teach patients to wear extra clothing in cold temperatures because of a cold intolerance seen in hypothyroidism.

- Teach patients to have thyroid levels checked once a year to make sure the thyroid supplement medication dose is adequate.

239

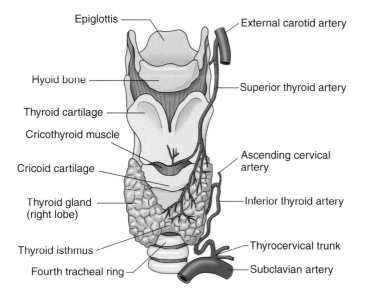

Epiglottis	External carotid artery
Hyoid bone	Superior thyroid artery
Thyroid cartilage	
Cricothyroid muscle	Ascending cervical artery
Cricoid cartilage	
Thyroid gland (right lobe)	Inferior thyroid artery
Thyroid isthmus	Thyrocervical trunk
Fourth tracheal ring	Subclavian artery

The thyroid gland is a butterfly-shaped structure located on the anterior portion of the trachea. The isthmus connects the right and left lobes of the thyroid. Lack of secretion of thyroid hormone from the thyroid gland leads to hypothyroidism.

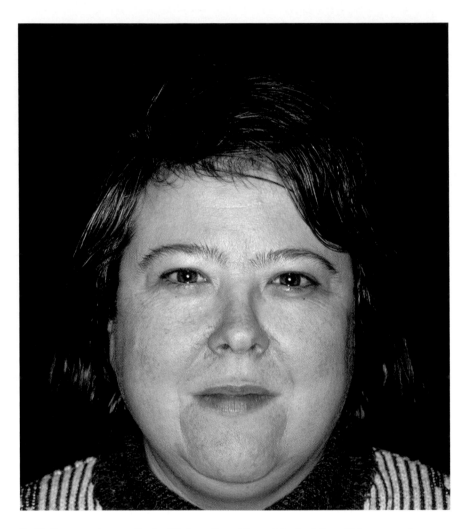

Puffy face seen in a patient with hypothyroidism. A lack of thyroid hormone slows down metabolism and leads to symptoms such as puffy face, cold intolerance, weight gain, and constipation. Once thyroid replacement is started, these symptoms begin to subside. (Courtesy of Viewing Medicine)

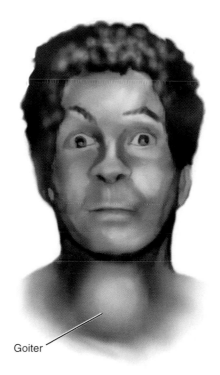

Goiter

An enlarged thyroid gland or goiter seen in hypothyroidism. When thyroid levels are low, the thyroid gland is being constantly stimulated to release thyroid hormones, and this causes the thyroid gland to enlarge. The patient needs to be assessed for an adequate airway as this may compress the trachea, and assessed for ability to swallow, as the enlarged thyroid gland may compress the esophagus.

LUNG CANCER

Lung cancer is malignancy of the lungs caused by a malignant neoplasm in which cells mutate and invade the tissue; these cells can travel via the lymphatic system and blood vessels to other sites.

Assessment

- Cough, blood sputum
- Wheezing
- Shortness of breath
- Weight loss
- Difficulty swallowing
- Change in voice

Planning and Implementation

- Oxygen administration
- Frequent vital signs including pulse oximetry
- Provide adequate pain relief
- Administer medications to treat nausea
- Encourage frequent oral care
- Provide frequent rest periods
- Prevent infections
- Encourage adequate fluid and nutritional intake
- Monitor CBC and platelets

Evaluation and Outcomes

The patient will:

- Verbalize understanding of therapy, including surgery, chemotherapy, and radiation
- Maintain adequate oxygenation status
- Maintain skin integrity
- Stop smoking

Nursing Considerations

- Instruct patient to eliminate tobacco use.

- Teach patients that supplemental oxygen may be needed to help relieve shortness of breath.

- Teach patients to sit up in a lounge chair or recliner to help alleviate shortness of breath.

- Instruct patients on side effects of pain medicine, including depression of respirations, constipation, and drowsiness.

- Refer the terminally ill patient to hospice.

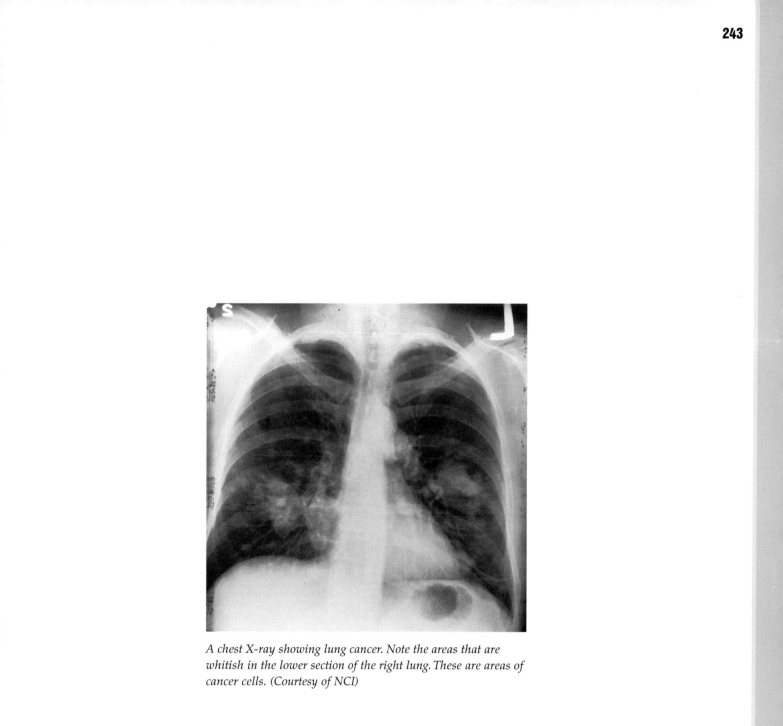

A chest X-ray showing lung cancer. Note the areas that are whitish in the lower section of the right lung. These are areas of cancer cells. (Courtesy of NCI)

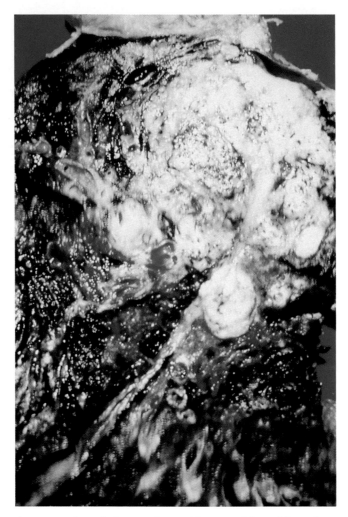

A cross section of a human lung with cancer. Normal lung tissue is pink in color. The white area in the upper portion is the cancer. The black areas indicate the patient was a smoker. The cancerous area will need to be surgically removed. (Courtesy of NCI)

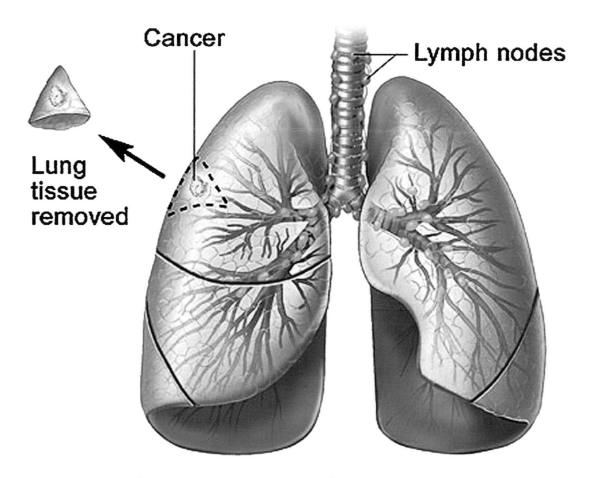

Cancer

Lymph nodes

Lung tissue removed

A surgical treatment for lung cancer is a wedge resection where only the tumor and surrounding lung tissue are removed. This requires a thoracotomy (opening of the chest) and patients will have much pain after the surgery. Since only a section of the lung is removed, patients should do well postoperatively. (Courtesy of NCI)

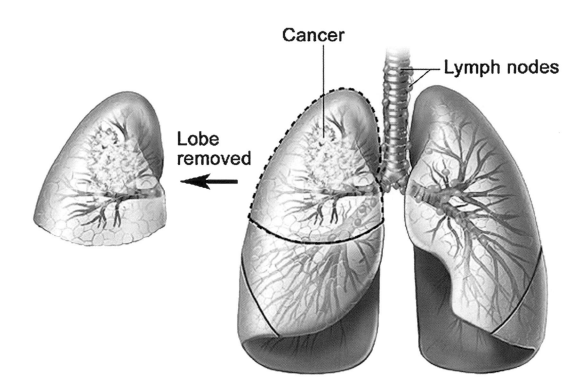

A lobectomy may also be a surgical treatment for lung cancer. In a lobectomy, only the lobe of the lung is removed. This requires a throacotomy approach and patients will be in the hospital for up to a week. Since a lobe of the lung is removed, the patient may have difficulty oxygenating. (Courtesy of NCI)

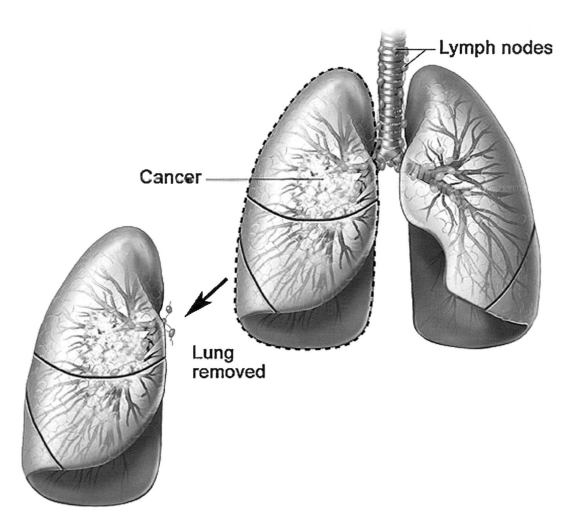

Lymph nodes

Cancer

Lung removed

Another surgical treatment for lung cancer is a pneumonectomy or the removal of an entire lung. This is a major operation requiring a thoracotomy. Since the entire lung is removed, patients may have trouble oxygenating and must be monitored for symptoms of hypoxia. (Courtesy of NCI)

LUPUS ERYTHEMATOSUS

Lupus erythematosus is a chronic and potentially fatal autoimmune disease characterized by spontaneous remissions and exacerbations. Lupus erythematosus involves changes in the skin, kidneys, joints, heart, lungs, and brain.

Assessment

- Dry, scaly raised rash on the face or upper body
- Myalgia
- Fever
- Fatigue and weakness
- Diminished urinary output

Planning and Implementation

- Assess skin
- Monitor urine output
- Assess joint pain and range of motion
- Assess breath sounds

Evaluation and Outcomes

The patient will:

- Be able to maintain activities of daily living
- Be free of pain
- Maintain adequate organ function
- Understand there will be periods of exacerbation and remission

Nursing Considerations

- Teach patients to avoid exposure to sunlight by wearing long sleeves or use sun-blocking agents of SPF of 30 or higher when in the sun.

- Teach patients to use cosmetics with moisturizers.

- Teach patients to use a mild shampoo and avoid hair permanents and hair coloring.

- Instruct patients to use mild soaps.

- Teach patients to monitor for fever, which is the first sign of an exacerbation of the disease.

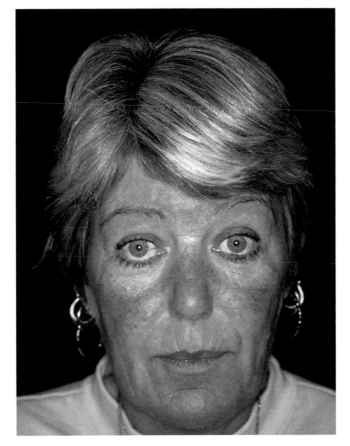

The patient has a butterfly rash on the face. This is a common finding in lupus erythematosus because the disease affects the collagen network of the skin, causing the skin to become dry and reddened. The patient should use cosmetics with moisturizers and avoid harsh soap and soap with a lot of perfume. (Courtesy of Viewing Medicine)

MACULAR DEGENERATION

Macular degeneration is the deterioration of the macula, which is the part of the retina that is responsible for the central vision needed to read, write, and drive. It is characterized by sclerosing of the retinal capillaries. It is diagnosed as either dry (non-neovascular) or wet (neovascular).

Assessment

- Blurred vision
- Distorted vision
- Loss of vision
- Amsler grid vision check (specific visual test for macular degeneration)

Planning and Implementation

- Assess visual acuity
- Assess visual fields
- Provide safe environment

Evaluation and Outcomes

The patient will:

- Maintain adequate vision
- Receive routine eye examinations
- Be free from injury

Nursing Considerations

- Instruct patients to stop smoking, as smoking has been associated with macular degeneration.

- Instruct patients that use of phenothiazines has been shown to induce macular degeneration.

- Instruct patients on safety, as macular degeneration leads to loss of central vision and patients may not be able to drive.

- Teach patients they may need help with reading and writing.

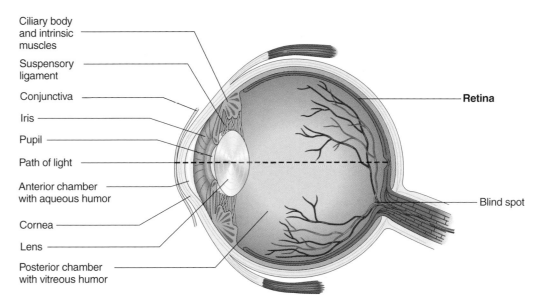

Ciliary body and intrinsic muscles

Suspensory ligament

Conjunctiva

Iris

Pupil

Path of light

Anterior chamber with aqueous humor

Cornea

Lens

Posterior chamber with vitreous humor

Retina

Blind spot

In macular degeneration, the macula, which is part of the retina, is destroyed. This leads to loss of central vision.

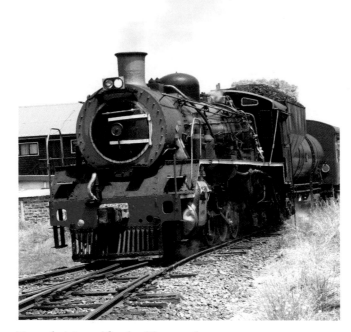

Normal vision with a healthy macula.

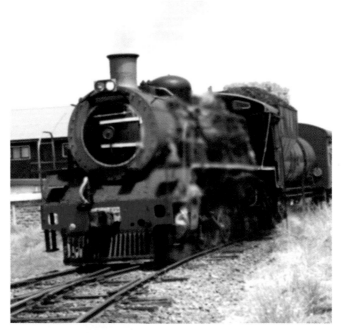

Vision for a patient with macular degeneration. Note how the center of the image is blurry. This is from the loss of the function of the macula. The patient will have trouble reading, writing, and driving.

MUSCULAR DYSTROPHY

Muscular dystrophy is a term that refers to over 30 genetic diseases characterized by progressive weakness and degeneration of the skeletal muscles. The more common types of muscular dystrophy are Duchenne, Becker, Llimb-girdle, and myotonic. A suspected cause is the genetic deficiency of the muscle protein dystrophin.

Assessment

Muscle weakness
Muscle spasms
Coordination
Frequent falls

Planning and Implementation

Assess muscle strength
Assess coordination
Assess gait

Evaluation and Outcomes

The patient will:

Be free of injury
Be able to complete activities of daily living
Understand the disease process and treatments

Nursing Considerations

Teach patients that there are no specific therapies to reverse or slow the disease.

Refer to support groups in the community that are available for families.

Instruct patient on injury prevention, especially fall prevention with the loss of muscle strength.

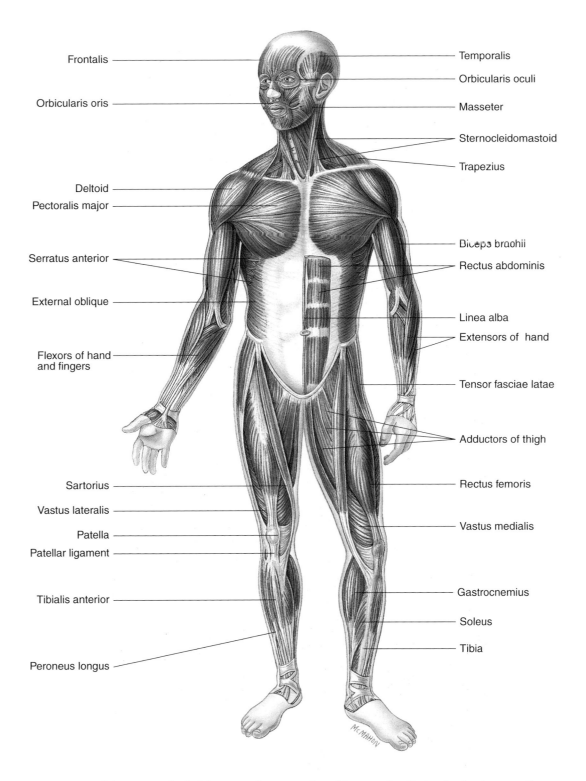

Frontalis

Orbicularis oris

Deltoid

Pectoralis major

Serratus anterior

External oblique

Flexors of hand
and fingers

Sartorius

Vastus lateralis

Patella

Patellar ligament

Tibialis anterior

Peroneus longus

Temporalis

Orbicularis oculi

Masseter

Sternocleidomastoid

Trapezius

Biceps brachii

Rectus abdominis

Linea alba

Extensors of hand

Tensor fasciae latae

Adductors of thigh

Rectus femoris

Vastus medialis

Gastrocnemius

Soleus

Tibia

The muscles of the anterior body. These muscles are weakened in muscular dystrophy due to a genetic alteration. The exact mechanism of how the disease progresses is unknown.

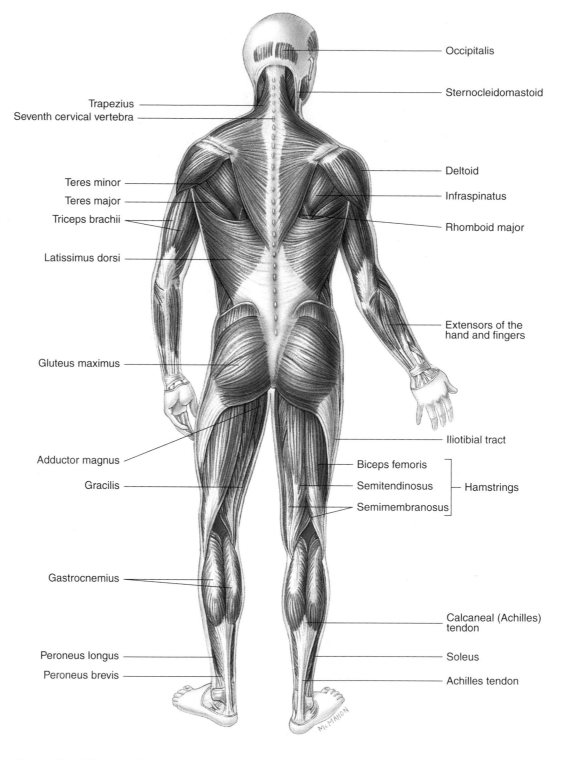

Trapezius
Seventh cervical vertebra

Teres minor
Teres major
Triceps brachii

Latissimus dorsi

Gluteus maximus

Adductor magnus

Gracilis

Gastrocnemius

Peroneus longus
Peroneus brevis

Occipitalis

Sternocleidomastoid

Deltoid
Infraspinatus
Rhomboid major

Extensors of the
hand and fingers

Iliotibial tract

Biceps femoris
Semitendinosus   Hamstrings
Semimembranosus

Calcaneal (Achilles)
tendon

Soleus

Achilles tendon

The muscles of the posterior body. These muscles are weakened in muscular dystrophy.

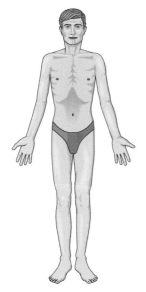

The picture shows atrophy of muscles, which occurs in muscular dystrophy.

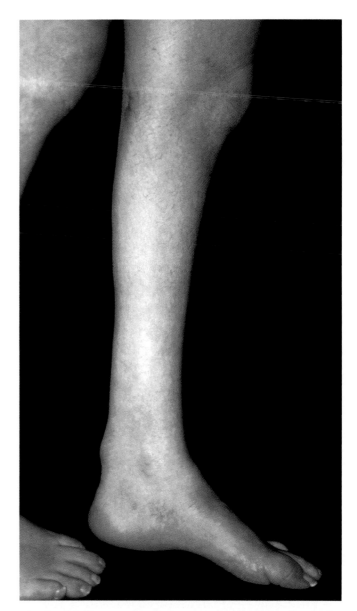

An atrophied lower extremity seen in muscular dystrophy. As the muscles are destroyed, the limb becomes atrophied or smaller in size, and there is no muscle tone. The patient is unable to bear weight and after time will no longer be able to walk.

MYASTHENIA GRAVIS

Myasthenia Ggravis (MG) is a chronic, progressive neuromuscular disease and is theorized to be caused by an autoimmune process. There is destruction and blockage of acetylcholine receptor sites, andas well as structural changes that diminish acetylcholine at the post-synaptic muscle junction. The loss of acetylcholine results in decreased muscle strength and profound fatigue.

Assessment

- Ptosis (eye lid drooping)
- Diplopia (double vision)
- Muscle weakness
- Loss of facial expression
- Slurred speech
- Difficulty swallowing/eating
- Respiratory difficulty

Planning and Implementation

- Monitor airway and respiratory status
- Monitor the ability to swallow
- Monitor fluid and nutritional intake
- Promote frequent oral care
- Monitor gag reflex
- Utilize nonverbal techniques and the use of communication boards
- Monitor for pulmonary infections (productive cough, fever)
- Provide frequent rest periods
- Assist with ADLs
- Keep emergency airway equipment available in case of respiratory distress
- Implement safety measures

Evaluation and Outcomes

The patient will:

- Be able to perform activities of daily living.
- Maintain adequate oxygenation status.
- Understand medical treatment and course of the disease.

Nursing Considerations

- Instruct patients to space activities of daily living to conserve energy.

- Ensure adequate nutrition by teaching the patients to consume small, frequent meals, since swallowing may be difficult.

- Refer patient and family to community support groups.

- Refer to speech therapist to assist with speech.

- Collaborate with physical and occupational therapy to maximize independence and assess for need for assistive devices.

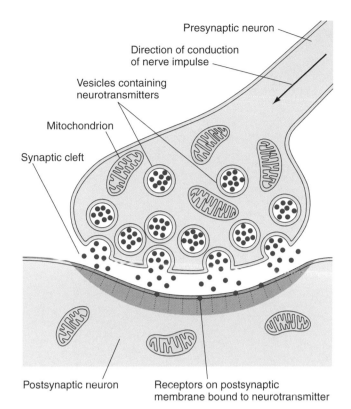

Presynaptic neuron

Direction of conduction
of nerve impulse

Vesicles containing
neurotransmitters

Mitochondrion

Synaptic cleft

Postsynaptic neuron

Receptors on postsynaptic
membrane bound to neurotransmitter

In myasthenia gravis, there is a disruption of the neurotransmitter molecules at the synaptic level.

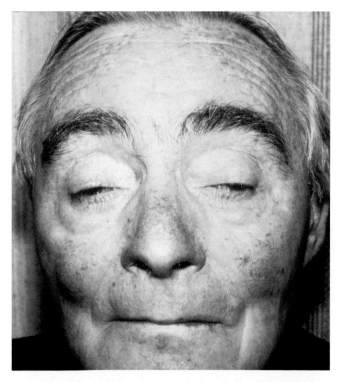

Drooping of the eyelids or ptosis seen in myasthenia gravis. The drooping of the eyelid occurs due to the loss of muscular function (Courtesy of Viewing Medicine).

MYOCARDIAL INFARCTION

Myocardial infarction occurs when the muscular layer of the heart or myocardium is deprived of adequate blood and oxygen supply. As a result, there is ischemia of muscle tissue and eventual infarction or death of myocardial tissue.

Assessment

- Angina (onset, duration, intensity, location)
- Tachycardia and hypertension
- Nausea and vomiting
- Shortness of breath

Planning and Implementation

- Vital signs
- Cardiac arrhythmias
- Description of angina
- Family history
- Prior history of cardiac events

Evaluation and Outcomes

The patient will:

- Be free of angina
- Understand lifestyle modifications, such as decreaseding dietary fat intake, and increaseing exercise.
- Quit smoking

Nursing Considerations

- Nurses must be aware that women have atypical angina, experiencing a more choking sensation or more jaw pain than men.

- Teach patients to seek medical help (call 911) as soon as they begin to experience chest pain.

- Instruct patients that they may resume sexual activity following a myocardial infarction when they can climb one flight of stairs without feeling shortness of breath.

- Nurses must be aware that women have higher morbidity and mortality rates following myocardial infarction than do men.

- Teach patients after a myocardial infarction to stop smoking.

- Instruct patients following a myocardial infarction onabout a low -fat diet.

- Refer patients for cardiac rehabilitation.

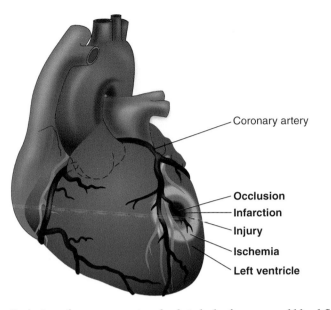

Coronary artery

Occlusion
Infarction
Injury
Ischemia
Left ventricle

Occlusion of a coronary artery leads to lack of oxygen and blood flow to the myocardium distal to the artery that is blocked. This leads to the areas of ischemia, injury, and infarction of the myocardium. The patient will present with chest pain and may have shortness of breath. The areas of ischemia and injury are reversible. If the patient does not receive early treatment, infarction results and the heart tissue is permanently dead.

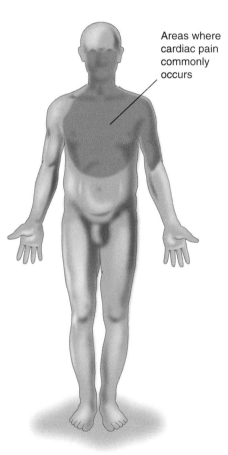

Areas where cardiac pain commonly occurs

Ischemia of the myocardium leads to chest pain or angina which commonly occurs over the anterior chest. Any pain that occurs from the nose to the navel should be considered heart-related. Patients typically describe the feeling as a"tightness" or "squeezing" over the anterior chest.

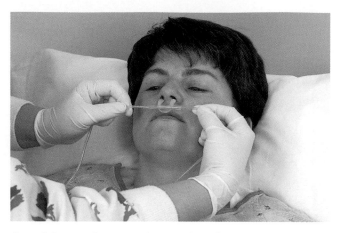

One of the most important interventions for a patient experiencing chest pain is the application of oxygen, usually via a nasal cannula.

Classic Myocardial Infarction

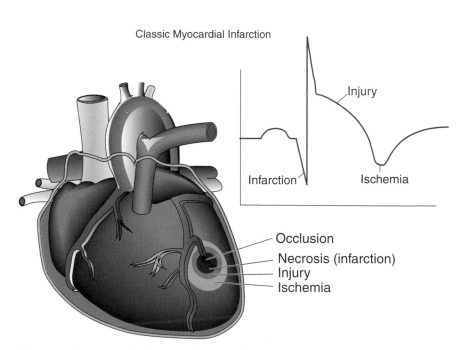

There are changes on the electrocardiogram when a patient is experiencing a myocardial infarction. Ischemia is represented by an inverted T wave. Injury is represented by an elevated S-T segment. Infarction is represented by the development of a Q wave.

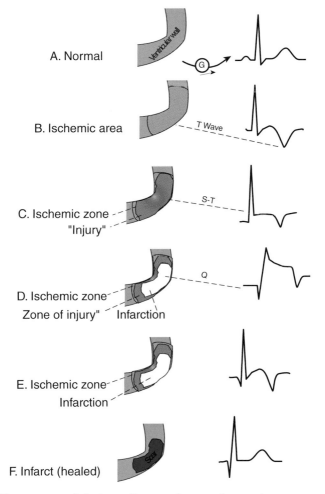

A. Normal

B. Ischemic area

C. Ischemic zone
"Injury"

D. Ischemic zone
Zone of injury"   Infarction

E. Ischemic zone
Infarction

F. Infarct (healed)

The sequence of electrocardiogram changes of an acute myocardial infarction.

OBESITY

Obesity is a weight greater than 30 percent of ideal body weight. Obesity is a complex condition with multifactor causes, including genetic, societal, nutritional, and hormonal issues. Obesity is a national problem that is associated with other diseases, including diabetes mellitus and cardiac disease. Bariatric medicine is the study of the cause, prevention, and treatment of obesity.

Assessment

- Body mass index of greater than 30
- Weight circumference greater than 35 inches in females and 40 inches in males
- Hypertension
- Cholesterol and triglycerides

Planning and Implementation

- Psychological support and counseling
- Diet history
- Calorie count
- Implement safety measures

Evaluation and Outcomes

The patient will:

- Acquire knowledge on how to prevent and treat obesity
- Exhibit a body mass index of 30
- Maintain a safe environment
- Detect or prevent cardiovascular disease and diabetes mellitus

Nursing Considerations

- Utilize bariatric equipment designed for the obese patient to maintain safety.

- Ensure the equipment will support the patient's weight prior to sending an obese patient for testing.

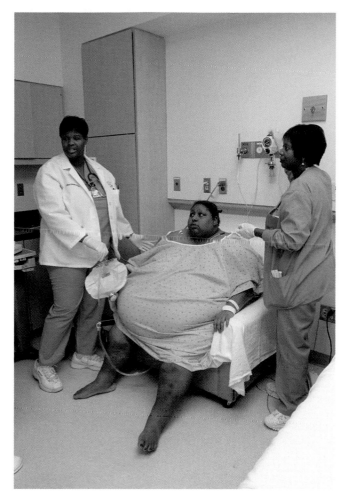

The patient exhibits signs of obesity with increased body weight and a weight circumference greater than 35 inches. Notice the use of appropriate sized gowns and a chair designed for the obese patient.

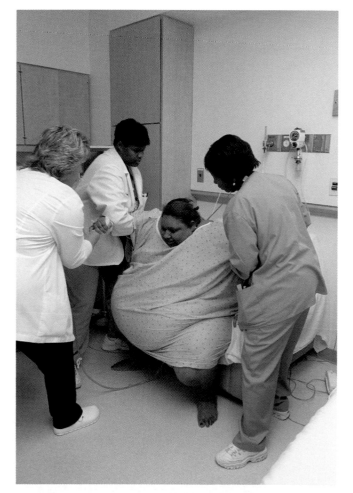

The nurses use an appropriate amount of staff to maintain safety while assisting the obese client with ambulation.

OROPHARYNGEAL CANCER

Oropharyngeal cancer is an uncommon cancer involving any structure in the oropharyngeal area, including the base of the tongue, tonsils, soft palate, or the oropharynx. Significant risk factors include tobacco and alcohol use. Men are affected 3–5 times more frequently than are women, and the disease occurs in the 5th to 7th decades of life.

Assessment

- Dysphagia
- Weight loss
- Pain in neck and ears
- Enlarged cervical lymph nodes

Planning and Implementation

- Surgery and chemotherapy is usually indicated
- Anticipate nutritional deficiencies
- Implement alternative communication techniques
- Maintain adequate pain control
- Monitor airway

Evaluation and Outcomes

The patient will:

- Maintain adequate caloric and fluid intake
- Effectively communicate
- Adequately control pain
- Communicate understanding of treatments

Nursing Considerations

- Preoperatively assess the patient's ability to nonverbally communicate (such as reading and writing) to establish post-operative communication techniques.

- Profuse post-operative bleeding around the tracheostomy site may be indicative of tracheoinnominate artery bleeding, and is considered a medical emergency.

- Discuss alternative eating methods (percutaneous gastric feedings or nasoduodenal) with the patient if long-term oral eating difficulties are anticipated due to surgery.

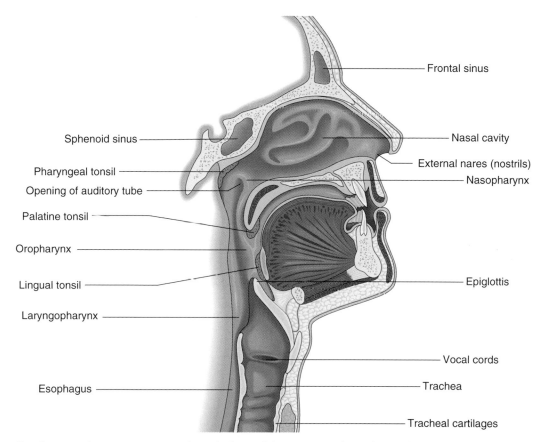

Frontal sinus

Sphenoid sinus

Pharyngeal tonsil

Opening of auditory tube

Palatine tonsil

Oropharynx

Lingual tonsil

Laryngopharynx

Esophagus

Nasal cavity

External nares (nostrils)

Nasopharynx

Epiglottis

Vocal cords

Trachea

Tracheal cartilages

Oropharyngeal cancer may occur from the base of the tongue to above the epiglottis. These structures are vital in the ability to speak and swallow.

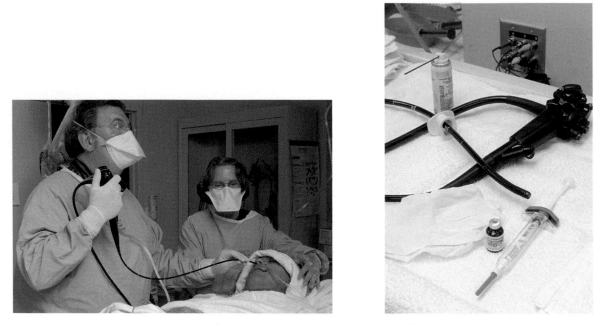

Endoscopic evaluation and biopsy help diagnose oropharyngeal cancer. The endoscope allows the physician to directly visualize any abnormality in the oropharyngeal area and obtain biopsies of the tissue.

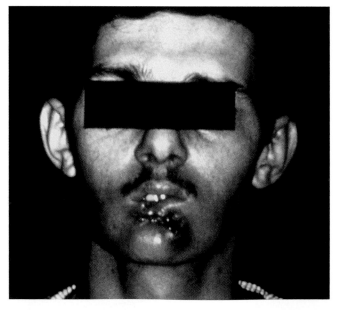

Oropharyngeal tumors as shown may cause pain and difficulty with eating and swallowing. (Courtesy of NCI)

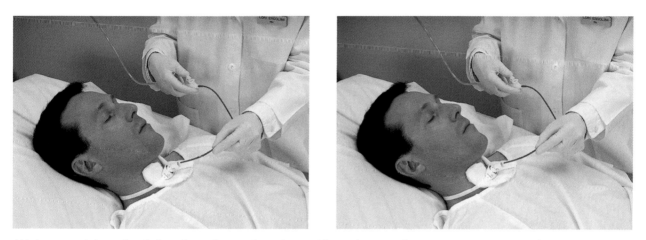

(A) A portacath is used to infuse chemotherapy in patients with oropharyngeal cancer, in conjunction with surgery.
(B) Tracheostomy placement may be necessary depending on the location and extent of the oropharyngeal cancer.

OSTEOMYELITIS

Osteomyelitis is a bone infection resulting from a soft tissue infection that spreads to the bone, open bone fracture, or bone made accessible by surgery. Patients with diabetes mellitus and vascular insufficiency are at higher risk for contracting osteomyelitis.

Assessment

- Pain
- Soft tissue swelling and redness
- Purulent draining
- Fever

Planning and Implementation

- Treat pain with analgesics
- Wound care as prescribed
- Elevate affected area
- Administer appropriate antibiotics (expect 4–6 week antibiotic course)

Evaluation and Outcomes

The patient will:

- Experience adequate pain control
- Be free of infection
- Possess intact skin without redness, drainage, or swelling

Nursing Considerations

- Ensure glycemic control in diabetic patients to promote healing.

- Monitor the patient for complications of long-term antibiotic therapy, such as kidney failure.

- Date, time, and initial all dressings.

- Inspect wounds daily and have the patient use a mirror if they cannot visualize the area directly.

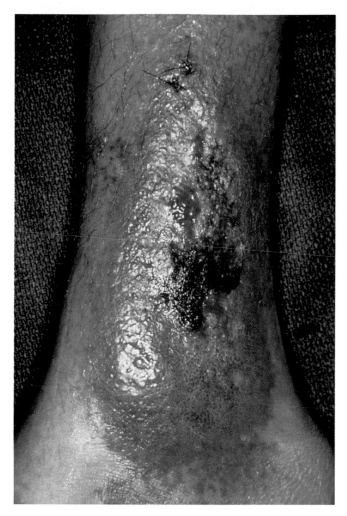

Osteomyelitis in patients with peripheral vascular insufficiency often begins with an infected venous ulcer. The infection may progress to the bone if not treated promptly and effectively. (Courtesy of the CDC, Dr. Steve Kraus)

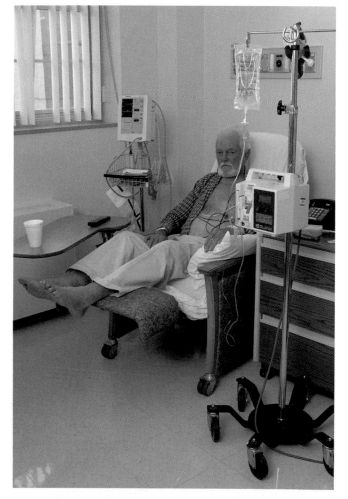

Elevate the extremities when peripheral edema is present to help decrease the edema. Peripheral edema decreases the tissue perfusion and slows healing.

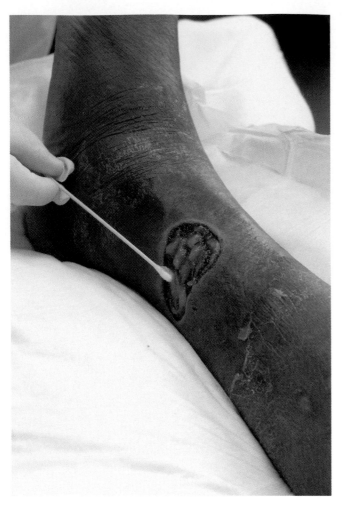

Meticulous wound care promotes healing. (A) The nurse applies prescribed antibacterial ointment to the venous ulcer on this patient. The nurse is simultaneously providing wound care and assessing the wound appearance for documentation.

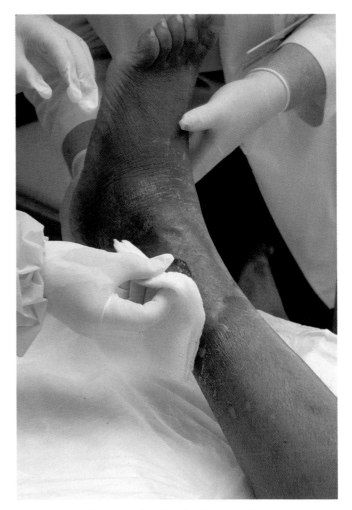

(B) The wound is covered with a sterile gauze dressing.

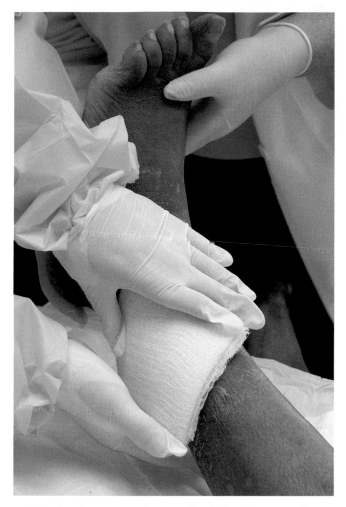

(C) The dressing protects the wound and absorbs any exudate from the site.

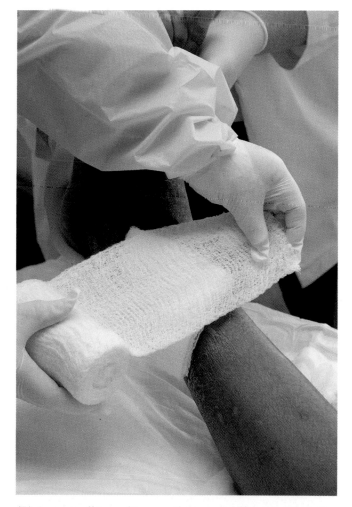

(D) A gauze roll is used to cover the wound and make ambulation possible without disrupting the dressing.

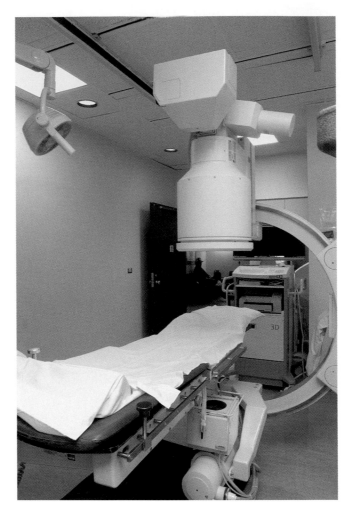

A bone scan is a painless, noninvasive diagnostic tool for osteomyelitis. The patient is injected with a radioactive isotope that will accumulate in any infected bone area. The patient lies on the table as the affected area is scanned. The scan usually takes thirty to sixty minutes.

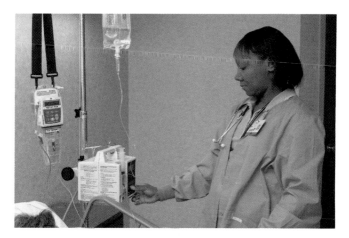

Six to eight weeks of IV antibiotic therapy administered by an IV pump is often necessary to treat osteomyelitis. Treatment usually begins in the hospital setting and continues at home through a home health agency. The agency will bring the equipment and medication prescribed into the patient's home.

OSTEOPOROSIS

Osteoporosis decreaseds bone mass and strength and is the most frequently diagnosed bone disease. It is often undetected until a fracture occurs. Osteoporosis is most common in elderly females.

Assessment

- Decrease in height
- Kyphosis (hunchback)
- Back pain
- Elderly, post-menopausal female

Planning and Implementation

- Administer bisphosphonates, selective estrogen receptor modulators, and calcium supplements as prescribed
- Encourage regular weight-bearing exercise
- Prevent falls

Evaluation and Outcomes

The patient will:

- Ingest adequate calcium intake
- Maintain a safe environment
- Experience adequate pain control
- Prevent falls

Nursing Considerations

- Encourage patients to remove loose rugs and keep hallways illuminated to prevent falls.

- Have patients sit upright when taking bisphosphonates.

- Encourage patients with osteoporosis to seek medical attention if they fall, because of the high risk of fractures.

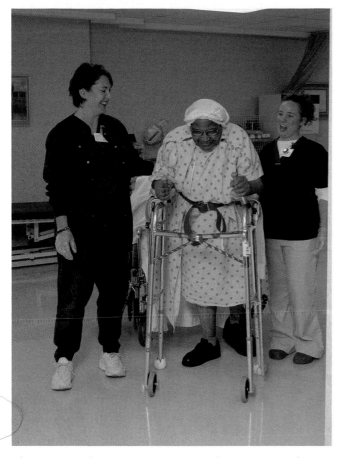

The patient with severe osteoporosis needs assistance with ambulation. Note the curvature of the spine and how the head leans forward.

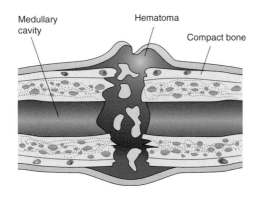

A. A hematoma forms from blood from ruptured vessels.

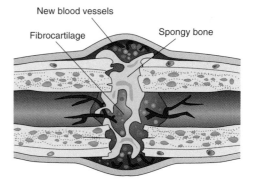

B. Spongy bone forms close to developing blood vessels; fibrocartilage forms away from new blood vessels.

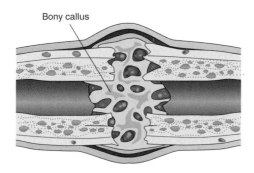

C. Bony callus replaces fibrocartilage.

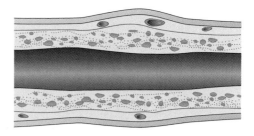

D. Excess bony tissue is removed by osteoclasts.

Fractures occur more frequently in patients with osteoporosis because of the decreased bone mass. Fractures decrease the patient's mobility, take months to heal, and are painful.

OVARIAN CANCER

Ovarian cancer is the fifth most common cancer in women, and 85% of ovarian cancers are epithelial. Risk factors include increased age, early menstruation, late menopause, no children or first child after age of 30, and family history of breast, ovarian, or colorectal cancer.

Assessment

- Abdominal pain and swelling
- Bloating
- Nausea and vomiting
- Change in bowel and bladder habits
- Leg and back pain

Planning and Implementation

- Surgical removal of the ovaries and uterus. Chemotherapy and radiation may be indicated
- Maintain adequate pain control
- Promote adequate fluid and nutritional intake
- Monitor for complications of radiation therapy and chemotherapy

Evaluation and Outcomes

The patient will:

- Experience adequate pain control
- Communicate understanding of treatments
- Have minimal side effects related to treatments

Nursing Considerations

- Discuss sexuality and reproductive concerns with the patient.

- Ovarian cancer may have extensive metastasis by the time it is diagnosed, making outcomes less favorable.

- Quality of life issues should be discussed when treatment decisions are being made.

- End of life issues, such as living wills, should be discussed prior to treatment.

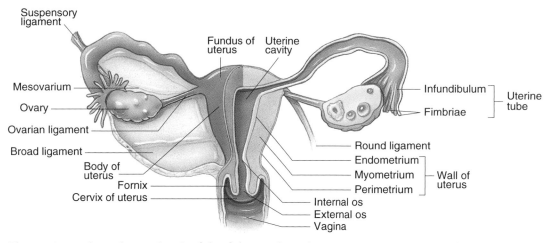

The ovaries are located on each side of the abdomen above the vagina. Ovarian cancer enlarges the ovary, causing pain and bloating.

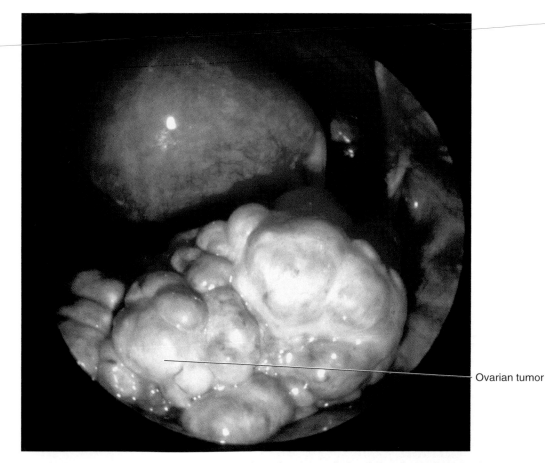

Ovarian tumor

Ovarian tumors may grow quickly and spread to other organs before being detected. Annual women's health exams include palpating ovaries to detect abnormalities. (Courtesy of Viewing Medicine)

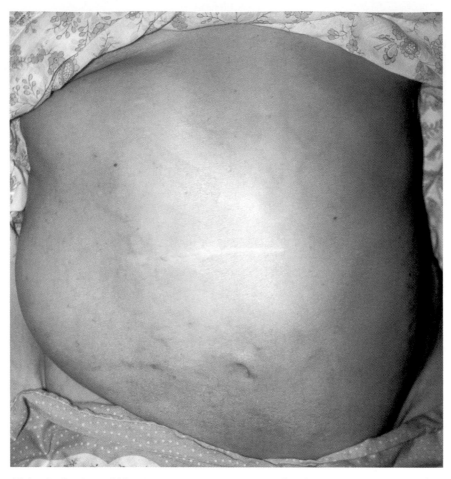

Abdominal pain and bloating are symptoms associated with ovarian cancer. Note the distention is more pronounced on the patient's left side and the veins are engorged as well. (Courtesy of Viewing Medicine)

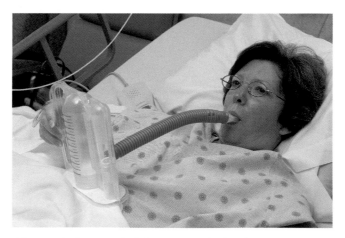

After surgical removal of the ovary and related structures, prevention of postoperative complications is necessary. Incentive spirometry promotes deep breathing and prevents atelectasis.

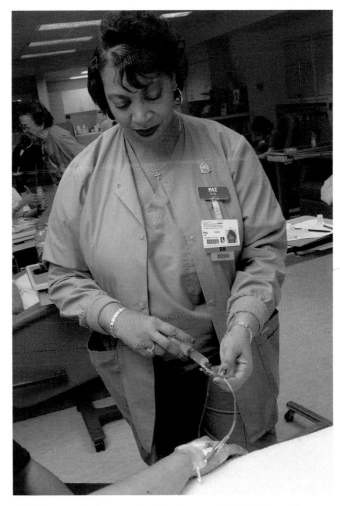

(A) *After surgical removal of the tumor, outpatient chemotherapy treats and prevents the spread of ovarian cancer.*

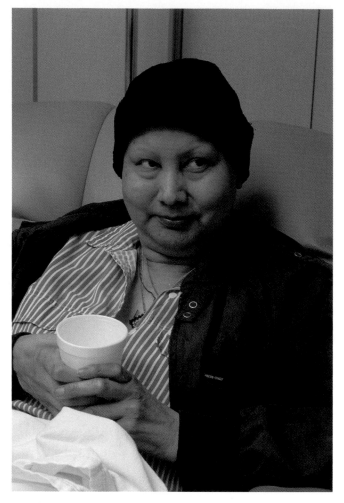

(B) This patient's length of chemotherapy and other associated treatments, such as radiation, depends on the size and extent of the tumor and if metastasis has occurred. Side effects of chemotherapy may include hair loss, as shown, nausea and vomiting, weight gain or loss, and fatigue.

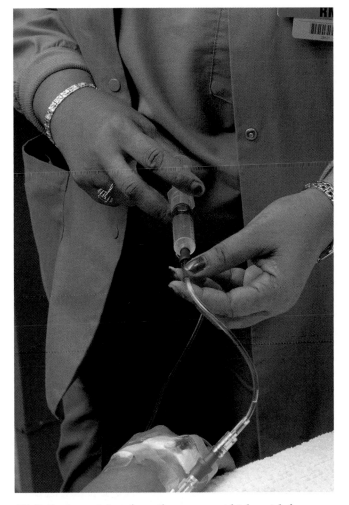

(C) Patients receiving chemotherapy are at higher risk for infection because chemotherapy kills healthy as well as cancer cells. Encourage patients to wash their hands, use germicidal lotions, and stay away from sick people.

PARKINSON'S DISEASE

Parkinson's disease is a progressively degenerative neurological disorder caused by the loss of nerve cell function in the basal ganglia. The loss of the nerve cells results in reduced dopamine production. The reduction in dopamine, a neurotransmitter essential for functions such as controlling posture and voluntary motions, causes the clinical symptoms.

Assessment

- Rigidity of muscles
- Akinesia (lack of movement)
- Bradykinesia (slow movement)
- Shuffled gait
- Mask-like face
- Difficulty with fine motor activities

Planning and Implementation

- Implement safety measures
- Monitor the patient's ability to swallow effectively
- Place patient in high Fowler's position when feeding
- Monitor fluid and nutritional intake
- Monitor bowel and bladder function
- Assist with ADLs
- Adhere strictly to medication administration regimes

Evaluation and Outcomes

The patient will:

- Maintain safety
- Adhere to medication regimes
- Experience adequate nutritional intake

Nursing Considerations

➡ In the early stages of the disease, encourage the patient to address long-term issues such as advanced directives, estate planning, and care options.

➡ Reinforce medication, nutrition, and safety teaching

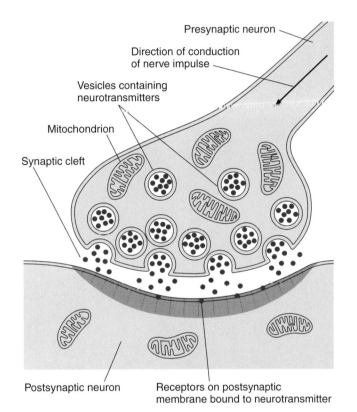

Presynaptic neuron

Direction of conduction
of nerve impulse

Vesicles containing
neurotransmitters

Mitochondrion

Synaptic cleft

Postsynaptic neuron

Receptors on postsynaptic
membrane bound to neurotransmitter

The loss of nerve cells causes a reduction in dopamine, a neu-rotransmitter essential for voluntary movements. Nerve impulses are altered, causing problems with walking, posture, eating, and facial expressions.

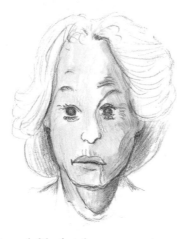

A mask-like facial appearance is a physical finding in patients with Parkinson's disease.

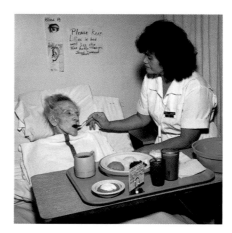

As Parkinson's disease progresses, eating becomes increasingly difficult. Assisting the patient with feeding and observing for any signs of aspiration are necessary for adequate nutritional intake and safety. Notice the patient is in high Fowler's position to help facilitate swallowing and prevent aspiration.

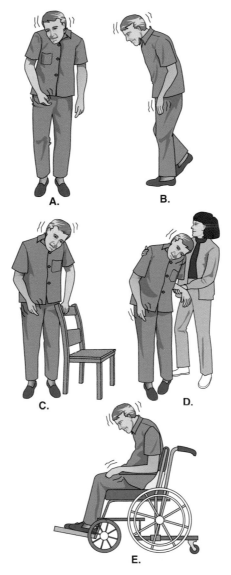

(A, B) Initially, Parkinson's disease may cause arm flexion and a shuffled gait. (C, D) As the disease progresses, the need for support to stand and ambulate is necessary. (E) Finally, the patient is unable to ambulate and requires assistance with all functions.

PEPTIC ULCERS

Peptic ulcers, or peptic ulcer disease (PUD), is inflammation of the mucosal lining of the gastric or duodenal portion of the gastrointestinal tract. Infection with Helicobacter pylori is the leading cause of PUD; other causes include ingestion of nonsteroidal medications, alcohol consumption, and stress.

Assessment

- Epigastric pain relieved by food or antacids
- Weight loss
- Poor appetite
- Bloating
- Nausea and vomiting

Planning and Implementation

- Treat nausea and vomiting
- Discontinue nonsteroidal medications
- Administer antacids, H_2 receptor antagonists (e.g., famotidine), and proton pump inhibitors (e.g., ompeprazole)
- If H. pylori is present, anticipate administering antibiotics (bismuth subsalicylate, metronidazole, and tetracycline)
- Offer small, frequent meals

Evaluation and Outcomes

The patient will:

- Experience adequate pain control
- Be free of nausea and vomiting
- Prevent gastric hemorrhage or perforation

Nursing Considerations

- After endoscopic procedures, check for the return of gag reflex on patients before administering oral liquids or medications.

- Target admission histories for signs and symptoms of PUD in elderly patients and those who smoke, because they are more likely to develop peptic ulcers.

- Smoking cessation materials should be offered to patients with PUD who smoke.

- Explain the reason for antibiotic therapy in patients with PUD who are positive for Helicobacter pylori infections.

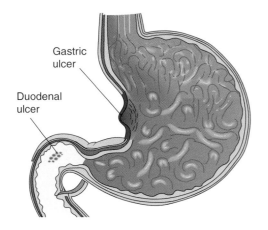

Peptic ulcers may occur in either the gastric or duodenal portions of the gastrointestinal tract.

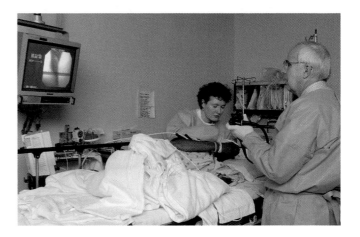

Endoscopic procedures allow the physician to directly visualize the mucosa of the stomach and duodenum. The patient is sedated and monitored by the nurse, while the physician advances the scope and visualizes the gastrointestinal tract for evidence of peptic ulcer disease.

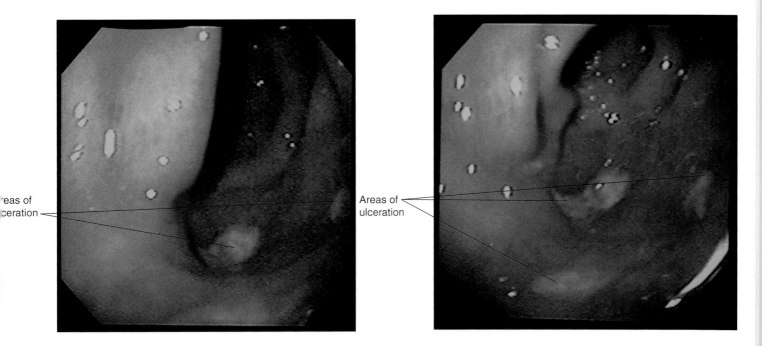

eas of ceration

Areas of ulceration

, B Ulcerations are present in white patches and inflammation (deeper pink areas) surrounds the ulcerations.

PERIPHERAL VASCULAR DISEASE (PVD)

Peripheral vascular disease (PVD), also known as arteriosclerosis obliterans, is primarily the result of athero-sclerosis causing narrowing of arteries of the legs, resulting in inadequate blood flow. Acute embolic syndrome, loss of arterial blood flow to an extremity, is an emergent condition that must be reported to the physician immediately to prevent the loss of a limb.

Assessment

- Intermittent claudication (pain occurring during activity that is relieved with rest)
- Nocturnal pain and pain at rest
- 5 Ps- pain, pallor, pulse, paresthesia, paralysis
- Delayed capillary refill
- Cool to touch

Planning and Implementation

- Monitor and treat pain
- Monitor temperature, color, pulse, sensation, movement
- If unable to palpate a posterior tibial or dorsalis pedis pulse, use a Doppler ultrasound to locate the pulse
- Monitor for the development of acute embolic syndrome

Evaluation and Outcomes

The patient will:

- Experience adequate pain control
- Maintain adequate tissue perfusion

Nursing Considerations

- Promote mild exercise and encourage rest when pain increases in the legs.

- If the patient agrees, mark pulse signals with a marker to assist others to quickly locate pulses in the feet.

- Encourage smoking cessation to patients that smoke.

- Teach patients to wear shoes that fit properly to avoid skin breakdown.

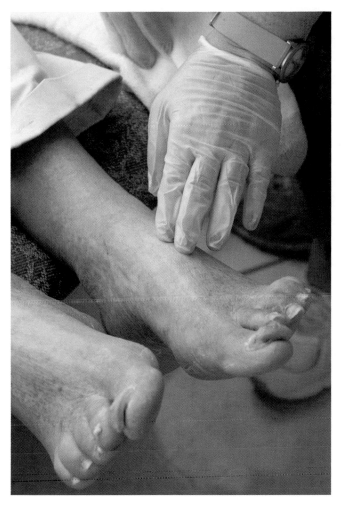

A) Palpating the dorsalis pedis pulse. The skin is pale and dry, and the toe nails are thick from poor perfusion.

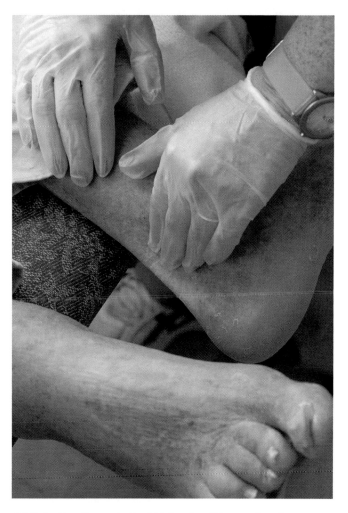

(B) Palpating the posterior tibial pulse. Observe the pigment changes from chronic PVD.

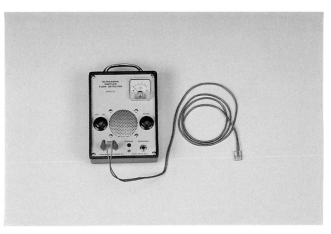

(C) Doppler ultrasound may be used to locate a pulse if unable to palpate one. If unable to locate a pulse with a Doppler, notify the physician promptly because the patient may be experiencing acute embolic syndrome, and notification and subsequent treatment may preserve the limb.

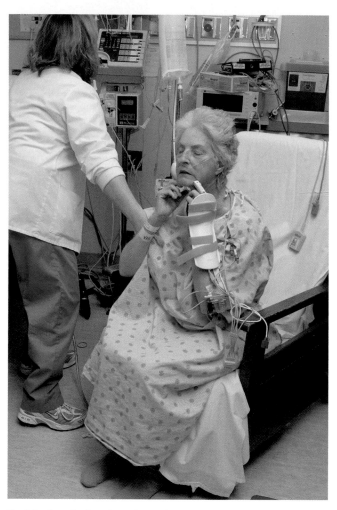

Positioning the legs in a dependent position may alleviate pain and promote perfusion to the lower extremities. Elderly patients with evidence of atherosclerosis, as in this woman after open heart surgery, are at risk for peripheral vascular disease.

PHEOCHROMOCYTOMA

Pheochromocytoma is a tumor of the adrenal gland that secretes catecholamines. Pheochromocytomas occur more frequently in men during the 4th or 5th decade of life. One third of pheochromocytomas cause fatal cardiac arrhythmias or strokes prior to diagnosis. Surgical removal of the tumor is the treatment of choice.

Assessment

- Hypertension
- Headache
- Abdominal pain
- Palpitations, chest pain
- Severe anxiety

Planning and Implementation

- Anticipate surgical removal of tumor
- Monitor vital signs
- Administer antihypertensive medications (alpha-adrenergic blockers)
- Do not palpate the abdomen

Evaluation and Outcomes

The patient will:

- Remain free of complications from pheochromocytoma
- Maintain a blood pressure within normal limits
- Understand cause of symptoms and the associated treatments

Nursing Considerations

- Blood pressure is considerably lower post-operatively and must be checked prior to medication administration.

- Reassure the patient that anxiety is related to the tumor.

- Teach patients to avoid any stimulant, including caffeine and nicotine, until the tumor is removed.

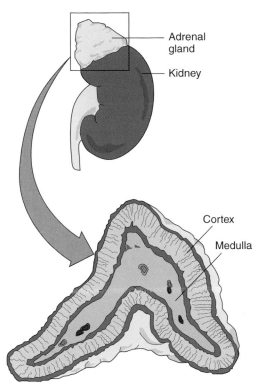

Pheochromocytoma occurs in the adrenal gland located on the top of each kidney. Most pheochromocytomas are unilateral and benign.

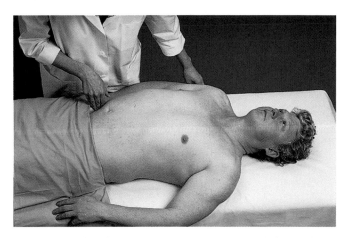

Patients with pheochromocytoma may experience abdominal pain from the tumor growing and pressing on the adrenal gland. Do not palpate the abdomen on a patient who has or is suspected of having pheochromocytoma, because increased pressure may cause the tumor to secrete more epinephrine, increasing the blood pressure and heart rate.

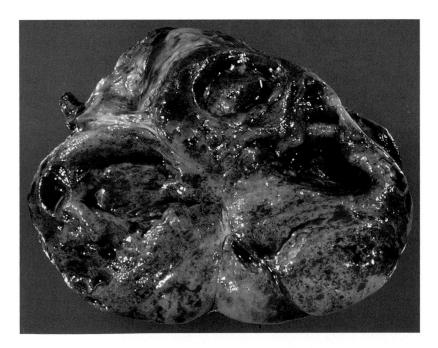

The treatment for pheochromocytomas is surgical removal. Notice the yellow-brown color of this resectioned pheochromocytoma. Symptoms associated with pheochromocytomas subside after removal. (Courtesy of Dharam M. Ramnani)

PICKWICKIAN SYNDROME

Pickwickian syndrome is chronic hypoventilation and obstructive sleep apnea related to obesity. The excess fat places a strain on the heart, lungs, and diaphragm of the patient, making it difficult to breathe. Long-term consequences include right-sided heart failure.

Assessment

- Enuresis
- Snoring and irregular breathing patterns at night
- Daytime sleepiness
- Poor concentration
- Cyanosis

Planning and Implementation

- Monitor breathing patterns
- Implement weight reduction diet
- Monitor oxygenation status
- BiPAP (continuous positive airway pressure with both inspiration and expiration) assistance with respirations

Evaluation and Outcomes

The patient will:

- Experience regular breathing patterns
- Avert right-sided heart failure, a long-term consequence
- Decrease body weight

Nursing Considerations

- Teach patients that Pickwickian syndrome can be aggravated by the use of alcohol, antihistamines, and over-the-counter cold preparations.

- Closely monitor the patient's breathing patterns and pulse oximetry during sleep and anticipate BiPAP use at night.

- Monitor intake and output for signs of fluid deficit during BiPAP mask use.

- Collaborate with social service if BiPAP use at home will be required.

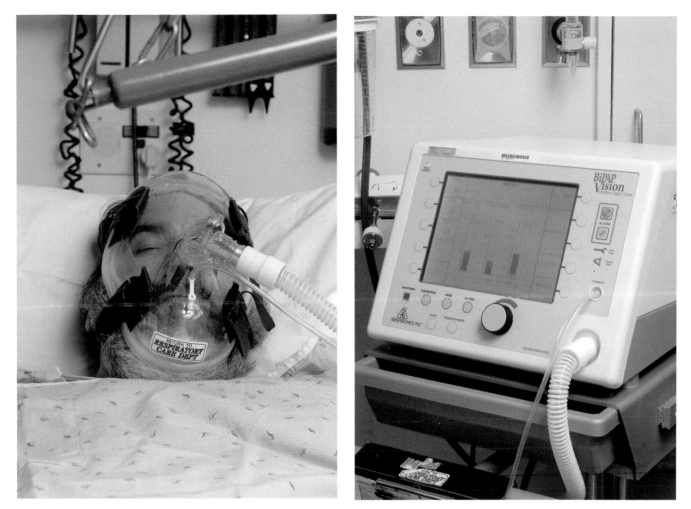

Figure 5 P-1 A, B (A) Sleep apnea associated with Pickwickian syndrome may be treated with a BiPAP mask. BiPAP assists with respirations in the obese patient by providing positive airway pressure during inspiration and expiration, increasing the volume inhaled and exhaled, and increasing oxygenation. The mask provides a seal to maintain the pressure. (B)The BiPAP machine monitors inhaled and exhaled volumes and pressures. The settings are prescribed by the health care provider.

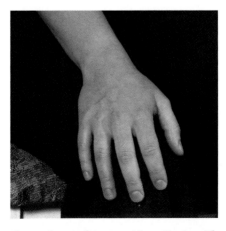

Cyanosis may be present in patients with Pickwickian syndrome, due to hypoventilation and subsequent hypoxia associated with the syndrome.

PNEUMOTHORAX

A pneumothorax is a collection of air in the pleural cavity that leads to a partial or full collapse of the lung and interferes with normal oxygenation. Causes of pneumothorax include trauma, surgery, and central line placement, and they may occur spontaneously.

Assessment

- Dyspnea
- Anxiety
- Tracheal deviation
- Absence of breath sounds over affected area
- Decreased pulse oximetry

Planning and Implementation

- Position in high Fowler's position if blood pressure is stable
- Administer oxygen therapy
- Treat pain and anxiety
- Anticipate chest tube insertion

Evaluation and Outcomes

The patient will:

- Oxygenate effectively
- Experience adequate pain control

Nursing Considerations

- If the chest tube tubing becomes disconnected from the container, place the open end in a bottle of sterile water to create a water seal.

- If an air leak is detected in the water seal chamber, ensure all connections are secure. If connections are secure and the air leak persists, notify the physician immediately because the patient may have a new pneumothorax.

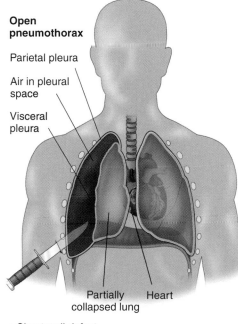

Open pneumothorax

Parietal pleura

Air in pleural space

Visceral pleura

Partially collapsed lung   Heart

- Chest wall defect
- Collapsed lung
- Ball valve effect

Air in the pleural space partially collapses the lung and interferes with oxygenation because the tissue cannot exchange oxygen at the capillary level.

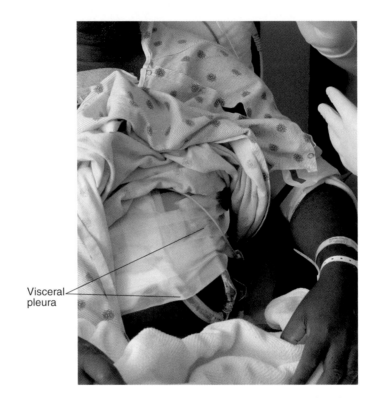

Visceral
pleura

*Chest tubes are covered with a sterile dressing and secured with
tape.*

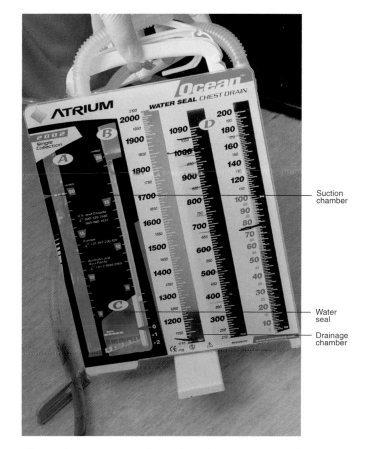

Chest tubes are connected to a chest drainage system. The nurse monitors the suction chamber, observing for the presence and amount of continual suction or the absence of suction (as ordered by the physician). Observe the water seal chamber for bubbling, indicating an air leak. If present, check connections and notify the physician, since there is a potential of a new pneumothorax. Monitor the color and amount of drainage in the drainage chamber. Copious bright red blood indicates new bleeding and should be reported immediately, due to active blood loss, scant to moderate amount of serosangenous drainage in normal and any amount of yellow- or green-tinged drainage may reflect the presence of infection.

POLYCYTHEMIA

Polycythemia is an increased amount of red blood cells, with a hematocrit level of greater than 55% in males and 50% in females. Polycythemia may be genetically acquired, caused by pulmonary disorders, neoplasm, or from living in high altitudes. The excessive amount of red blood cells causes a thickening of the blood, and associated complications include stroke or myocardial infarction.

Assessment

- Hypertension
- Fatigue
- Headache, paresthesia
- Ruddy complexion
- Erythromelalgia, burning sensation in the digits

Planning and Implementation

- Encourage fluid intake
- Monitor neurological status
- Monitor vital signs
- Phlebotomy or chemotherapeutics may be ordered to maintain hematocrit within normal levels

Evaluation and Outcomes

The patient will

- Maintain a normal hemoglobin and hematocrit
- Be free of complications of polycythemia (stroke, myocardial infarction).
- Nursing Considerations
- Often patients with polycythemia are asymptomatic and require teaching concerning complications of the disorder.
- Explain to patients that polycythemia is often a genetic trait and other family members should be tested for the disorder.

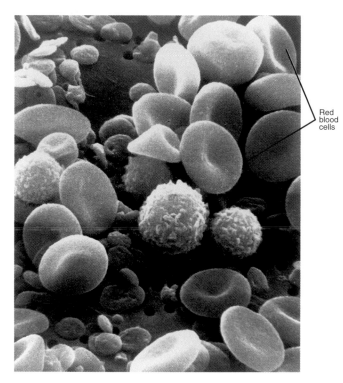

Red
blood
cells

Polycythemia occurs when the blood has an abnormally high amount of red blood cells. The excess red blood cells cause the blood to become thicker, which causes many symptoms ranging from headaches to stroke. (Courtesy of NCI)

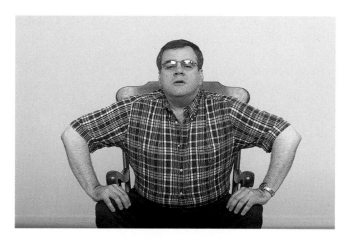

Patients with polycythemia experience shortness of breath. The leaning position is indicative of shortness of breath and may help alleviate symptoms. If a polycythemia patient experiences shortness of breath, thoroughly assess the patient for complications such as myocardial infarction or stroke. Observe the patient's complexion, as a ruddy or reddish complexion is common in polycythemia.

PRESSURE ULCERS

Pressure ulcers, also referred to as decubitus ulcers, bedsores, and pressure sores, refer to damage to the skin and underlying tissue from excessive pressure, and range from stage 1 to stage 4 in severity. Immobility, poor nutritional status, and altered sensation put patients at higher risk for developing pressure ulcers.

Assessment

- Size, color, appearance of ulcer
- Presence of drainage
- Ulcer stage
- Perform and document a thorough skin assessment during each shift

Planning and Implementation

- Turn patients every 2 hours if immobile or experiencing limited mobility
- Check for incontinence or bowel movements and clean if necessary every 2 hours for patients that are incontinent and/or involuntary
- Minimize amount of linens and pads
- Promote adequate nutrition and hydration
- Wound care as ordered by wound care nurse or health care provider

Evaluation and Outcomes

The patient will:

- Exhibit signs of wound healing
- Not experience any further skin breakdown

Nursing Considerations

- Many scales are used to identify patients at risk for pressure ulcer development, including the Norton, Gosnell, and Braden scales.

- On the admission history, document the presence of any pressure ulcer.

- Patients at risk for pressure ulcers benefit from therapy mattresses to reduce pressure, which decreases the incidence of pressure ulcers.

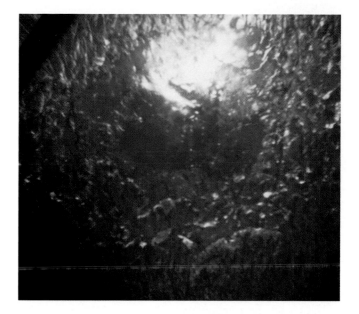

A stage 1 pressure ulcer has reddened skin and the skin is intact. If treated at this stage, further breakdown is prevented. (Courtesy of the CDC, Dr. Dancewicz)

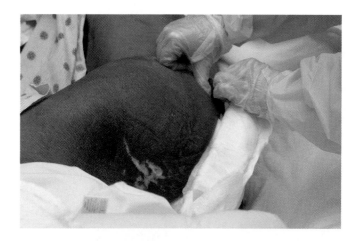

A stage 2 pressure ulcer has injury to the epidermal and dermal layers and the skin is no longer intact. These wounds are painful and at risk for infection.

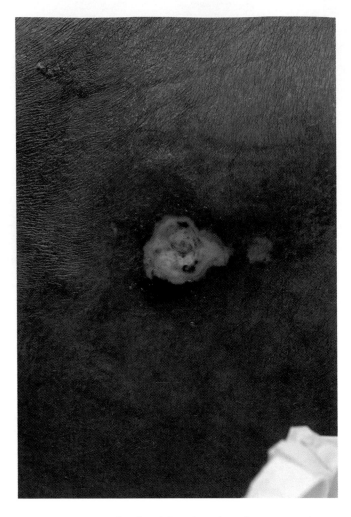

A stage 3 pressure ulcer has injury into the subcutaneous tissues below the dermis. Deeper wounds are more difficult to heal and prone to infection.

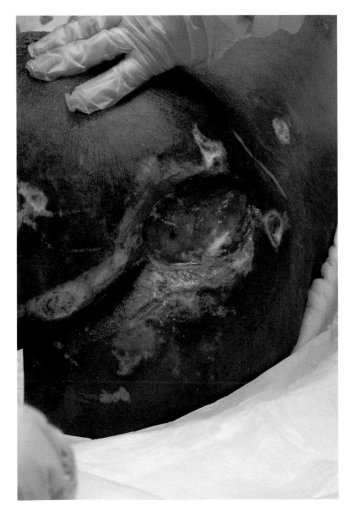

A stage 4 pressure ulcer has injury extending into the muscle tissue and may extend into the bone. These pressure ulcers take significant time with meticulous care to heal.

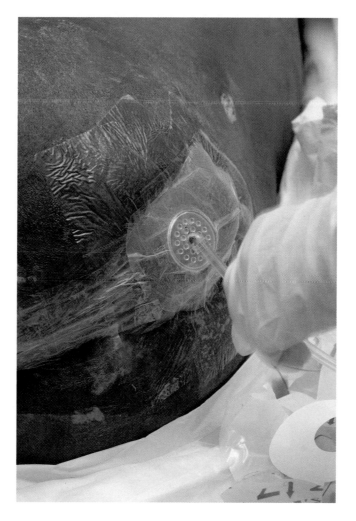

Treatment of pressure ulcers depends on the level of injury. A wound vacuum system is pictured for treating a stage 4 pressure ulcer. The device removes exudates and promotes granulation.

PULMONARY FIBROSIS

Pulmonary fibrosis is scarring throughout the lungs. Pulmonary fibrosis can be caused by many conditions, including chronic inflammatory processes, infections, environmental agents, exposure to ionizing radiation, and chronic conditions. The disease is chronic and there is no cure.

Assessment

- Shortness of breath
- Dry cough
- Unintended weight loss
- Fatigue
- Clubbing of the extremities

Planning and Implementation

- Administer oxygen
- Space activities
- Promote adequate oral and nutritional intake

Evaluation and Outcomes

The patient will:

- Experience less fatigue and shortness of breath
- Maintain adequate body weight
- Not experience pulmonary infections

Nursing Considerations

- Discuss long-term decisions, such as "do not resuscitate orders" and possible long-term placement before the necessity of such decisions is imminent.

- Lung transplantation is a treatment option for patients with severe pulmonary fibrosis.

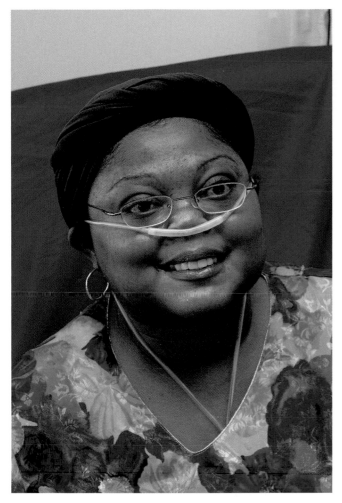

A patient with a pulmonary fibrosis utilizes oxygen to improve breathing. Pulmonary fibrosis patients are prescribed steroid therapy and may cause a rounding of the face or "moon face."

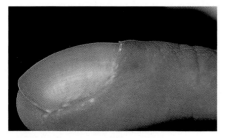

Note the severe clubbing in this image. Clubbing is most often the result of long-term hypoxia in patients with pulmonary fibrosis. (Courtesy of Dr. Robert Silverman, MD, Clinical Associate Professor, Department of Pediatrics, Georgetown University)

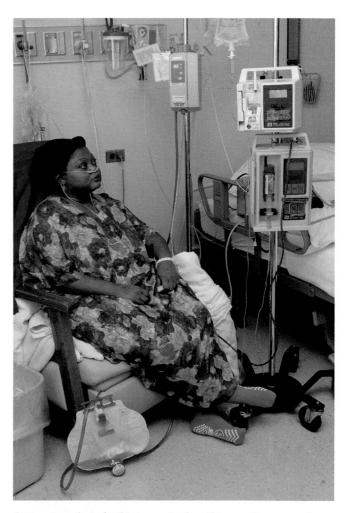

Sitting in a chair facilitates easier breathing and promotes better oxygenation.

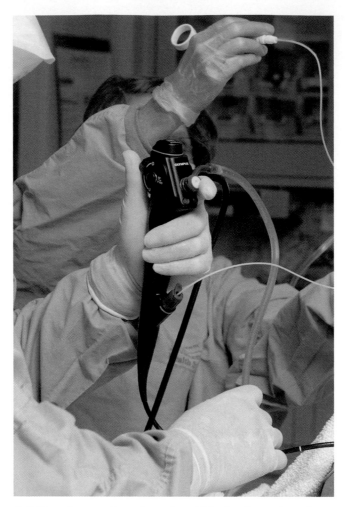

A, B Bronchoscopy is performed to aid in the diagnosis and treatment in patients with pulmonary fibrosis. The physician inserts the flexible tube into the bronchus.

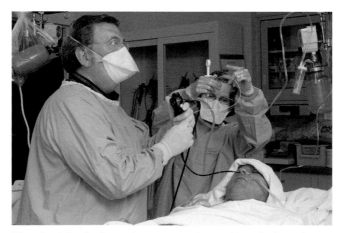

The physician looks at the screen and visualizes the bronchus as the nurse monitors the patient.

RASHES

A rash is any abnormal redness of the skin and may be associated with flat or raised bumps. Itching and pain may be present. A rash may be contained[EB1] to an area of the body or may be generalized. The etiology of rashes may be allergic, infectious, or the result of an insect bite.

Assessment

- Red, raised skin on part or all of skin
- Pruritis
- Pain

Planning and Implementation

- Treat rash based on cause
- Document skin assessments
- Meticulous skin care
- Treat pain and pruritis

Evaluation and Outcomes

The patient will:

- Experience an improvement in the rash
- Experience adequate pain and pruritis relief
- Understand cause of rash and how prevent

Nursing Considerations

- Severe allergic reactions with hives and difficulty breathing may be indicative of an anaphylactic reaction, and the patient will need emergency care.

- Use mitts on children to prevent further skin irritation from scratching.

- Attempt to find the etiology of any rash by careful taking of history, including asking the patient about any new medications, foods, or detergents recently used.

- Side effects of antipruritis medications may include drowsiness, and patients should avoid driving once such medications have been taken.

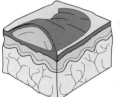

Wheal:
Localized edema in the epidermis causing irregular elevation that may be red or pale
Example:
Insect bite, hive, angioedema

Vesicle:
Accumulation of fluid between the upper layers of the skin; elevated mass containing serous fluid; less than 0.5 cm
Example:
Herpes simplex, herpes zoster, chickenpox, scabies

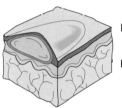

Bullae:
Same as a vesicle only greater than 0.5 cm
Example:
Contact dermatitis, large second-degree burns, bullous impetigo, pemphigus

Common skin lesions associated with rashes include wheals, vesicles, and bullae. The rash appearance is related to the etiology. (Courtesy of the CDC)

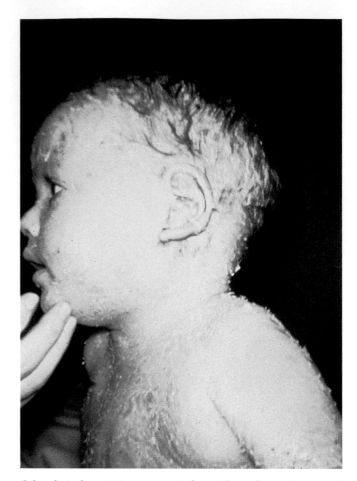

Seborrheic dermatitis occurs in infants. The rash may be present anywhere sebaceous glands are present. (Courtesy of the CDC)

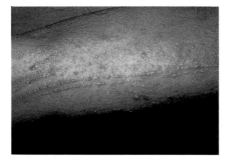

Contact dermatitis from contact with an allergen such as laundry detergent or perfumes. (Courtesy of the CDC)

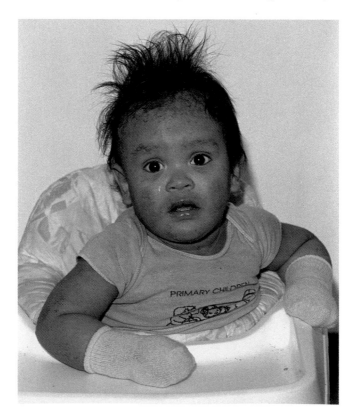

Atopic dermatitis in children is associated with severe itching. The scratching may cause lesions and topical skin infections, so mitts are often used to protect the skin.

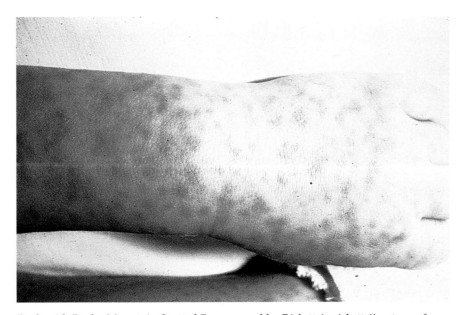

Rash with Rocky Mountain Spotted Fever caused by Rickettsia rickettsii, a type of bacteria that is spread to humans by tick bites. The rash is associated with fever, headache, and muscle pain. (Courtesy of the CDC)

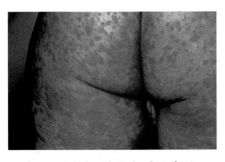

Rash associated with Rubeola infection. The rash is associated with fever, cough, and runny nose. (Courtesy of the CDC)

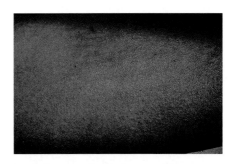

Rash from scarlet fever caused by a group A streptococcus infection. The rash begins on the chest and abdomen and is accompanied by a sore throat and fever. (Courtesy of the CDC)

RAYNAUD'S DISEASE

Raynaud's disease is the presence of bilateral arterial spasms of the extremities. The etiology is unknown, but may be related to other diseases, such as systemic lupus erythematosus, progressive systemic sclerosis, and connective tissue diseases. Episodes of exacerbation can be generated by stress and cold.

Assessment

- Pain to extremity
- Cyanosis followed by redness
- Decreased peripheral pulses
- Presence of infection or ulcerations

Planning and Implementation

- Provide warm environment
- Treat pain
- Monitor pulses and capillary refill
- Wound care for ulcers present

Evaluation and Outcomes

The patient will:

- Maintain adequate circulation to the extremities
- Understand ways to avoid exacerbations, including avoiding cold temperatures
- Experience adequate pain control

Nursing Considerations

- Women are affected by Raynaud's disease more frequently than are men.

- Offer assistance to patients experiencing exacerbations of Raynaud's disease.

- Encourage the patient to wear clothes that are easy to put on and remove.

- If a patient with Raynaud's goes for testing, encourage them to bring gloves in case of temperature fluctuation.

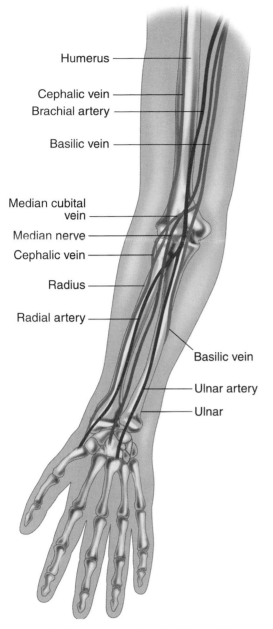

Humerus

Cephalic vein

Brachial artery

Basilic vein

Median cubital vein

Median nerve

Cephalic vein

Radius

Radial artery

Basilic vein

Ulnar artery

Ulnar

Raynaud's disease is associated with arterial spasms of the extremities. Assess radial and ulnar pulses for strength and the extremity for pallor, coolness, and pain.

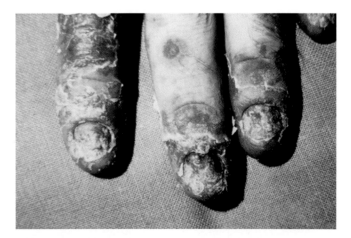

Ulcerations and skin sloughing may be present in the patient with Raynaud's disease from a lack of blood flow to the extremity.

SCABIES

Scabies is the infestation of the skin with a microscopic mite, sarcoptes scabiei, causing intense itching. Scabies infestation is via direct contact with an individual with scabies or close contact with an item they were recently in contact with (bedding or towels). Scabies spreads rapidly in crowded conditions, such as day care centers and large extended families living together.

Assessment

- Pimple-like irritations
- Burrows or rash of the skin in skin folds, between fingers, and perineum
- Intense itching, especially at night
- Sores on the skin from itching

Planning and Implementation

- Apply topical scabicides
- Prevent the spread of scabies to other patients
- Treat pruritis
- Wound care

Evaluation and Outcomes

The patient will:

- Prevent transmission of scabies to others
- Experience relief in pruritis
- Understand scabies treatment

Nursing Considerations

- Patients need to be assured that scabies infestation does not reflect cleanliness or socioeconomic status.

- Utilize contact precautions to prevent the spread of scabies.

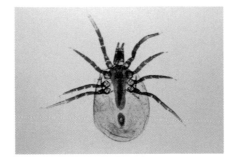

Scabies is caused by the infestation of a microscopic mite, sarcoptes scabiei. Attracted to odor and warmth, scabies will burrow into the skin of their human host. (Courtesy of the CDC)

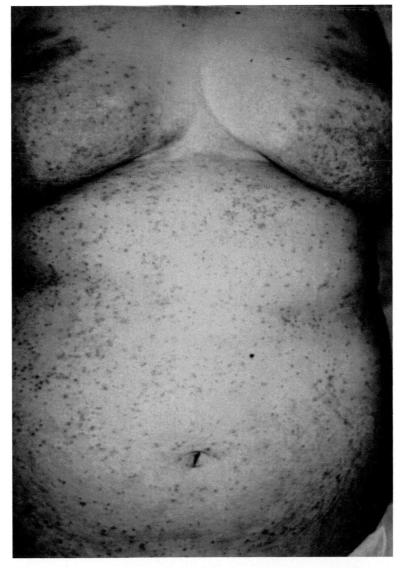

This severe case of scabies infestation causes intense itching of the skin and a red rash with pimple-like lesions. Notice the concentration of lesions on the breasts and breast folds. (Courtesy of the CDC)

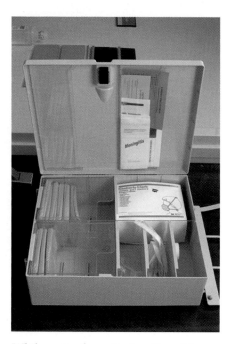

While caring for patients with scabies, nurses should observe and utilize contact isolation precautions to prevent spreading the infestation to themselves or other patients. Place patients in private rooms with isolation equipment outside the door for visitors and staff.

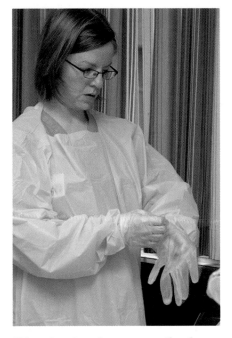

When donning gloves, ensure the gloves are under the gown cuff. This will prevent accidental scabies exposure to the wrist area.

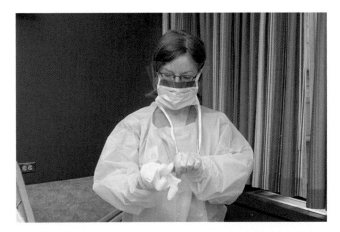

Masks are necessary with close contact with the patient and during linen changes. All items in the room making contact with the patient should be considered infectious and disposed of properly.

SCLERODERMA

Scleroderma is an autoimmune disease of the connective tissue causing fibrosis or scarring and may be considered diffuse or limited. Limited scleroderma affects the hands and face, while diffuse affects the entire body and organ dysfunction. The cause is unknown and treatment is supportive.

Assessment

- Calcinosis, calcium deposits it the skin
- Raynaud's disease (arterial spasms causing painful, cold hands)
- Esophagitis (inflammation or irritation of the esophagus causing heart burn and difficulty swallowing)
- Sclerodactyly, thickening and tightness of the skin
- Telangiectasias, red, dilated capillaries
- Cardiovascular, gastrointestinal and renal systems for organ involvement

Planning and Implementation

- Monitor disease progression
- Treat organ dysfunction, if present
- Treat hypertension, if present

Evaluation and Outcomes

The patient will:

- Maintain a normal blood pressure
- Limited disease progression
- Understand treatment and care

Nursing Considerations

- Women are affected more frequently with scleroderma than are males.

- Observe patients for organ dysfunction such as renal failure.

- Swelling and stiffness, especially in the morning may cause difficulties in performing everyday morning tasks such as bathing and eating.

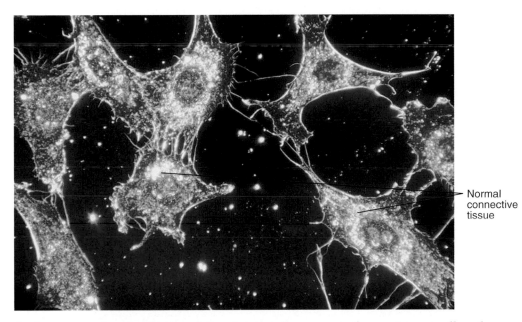

Normal
connective
tissue

As shown, normal connective tissue is found surrounding organs and supports nerve cells and blood vessels. Scleroderma causes inflammation of the connective tissue, causing scarring and organ dysfunction. (Courtesy of the NCI)

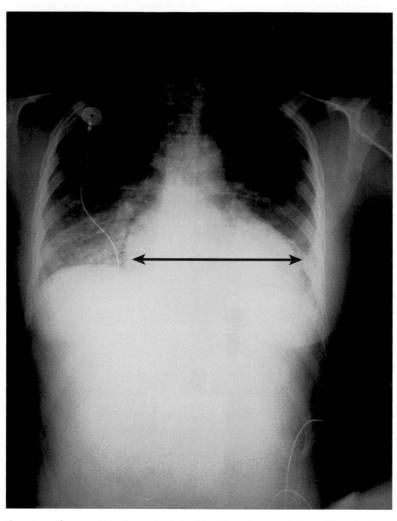

Scarring of connective tissue leads to fibrosis and organ failure. The chest radiograph exhibits an enlarged heart and heart failure from fibrosis and thickening of the heart muscle. (Courtesy of the CDC, Dr. Thomas Hooten)

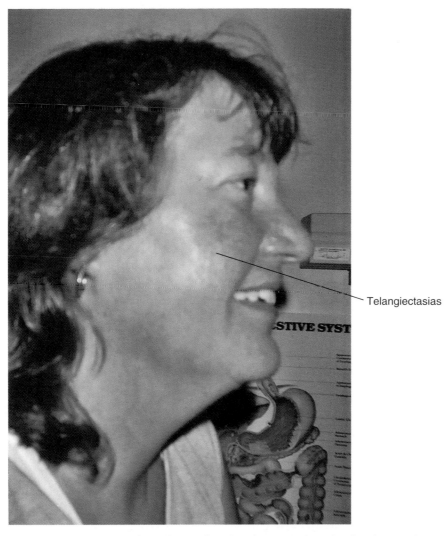

Telangiectasias

Telangiectasias are dilated capillaries often found in patients with scleroderma. They are painless and patient concerns are usually about cosmetic effects.

SCOLIOSIS

Scoliosis is an abnormal curvature of the spine, and its cause is unknown. Scoliosis is often diagnosed in childhood. Severe curvature may be associated with breathing difficulties. If untreated, scoliosis may cause degenerative changes in the spine with aging.

Assessment

- Uneven shoulders
- One shoulder blade is more prominent
- Uneven waist
- One hip higher than the other
- Difficulty breathing

Planning and Implementation

- Back brace or surgery to correct curvature
- Treat pain, if present

Evaluation and Outcomes

The patient will:

- Understand scoliosis treatments
- Experience a normally curved spine

Nursing Considerations

- Teach patients that carrying heavy objects during childhood, such as backpacks, does not contribute to the development of scoliosis.

- A back brace may be uncomfortable and a source of embarrassment for patients. Encourage them to discuss these feelings.

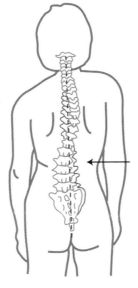

Scoliosis is an abnormal curving of the spine. It is usually found and treated in childhood.

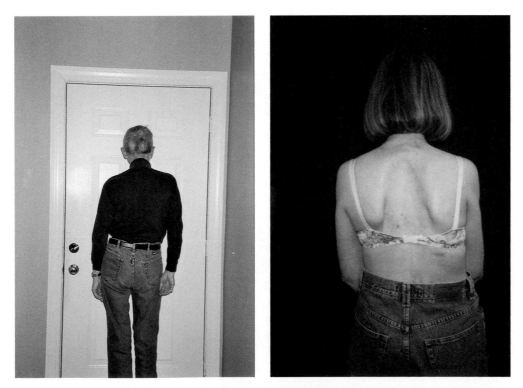

Scoliosis is present in these individuals. Observe the uneven shoulders and waists in each. In figure 2A, notice the finger tips are uneven and in 2B, the elbows are uneven.

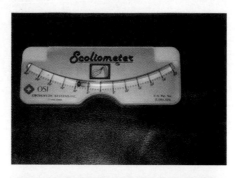

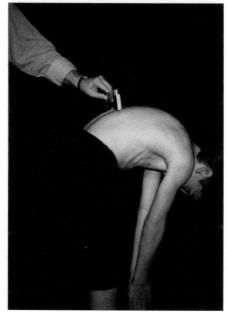

Scoliosis screening is common in school-age children. The nurse utilizes a scoliometer that measures the angle of trunk rotation. The child leans forward and the nurse places the scoliometer on the thoracic and lumbar vertebrae in the midspinal line to measure for the presence of lateral rotation of the spine. A lateral deviation greater than seven degrees is indicative of scoliosis.

SHINGLES

Shingles, or herpes zoster, is a painful condition caused by a previous infection, usually in childhood, with varicella zoster virus, commonly called chickenpox. The virus lays dormant in nerve cells until a patient ages or the immune system becomes weakened. Shingles, also called adult chickenpox, appear as a painful rash on the face, eyelids, or trunk.

Assessment

- History of chickenpox or vaccinated for chickenpox
- Red rash and blisters on trunk, face or eyelids
- Burning, severe pain to reddened area

Planning and Implementation

- Monitor and treat pain
- Minimize contact with affected area
- Administer antiviral medications

Evaluation and Outcomes

The patient will:

- Experience pain control
- Understand the cause of shingles
- Understand the treatment for shingles

Nursing Considerations

- A patient with shingles may transmit the virus to a patient that has never had chickenpox, and thus contact should be avoided by those without previous exposure to the virus.

- Patients with weakened immune function, such as oncology or AIDS patients, are at higher risk for shingle breakouts.

- Pregnant women should avoid patients with shingles until the scabs have dried, in order to prevent unintentional contact with the fetus.

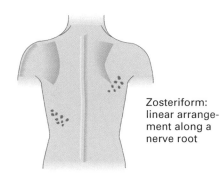

Zosteriform:
linear arrange-
ment along a
nerve root

*The rash associated with shingles usual-
ly follows along a nerve root, because
the herpes zoster virus emerges from
nerve cells.*

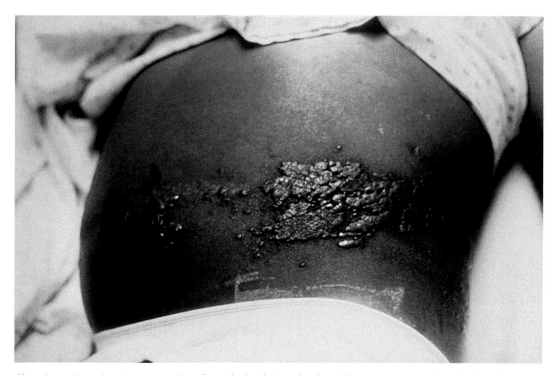

*Shingles rash and redness extending from the back into the chest. The pain associated with shingles can
be severe and debilitating. Contact even with clothing on the area intensifies pain.*

SKIN CANCER

Skin cancer is a malignancy found on the skin. Skin cancer includes basal cell carcinoma, squamous cell carcinoma, and melanoma. Most skin cancer is preventable by avoiding sunlight and use of sunblock lotion.

Assessment

- Change in the size or color of an existing freckle or mole
- Asymmetrical freckle or mole with an irregular border
- Dark brown, black, or bluish freckle or mole
- Any freckle or mole larger than ¼ inch

Planning and Implementation

- Perform skin assessments
- Teach how to avoid skin cancer

Evaluation and Outcomes

The patient will:

- Utilize sunblock
- Perform monthly skin assessments
- Seek a healthcare provider if any irregularity is noted

Nursing Considerations

- Melanoma, a deadly form of skin cancer, has increased dramatically in the last decade.

- Teach patients that using tanning beds also increases the risk of skin cancer.

- Encourage patients to inspect their skin monthly and to report changes.

- Anti-aging therapies (skin peels, laser treatments) decrease the incidence of skin cancer.

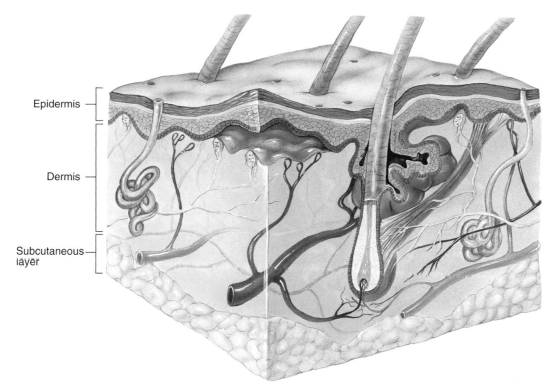

Epidermis

Dermis

Subcutaneous
layer

Skin cancers form in the outmost layer of the skin, the epidermis. If detected and removed before invading deeper layers, skin cancer is almost 100% curable. When assessing for skin cancer, all skin should be assessed with emphasis on any skin that has been exposed to sunlight.

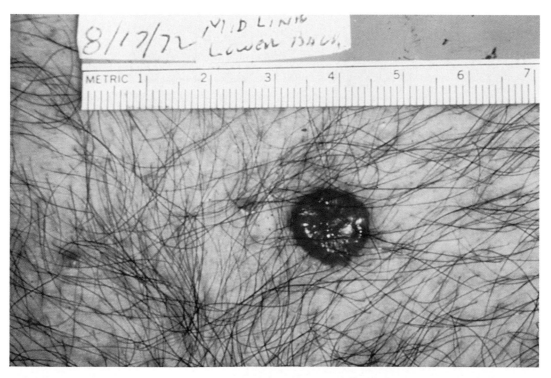

Basal cell skin cancer is the most common form of skin cancer, and the most common of all cancers. The lesions are characterized by a small, reddish-brown papule that may seem pearly in color. The center may be slightly depressed with raised edges, as shown in this picture. Chronic exposure to sunlight is the cause of most basal cell skin cancers. (Courtesy of the NCI)

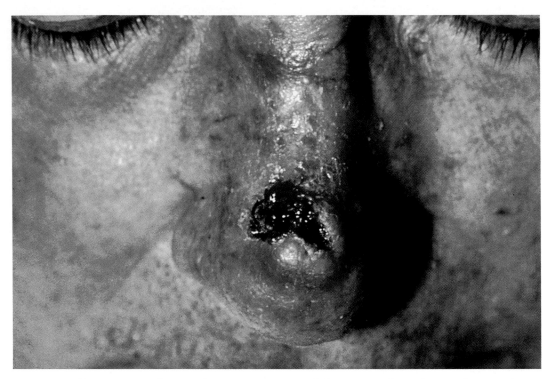

Squamous cell carcinoma is the second most common type of skin cancer. Shown here on the nose, the lesions appear as an ulcerated area with scaly edges. They may also be found on the lips and in mucous membranes. Chronic exposure to sunlight is the cause of most squamous cell skin cancers. (Courtesy of the NCI)

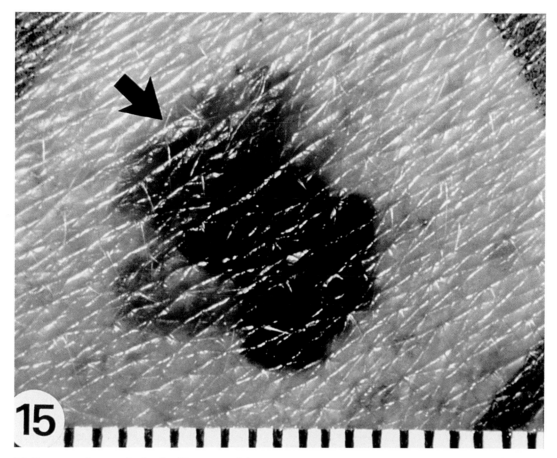

Malignant melanoma is the deadliest type of skin cancer. It originates in melanocytes, which produce the melanin that gives skin color. This accounts for the deep brown black or purple appearance of the tumor. If diagnosed and removed while in the epidermis, it is almost 100% curable. When melanoma metastasizes, it is difficult to treat and may be deadly. (Courtesy of the NCI)

SYPHILIS

Syphilis is caused by the bacteria *Treponema pallidum* and may be contracted through sexual contact, contact with a primary syphilis genital ulcer, also called a chancre, or syphilis-infected blood. It is often asymptomatic, but may produce a genital ulcer that heals. If not treated with antibiotics, it can progress to a secondary stage clinically noted by a rash on the hands and feet that disappears even without treatment. If untreated, the infection may lead to tertiary syphilis with internal organ damage and nervous system involvement that may lead to death.

Assessments

- Unprotected sexual contact
- Patients may be asymptomatic
- Vaginal, cervical, penile, anal lesions (chancre)
- Rash on body or on mucous membranes

Planning and Implementation

- Implement appropriate treatments
- Prevent spread
- Educate on transmission

Evaluation and Outcomes

The patient will:

- Undergo treatment for syphilis infection
- Understand safe sex practices
- Notify recent sexual partners of infection

Nursing Considerations

- Pregnant women should be tested for syphilis because an untreated infection may cause fetal death.

- Serology tests to confirm the diagnosis of syphilis frequently have false-positive results and repeated tests are often necessary.

- Universal precautions will prevent the spread of the infection to health care providers when caring for patients with tertiary syphilis.

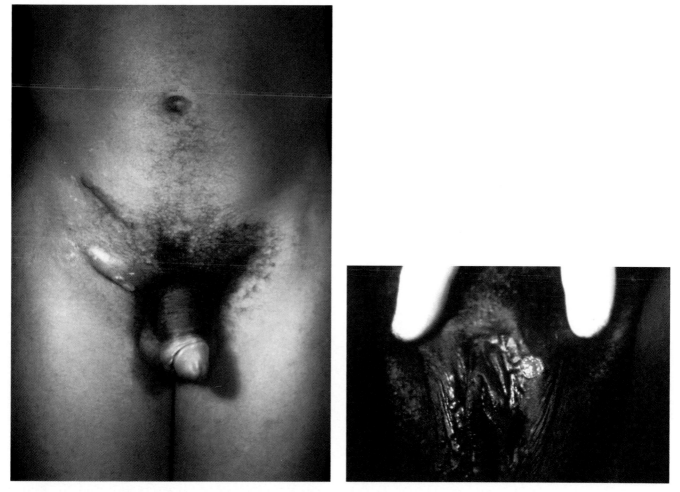

Chancre lesion on female and male genitals. A chancre lesion is found as a primary infection with syphilis. The chancre is infectious and contact with the lesion may cause syphilis. The lesions are painless and appear ten days to three months after contact with syphilis. The lesions normally heal with or without treatment. (Courtesy of the CDC, Renelle Woodhall)

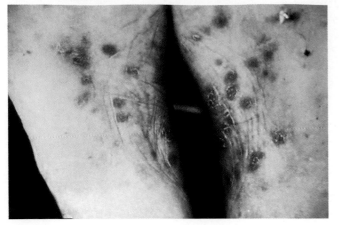

Untreated primary syphilis may lead to the secondary stage of syphilis infection. A rash on the body, genitals, mucous membranes, or feet as the image indicates is a vague, non-specific assessment finding. Other vague assessments such as hair loss, mild fever, and sore throat may be present. Often patients are unaware that they have a syphilis infection and may infect others. (Courtesy of the CDC, Dr. Gavin Hart)

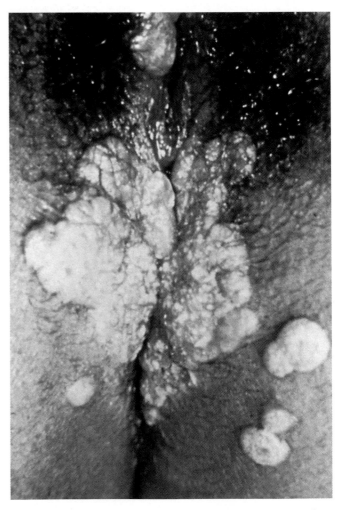

Condyloma latum are moist, genital warts; they are a sign of secondary syphilis infection, though they are not definitive in themselves for syphilis. After the secondary syphilis stage, patients may enter the latent phase where they do not harbor any symptoms, but remain infected. (Courtesy of the CDC)

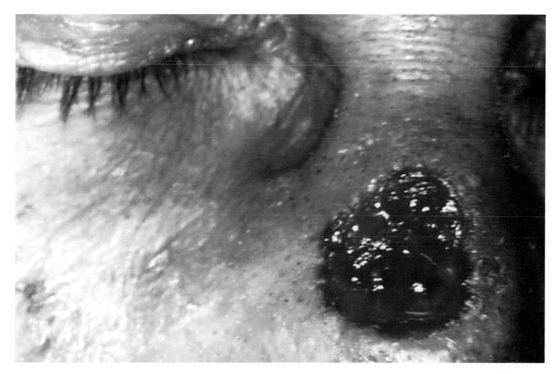

A gumma, a non-cancerous form of a granuloma, is a sign of tertiary syphilis infection. Shown on the face, a gumma can form anywhere, including the liver, lungs, and heart. Tertiary syphilis is associated with severe illnesses, including blindness, cardiac disease, mental illness, and death. (Courtesy of the CDC, J. Pledger)

THROMBOPHLEBITIS

Thrombophlebitis is the inflammation of a vein accompanied by the formation of a blood clot or thrombus, and is referred to as a deep vein thrombosis (DVT). DVTs occur most often in the deep veins of the lower extremities and if dislodged, may lead to pulmonary emboli. Virchow's triad (venous stasis, vessel injury, and altered blood coagulation) are key factors in the formation of thrombophlebitis.

Assessment

- Pain, warmth, redness, swelling at thrombus site
- Fever, malaise
- Fatigue
- Edema

Planning and Implementation

- Treat pain
- Elevate affected extremity
- Anticoagulation therapy
- Monitor distal pulses
- Monitor for pulmonary embolism

Evaluation and Outcomes

The patient will:

- Experience effective pain control
- Understand risk factors for thrombophlebitis
- Not experience dislodging of the thrombus

Nursing Considerations

- Educate patients concerning the need for early postoperative ambulation, the importance of using thromboembolic elastic stockings (TED hose), and pneumatic pulsation devices to prevent DVT formation.

- Instruct patients not to get out of bed while wearing pneumatic devices; the connected tubing may inadvertently cause a fall.

- If a patient experiences thrombophlebitis, do not apply a pneumatic device to the affected extremity.

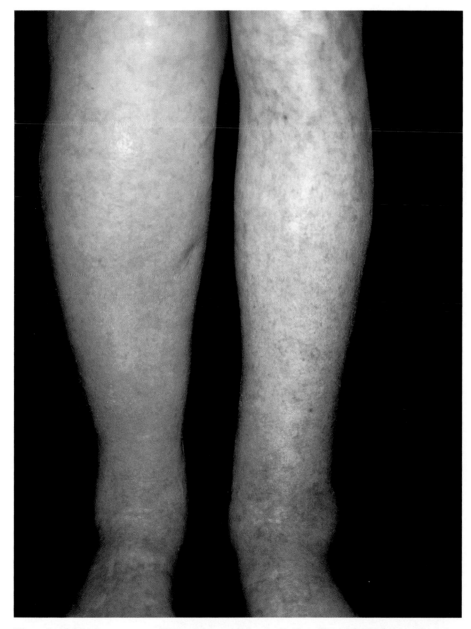

Thrombophlebitis causes swelling, redness, and pain in the affected limb. Notice the swelling in the right calf. (Courtesy of Viewing Medicine)

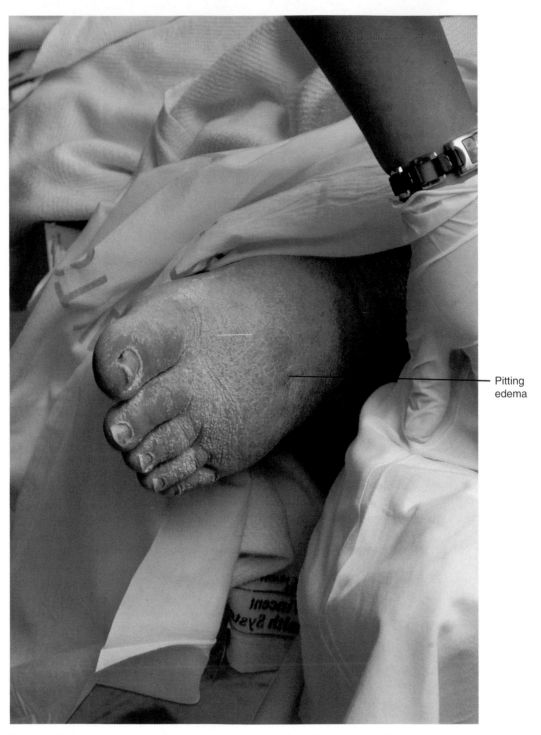

Pitting
edema

Thombophlebitis may cause pitting edema distal to the thrombus site. Note the imprints left in the patient's foot from the nurse's fingers while palpating the dorsalis pedis pulse.

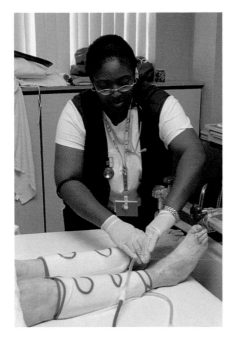

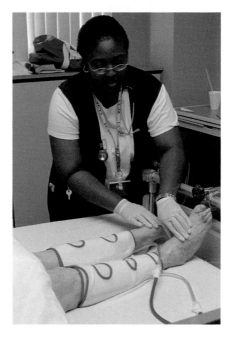

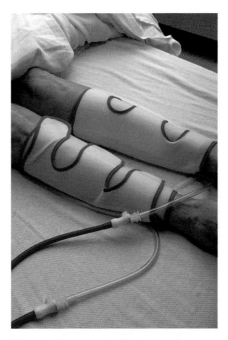

The use of pneumatic devices to the lower extremities lessens the chance of thrombus formation and subsequent thrombophlebitis. The nurse applies the pneumatic device when the patient is in bed. Notice how the device is connected with tubing. Lastly, the nurse palpates pedal pulses to assess the distal extremity circulation status.

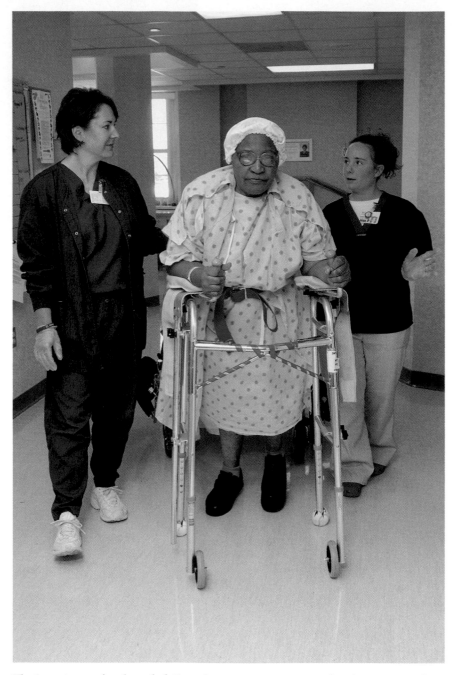

The importance of early ambulation after any surgery or procedure is paramount in preventing thrombophlebitis.

TRAUMA, BLUNT CHEST

Blunt chest trauma is any traumatic blow or force to any portion of the chest wall. Mortality from blunt chest trauma is high because of the subsequent damage to lungs, heart, or great vessels causing cardiogenic shock (myocardial damage), hypovolemic shock (blood loss), or hypoxia (lung injury).

Assessment

- ABCs—Airway, breathing, signs of circulation
- Mechanism of injury
- Shock (hypotension, tachycardia, evidence of blood loss)
- Pain

Planning and Implementation

- Support airway and administer oxygen
- Administer fluids
- Treat pain
- Treat specific injuries

Evaluation and Outcomes

The patient will:

- Maintain a patent airway
- Oxygenate effectively
- Maintain an adequate blood pressure
- Experience pain relief

Nursing Considerations

- The most significant cause of blunt chest injury is motor vehicle accidents. Promote wearing seatbelts and using good driving practices.

- Quick assessments and obtaining details about how patients sustained their injuries may aid in rapid treatment and ultimately save lives.

- Anticipate a team approach in caring for blunt trauma patients once they arrive in the emergency department. Severe injuries require many treatments and actions simultaneously.

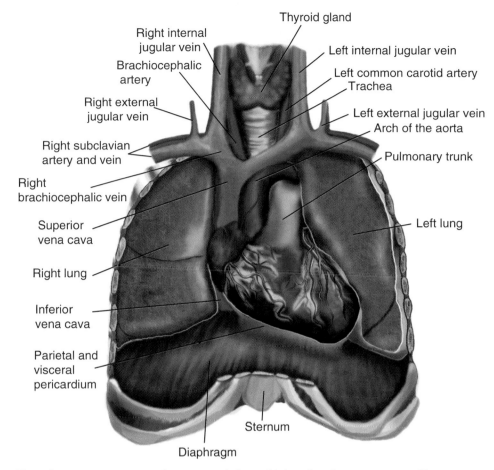

Right internal jugular vein
Brachiocephalic artery
Right external jugular vein
Right subclavian artery and vein
Right brachiocephalic vein
Superior vena cava
Right lung
Inferior vena cava
Parietal and visceral pericardium

Thyroid gland
Left internal jugular vein
Left common carotid artery
Trachea
Left external jugular vein
Arch of the aorta
Pulmonary trunk
Left lung

Sternum
Diaphragm

Blunt chest trauma may not show outward signs of injury, but the trauma may affect any component in the chest area, including the heart, lungs, and major blood vessels.

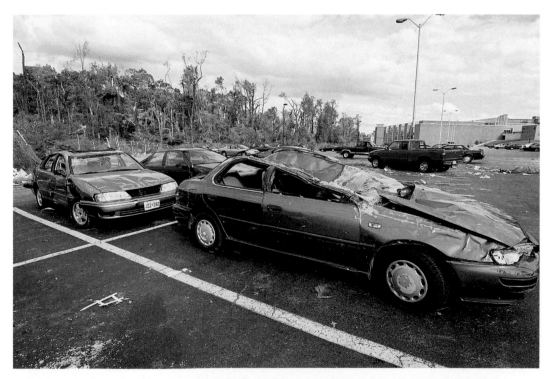

The person driving this vehicle most likely suffered blunt chest trauma from the steering wheel or dashboard. Motor vehicle accidents are major causes of blunt chest trauma. Wearing seatbelts can help reduce blunt chest trauma. (Courtesy of the FEMA)

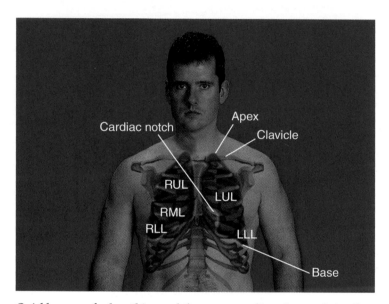

Quickly assess for breathing and the presence of breath sounds in all lung fields in any patient with blunt chest trauma. Pneumothorax and hemothorax may occur.

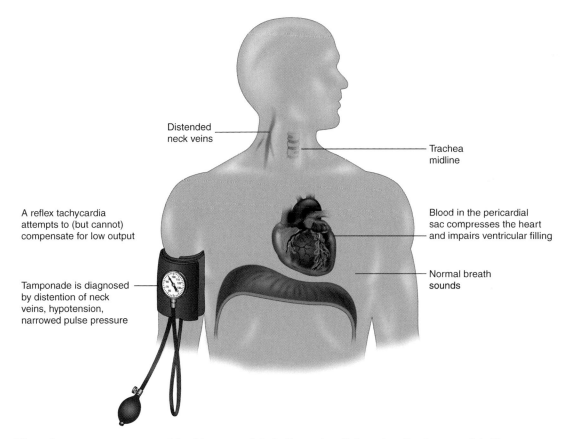

Distended neck veins

Trachea midline

A reflex tachycardia attempts to (but cannot) compensate for low output

Blood in the pericardial sac compresses the heart and impairs ventricular filling

Normal breath sounds

Tamponade is diagnosed by distention of neck veins, hypotension, narrowed pulse pressure

Blunt chest trauma may cause blood to accumulate in the pericardial sac (cardiac tamponade). Signs include distended neck veins, tachycardia, hypotension, and muffled heart tones.

TRAUMA, PENETRATING CHEST

Penetrating chest trauma is any trauma to the chest area from penetration with an object, such as bullets and knives. Mortality from penetrating chest trauma is significant, due to the subsequent damage to lungs, heart, or great vessels, causing cardiogenic shock (myocardial damage), hypovolemic shock (blood loss), or hypoxia (lung injury).

Assessment

- ABC's—Airway, breathing, signs of circulation
- Entrance and exit wounds (gunshot wounds)
- Pulsation of impaled object (knife wound)
- Shock (hypotension, tachycardia, evidence of blood loss)
- Pain

Planning and Implementation

- Support airway and administer oxygen
- Administer fluids
- Treat pain
- Apply dressing over entrance and exit wounds
- Support impaled object, never remove

Evaluation and Outcomes

The patient will:

- Maintain a patent airway
- Oxygenate effectively
- Maintain an adequate blood pressure
- Experience pain relief

Nursing Considerations

➡ Prompt, pre-hospital treatment of penetrating chest wounds significantly enhances the chances of patient survival.

➡ Obtain blood consents immediately and anticipate blood transfusions.

➡ If violence is suspected, notify hospital security and carefully screen visitors.

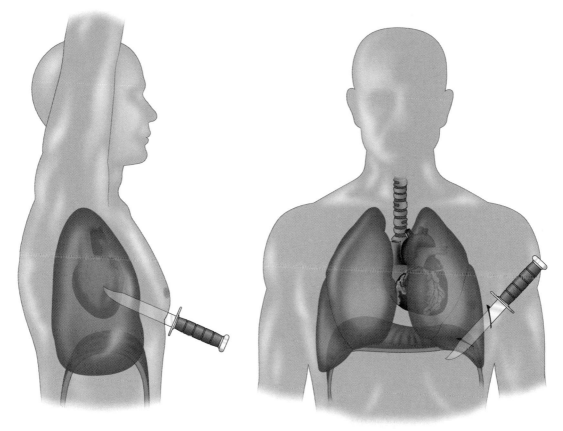

Stab wounds at nipple level or below frequently penetrate the abdomen

Penetrating chest wounds would have small external wounds, yet significant injury occurs to underlying organs and tissue. Injuries to the heart and lungs cause significant hypoxia and blood loss. Injuries to the spinal cord may cause paralysis.

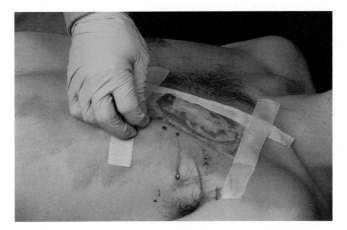

Wounds caused by a penetrating chest injury, such as an exit wound from a gunshot, may leave an open chest wound. The wound is covered with a sterile dressing that is secure on three sides with the fourth side left unsecured as a vent. This allows any air trapped in the pleural space to exit, and acts as a way to allow air to exit upon exhalation, as normal anatomy is disrupted.

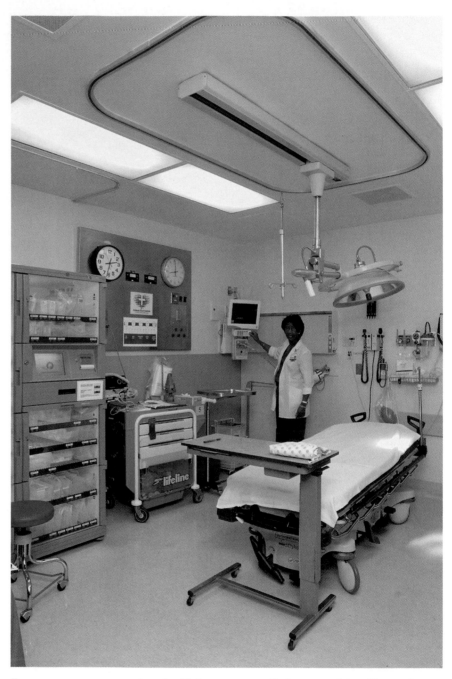

Emergency rooms are equipped with trauma rooms that are complete with any item required for a trauma patient. Defibrillators, chest tubes, artificial airways, proper lighting, and equipment for emergency surgery are types of equipment found in trauma rooms. Notice in the picture the blue "crash cart" used to house emergency medications, and the large clock used to document when medications and treatments are initiated.

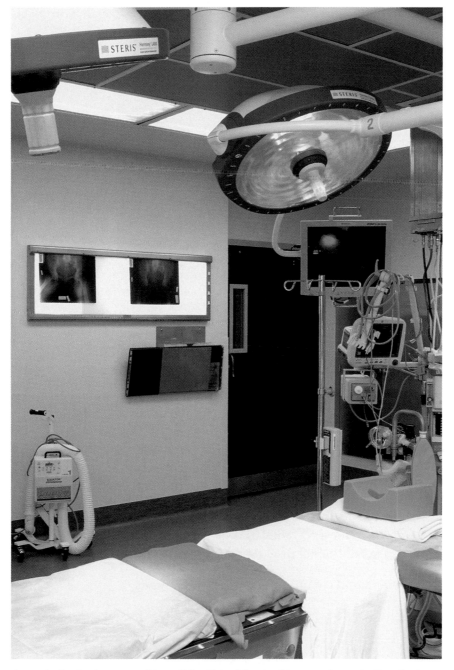

A surgical suite is prepared in anticipation of the need to correct penetrating chest trauma injuries after initial stabilization in the emergency room. Notice the chest radiographs in the surgical suite that allow surgeons to visualize damage before performing surgery.

TUBERCULOSIS

Tuberculosis (TB) is a chronic infection of the lung caused by a mMycobacterium infection, resulting in the development of tubercles in the lungs. Tubercles are the nodules seen on a chest xX-ray, and consist of lymphocytes and epithelioid cells. Mycobacterium enters the body through inhaled droplets.

Assessment

- Cough, hemoptysis
- Fever, chills
- Weight loss
- Night sweats
- Weakness

Planning and Implementation

- Place patient in a negative flow room
- Oxygen administration and chest physiotherapy
- Administer treatment regimes for TB
- Encourage adequate nutritional and fluid intake
- Encourage frequent rest periods

Evaluation and Outcomes

The patient will:

- Maintain adequate oxygenation
- Effectively overcome tuberculosis infection
- Maintain adequate nutritional and fluid intake
- Understand tuberculosis transmission and treatments

Nursing Considerations

- Patients with immunologic disorders, such as human immunodeficiency virus and cancer, are at higher risk for contracting tuberculosis.

- Multiple drug resistant tuberculosis (MDR-TB) is increasing; if a patient on proper drug therapy is not responding to therapy, non-traditional drug therapies may be necessary.

- Visitors need to understand and comply with droplet precautions.

- Health care workers require fit testing of particulate respirators to make certain droplets are not inhaled.

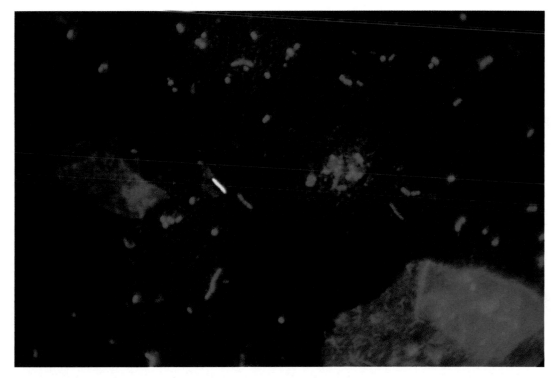

Tuberculosis is caused by an infection with Mycobacterium tuberculosis bacilli. Shown here as the bright orange, the bacilli are present in a sputum specimen, the most accurate type of specimen for diagnosing tuberculosis. (Courtesy of the CDC)

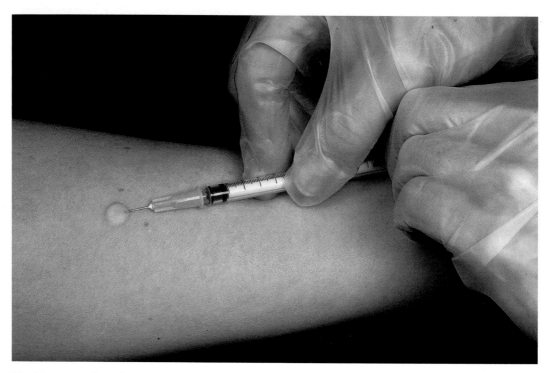

The Mantoux tuberculin skin test screens patients for tuberculosis. Notice the wheal created. If the test is positive, the injection site will become raised and red and will be followed up with a chest X-ray. (Courtesy of the CDC, Greg Knobloch)

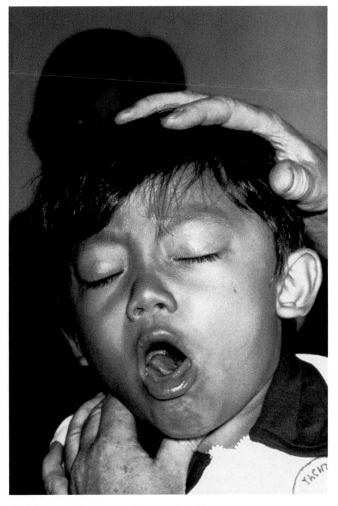

Coughing, night sweats, fever and chills are common assessment findings in patients with tuberculosis. If tuberculosis is suspected, anyone in close contact with the patient should be tested.

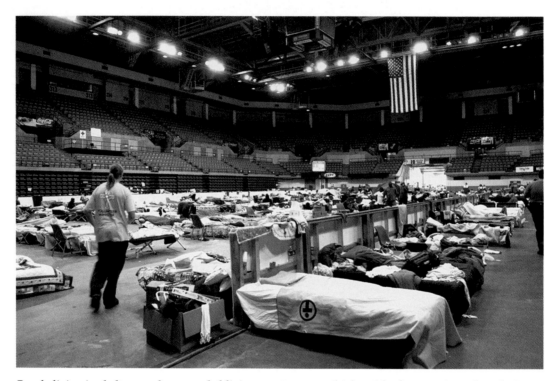

People living in shelters or close crowded living quarters are at higher risk of contracting tuberculosis, because it is an airborne disease caused by inhaling droplets from an infected person's cough. (Courtesy of the FEMA, W. Henderson)

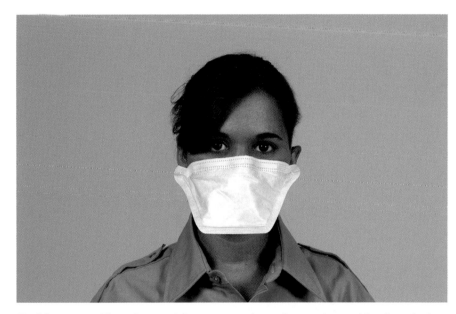

Health care providers observe airborne precautions; place patients with tuberculosis in reverse airflow rooms, and wear N 95 particulate respirator masks to protect themselves and other patients.

UTICARIA

Uticaria, commonly known as hives, consists of well-defined areas of raised redness and edema of the skin. Uticaria can be acute or chronic, and is the most benign form of anaphylaxis. It may occur independently, or be accompanied by more serious forms of anaphylaxis, including angioedema and anaphylactic shock (see anaphylactic shock).

Assessment

- Question patient concerning recent changes in topical products, food ingestion, medications, or bee stings
- Vital signs (hypotension and tachycardia, signs of anaphylactic shock)
- Area affected
- Presence of pruritis

Planning and Implementation

- Monitor vital signs and airway
- Anticipate diphenhydramine and possible epinephrine administration
- Treat pruritis by removal of allergen and cool baths

Evaluation and Outcomes

The patient will:

- Experience prompt treatment of uticaria
- Maintain an adequate blood pressure and airway
- Understand treatment and cause of uticaria

Nursing Considerations

- Patients experiencing uticaria and associated angioedema in response to an allergen (such as a bee sting) require an Epi-Pen to promptly treat uticaria outside the hospital setting.

- In the hospital setting, anytime a patient is introduced to a new medication they are at risk for uticaria and risk of anaphylactic shock.

- Admission histories include allergies and, additionally, the nurse should document the type of allergic reaction the patient experiences, such as uticaria, difficulty breathing, or headache.

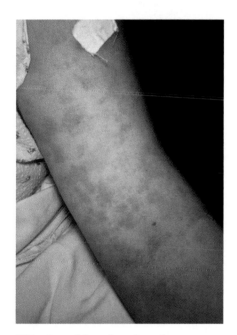

Uticaria, or hives, is a sign of a severe allergic response. Uticaria consists of red raised patches of skin. They may occur anywhere on the body and are accompanied by severe itching. The cause of the uticaria should be documented and reported as an allergy. (Courtesy of the CDC)

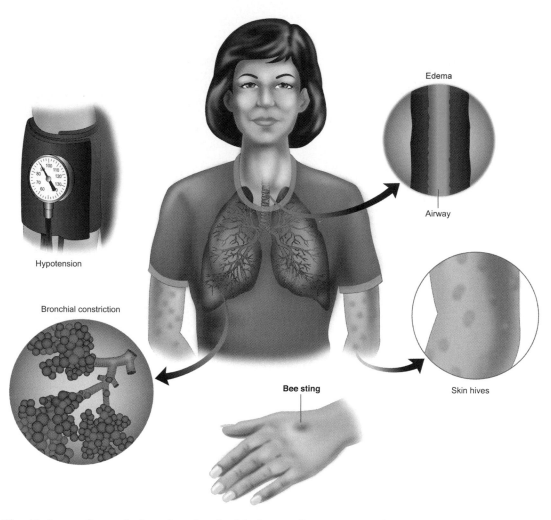

Hypotension

Bronchial constriction

Edema

Airway

Bee sting

Skin hives

The skin is one of many body systems involved during an allergic reaction. Severe reactions called anaphylaxis include uticaria, shortness of breath from airway edema and constriction, and hypotension. Death may ensue if not treated.

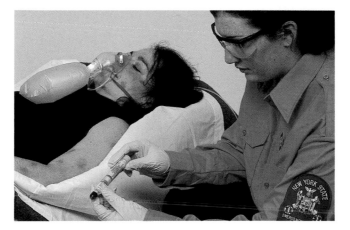

Observe the red, raised patches (uticaria) on the patient's arms and face. If a patient develops uticaria, they should receive prompt medical treatment. Medical treatment usually consists of diphenhydramine administration. If the patient is short of breath and anaphylaxis is suspected, oxygen and epinephrine will be administered as pictured.

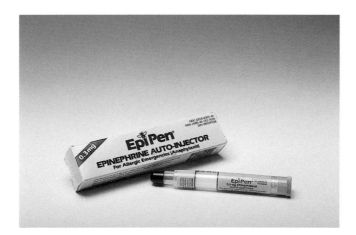

If a patient experiences a severe allergic reaction, an Epi-Pen is prescribed. An Epi-Pen is a single dose, self-injectable amount of epinephrine easily administered via an Epi-Pen auto injector. Once a patient experiences a severe allergic reaction, an Epi-Pen should be carried to promptly treat any future allergic reaction.

VARICOSE VEINS

Varicose veins are dilated veins that lack surrounding muscle support. The saphenous veins of the legs are commonly affected, and there is a familial tendency. Thrombophlebitis, obesity, prolonged standing, and pregnancy are risk factors.

Assessment

- Distended, torturous bluish veins
- Pain of the legs
- Prolonged capillary refill
- Family history of varicose veins

Planning and Implementation

- Weight loss
- Exercise
- Use of support hose
- Avoid prolonged standing

Evaluation and Outcomes

The patient will:

- Understand causes and treatments of varicose veins
- Experience less leg pain
- Utilize support hose when standing

Nursing Considerations

- Varicose veins affect approximately 60% of women. Concerns with varicose veins are predominantly in regard to cosmetic effects.

- Wearing support hose during prolonged standing periods decreases the incidence and severity of varicose veins.

- Measure calf circumference and length of leg for correct fit of support stockings.

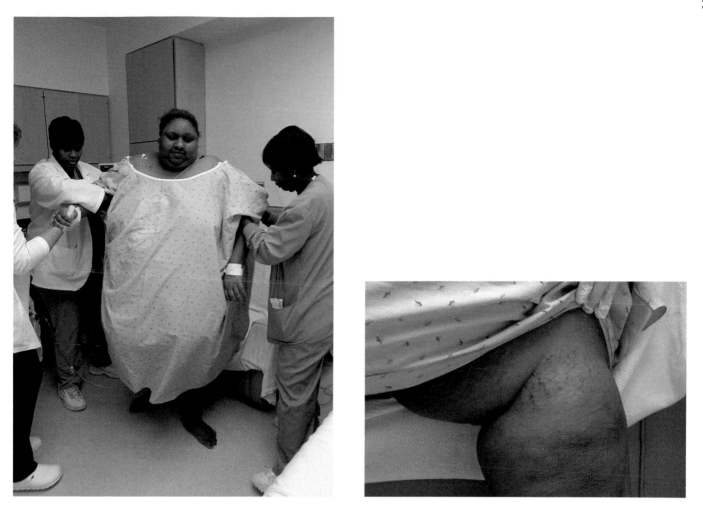

Varicose veins are prominent, distended, tortuous blue veins. Encourage weight loss to prevent further varicose veins. Observe the varicose veins on the calf of the obese patient.

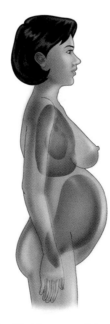

Anything that increases intra-abdominal pressure may cause varicosities. Varicose veins may occur during pregnancy from the abdominal pressure. Encourage pregnant women to avoid prolonged standing to help prevent varicose veins.

VENOUS STASIS ULCERS

A venous stasis ulcer is an erosion of the skin that may lead to skin necrosis, open wounds, and eschar formation. Approximately 75% of venous stasis ulcers are caused by chronic venous insufficiency. Other risks include diabetes, arterial insufficiency, neuropathy, burns, being elderly, and certain blood disorders.

Assessments

- Pain at ulcer site
- Edema of affected foot and ankle
- Open wound with or without the presence of infection
- Brown or purplish pigmentation of lower legs and feet

Planning and Implementation

- Wound care routine
- Provide adequate nutrition
- Treat pain
- Document wound assessment
- Debridement, a mechanical method of eliminating necrotic tissue, may be performed to promote healing

Evaluation and Outcomes

The patient will:

- Experience wound healing
- Experience adequate pain control
- Understand wound causes and treatments

Nursing Considerations

- Venous stasis ulcers are the most significant cause of chronic wounds. Many venous stasis ulcers require months of vigilant care to experience healing.

- The use of compression stockings reduces the incidence and severity of venous stasis ulcers.

- Monitor the patient's unilateral leg swelling or pain (signs of deep vein thrombosis). Venous stasis increases the risk for thrombophlebitis.

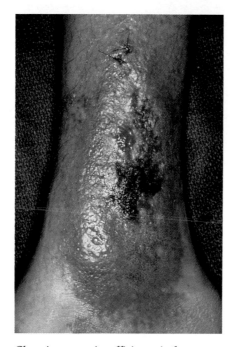

Chronic venous insufficiency is the cause of most venous stasis ulcers. They occur on the lower extremities. (A) Note the area is reddened with an area of breakdown. (Courtesy of the CDC)

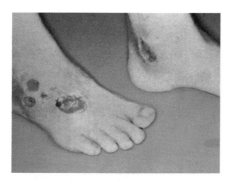

(B) Venous ulcers may have a circular appearance. Healing is difficult because of the poor circulation to the area.

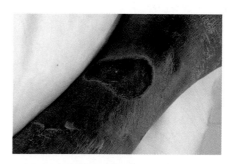

(C) Surgical debridement may be necessary to promote healing in venous stasis ulcers. Observe the clean wound edges in this venous ulcer.

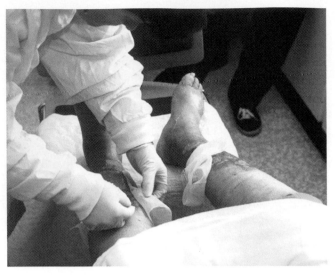

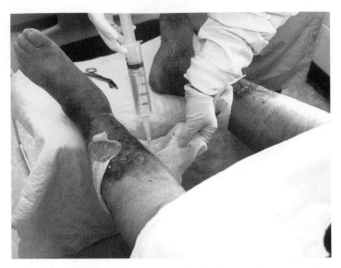

Meticulous wound care as prescribed promotes healing in venous ulcers. (A) Remove the previous dressing carefully. Bandages may dry and stick to the ulcer, causing further skin breakdown when removed.

(B) Cleanse the wound with prescribed solutions. Document the wound appearance and drainage, if present. Note the brownish pigment changes surrounding the ulcers. This discoloration is an assessment finding with chronic venous insufficiency.

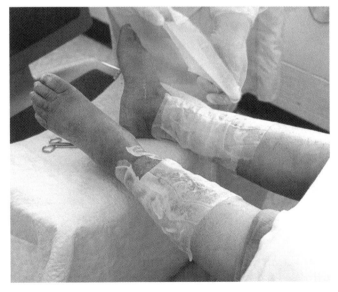

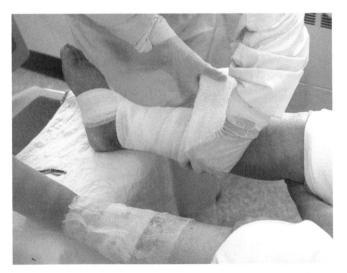

(C) Prescribed dressing and/or ointments are applied to the wounds.

(D) Apply dressings, allowing the patient the greatest mobility; notice the ankle movement is not restricted. The dressing allows toes and pedal pulses to be assessed for color, temperature, pulse, and for presence of edema.

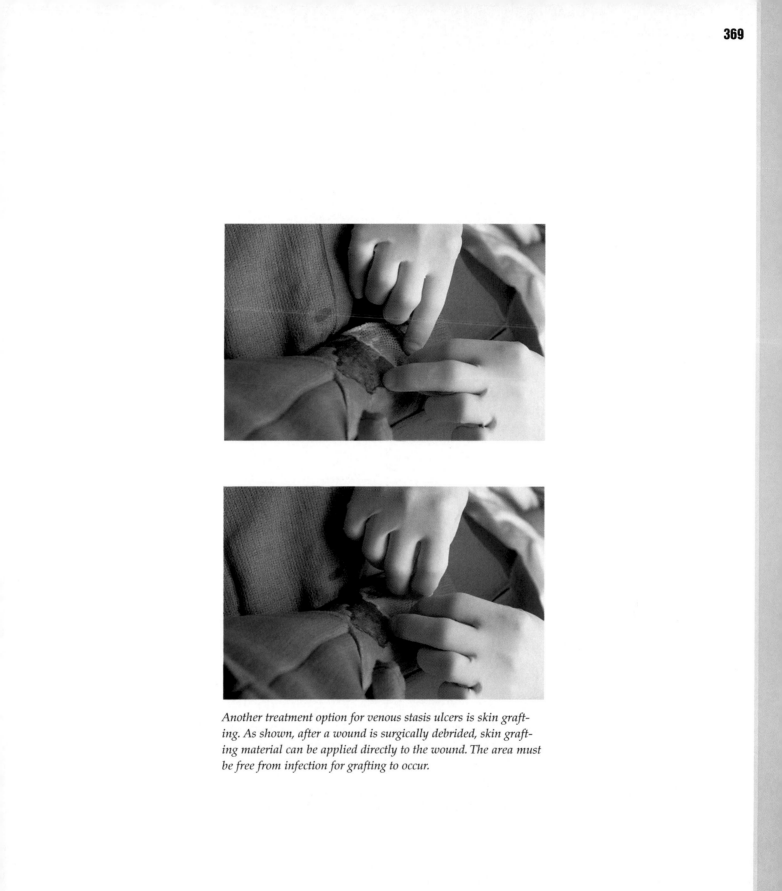

Another treatment option for venous stasis ulcers is skin graft-ing. As shown, after a wound is surgically debrided, skin graft-ing material can be applied directly to the wound. The area must be free from infection for grafting to occur.

WARTS

Warts are benign tumors of the epidermal layer of the skin, and are caused by a virus. The most common virus causing warts is the human papillomavirus (HPV). The transmission of warts includes via casual contact and sexual transmission. HPV infection may cause genital warts, and is the cause of cervical cancer in many women.

Assessment

- Small, firm raised area or areas on skin or mucous membrane
- Pain and possible bleeding when bumped

Planning and Implementation

- Promote hand washing
- Educate patient on etiology (casual and sexual contact) of warts
- Medical treatments may include cryosurgery, application of acid solutions, laser removal, and electrocautery
- Home remedies include the use of over-the-counter topical wart therapies, and the application of duct tape to the site until warts are gone
- Do not use home remedies to treat genital warts

Evaluation and Outcomes

The patient will:

- Understand wart treatments
- Effectively treat warts

Nursing Considerations

- Educate patients that warts are infectious, but not caused by handling frogs or small animals.

- A series of 3 HBV vaccines are now available for girls ages 9-13 to reduce the risk of cervical cancer caused by the HBV virus.

- Stress that abstinence is the only way to eliminate the chance of contracting sexually transmitted infections.

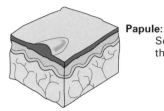

Papule:
Solid, elevated lesion less than 0.5 cm in diameter

A wart is a solid, elevated papule found on the epidermal layer of the skin, in the mouth, or genital region. Warts can form as a single papule or in clusters.

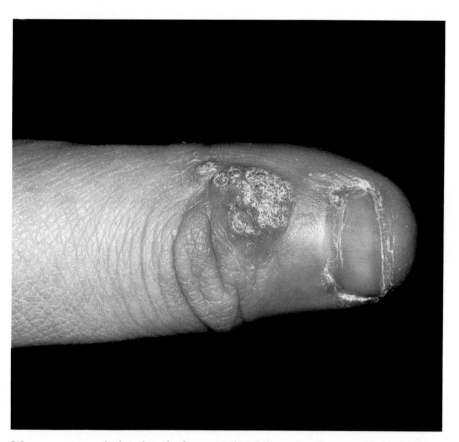

Warts are commonly found on the fingers or thumb (as pictured) of school-age children. The human papillomavirus may be spread from child to child in the school setting from casual contact. Warts respond to simple treatment, including over-the-counter products. (Courtesy of Viewing Medicine)

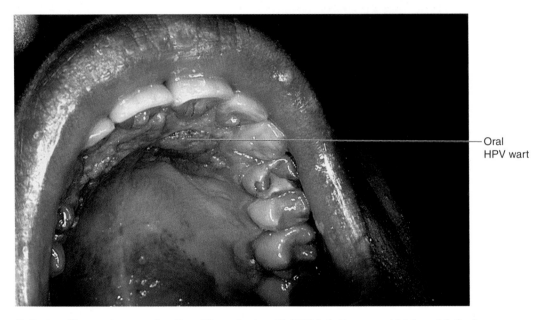

Oral
HPV wart

Patients with poor immune function, like patients with HIV infection, are at higher risk for human papillomavirus infection. Oral warts are rare and are treated by excision, laser, or cryotherapy. (Courtesy of the CDC, Sol Silverman Jr., DDS)

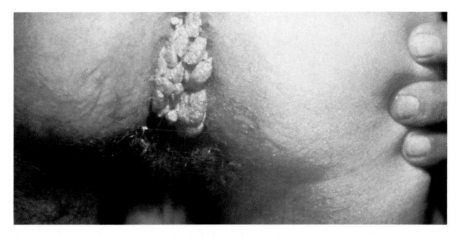

(A) Anal warts. Warts may be spread through sexual contact to the anal area, the penis, and the vagina. Many in infections to sexual organs are painless. The warts may disappear with treatment from the health care provider or on their own, but the virus remains and the person can still infect others. (Courtesy of CDC, Dr. Weisner)

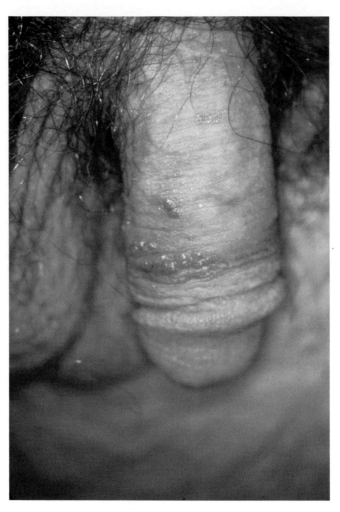

B) Penile warts. There is no known risk of cancers in men associated with the genital warts. (Courtesy of the CDC, Susan Lindsley)

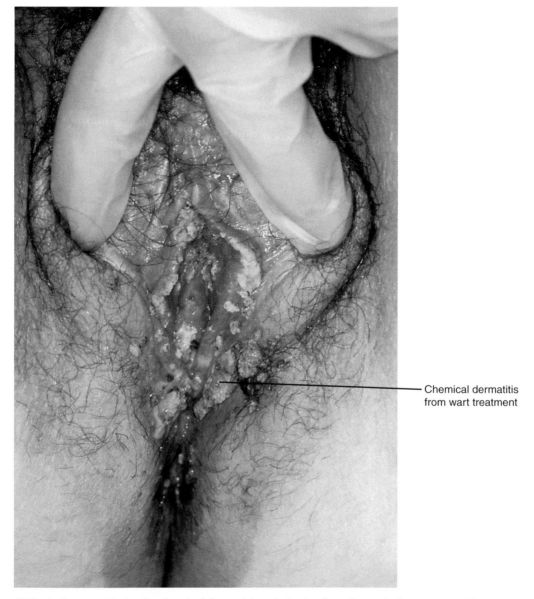

Chemical dermatitis from wart treatment

C) Vaginal warts. Notice the chemical dermatitis or irritation from the topical treatment of the vaginal warts. Many healthcare providers urge female patients to receive the human papillomavirus vaccine before they are sexually active to reduce the risk of cervical cancer in women. (Courtesy of the CDC, Joe Millar)

XANTHOMAS

Xanthomas are soft whitish-yellow painless papules occurring anywhere on the skin, but are most commonly found on the eyelids. Xanthomas are a cutaneous finding indicative of hyperlipidemia or a lipid disturbance.

Assessment

- Soft white or yellow painless lesions
- Hyperlipidemia
- Family history of xanthomas

Planning and Implementation

- Document findings
- Lipid profile
- Initiate low fat and cholesterol diet

Evaluation and Outcomes

The patient will:

- Experience a reduced lipid level
- Verbalize a low fat and cholesterol diet

Nursing Considerations

- Xanthomas are painless and are removed for cosmetic purposes.

- Familial history of xanthomas may indicate familial hyperlipidemia.

- The presence of xanthomas increases the risk for coronary artery disease and pancreatitis because of lipid disturbances.

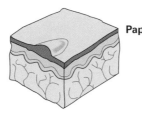

Papule:
Solid, elevated lesion less than 0.5 cm in diameter

Xanthomas are papules created from accumulation of lipid-laden macrophages, and reflect alterations in lipid metabolism.

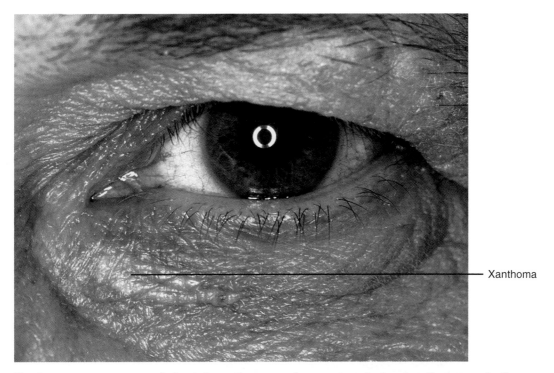

Xanthoma

Xanthomas are most commonly located near the eyes as shown, yet can be found on the face, neck, elbows, buttocks, and near tendons of the feet and hands. Xanthomas are often bilateral and most common in patients over the age of 50. (Courtesy of Viewing Medicine)

PART 2
PROCEDURES AND TREATMENTS

ANGIOGRAM

Angiogram or "catheterization" involves puncturing an artery, advancing a catheter towards the desired vascular area (i.e., heart, cerebral vessels, or distal extremities) and injecting a radiopaque contrast to visualize the arteries.

Assessment

- Pre-angiography
- Allergies (shellfish and iodine allergies must be reported)
- Presence of renal disease (contrast is nephrotoxic)
- Nothing by mouth for 8 hours prior to the procedure
- Assess and document pulses.
- Obtain written consent
- Post-angiography
- Assess puncture site for bleeding or hematoma formation
- Frequent vital signs for shock related to reaction or hemorrhaging
- Frequent assessment and documentation of distal pulses

Planning and Implementation

- Do not bend the punctured limb for 4-6 hours or as prescribed
- Monitor vital signs for signs of shock related to hemorrhage every 15 minutes for an hour and then as ordered
- Monitor neurological status every 15 minutes for an hour and then as ordered and call the physician if changes occur
- Monitor puncture site for evidence of bleeding or hematoma formation every 15 minutes for an hour and then as ordered
- Monitor distal pulses every 15 minutes for an hour and then as ordered
- Monitor urine output for a minimum output of 200 cc per shift or as specified per order

Evaluation and Outcomes

The patient will:

- Understand the angiogram procedure and purpose
- Understand restrictions after the angiogram
- Maintain adequate blood flow to extremities

Nursing Considerations

- If the extremity punctured for the angiogram becomes cold, painful and pulseless, contact the physician immediately. These symptoms may indicate arterial occlusion from a thrombus and an emergency embolectomy would be required to restore arterial flow to the extremity.

- Instruct the patient that for 4 to 6 hours after the procedure they should not change the elevation of the head of the bed without speaking to the nurse. Changing the head of bed will cause leg flexion and undue stress on the puncture site.

- Encourage the patient to drink plenty of liquids after the procedure. The angiogram contrast may be nephrotoxic and increasing liquids will help flush the contrast out of the patient's system.

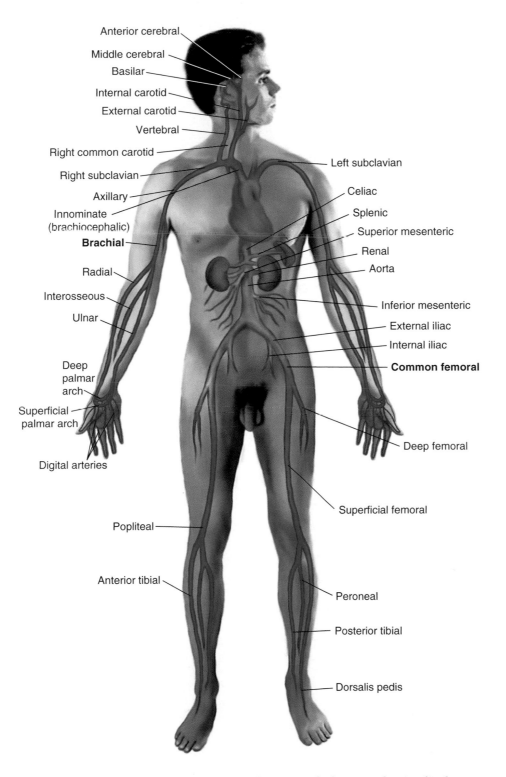

Anterior cerebral
Middle cerebral
Basilar
Internal carotid
External carotid
Vertebral
Right common carotid
Right subclavian
Axillary
Innominate
(brachiocephalic)
Brachial
Radial
Interosseous
Ulnar
Deep
palmar
arch
Superficial
palmar arch
Digital arteries
Popliteal
Anterior tibial

Left subclavian
Celiac
Splenic
Superior mesenteric
Renal
Aorta
Inferior mesenteric
External iliac
Internal iliac
Common femoral
Deep femoral
Superficial femoral
Peroneal
Posterior tibial
Dorsalis pedis

Arterial puncture is required to advance the catheter towards the area to be visualized. The most common site for arterial puncture is the femoral artery, followed by the brachial artery.

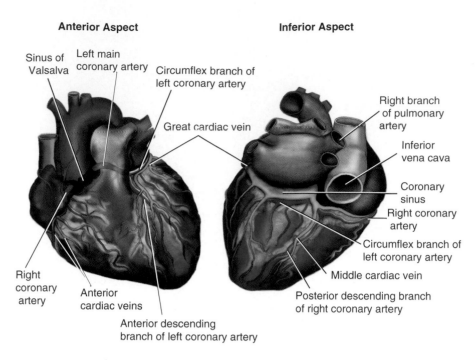

Anterior Aspect

Sinus of Valsalva

Left main coronary artery

Circumflex branch of left coronary artery

Great cardiac vein

Right coronary artery

Anterior cardiac veins

Anterior descending branch of left coronary artery

Inferior Aspect

Right branch of pulmonary artery

Inferior vena cava

Coronary sinus

Right coronary artery

Circumflex branch of left coronary artery

Middle cardiac vein

Posterior descending branch of right coronary artery

Angiogram is performed to visualize the patency and blood flow through arteries. Coronary angiogram is the most common type of angiogram, and visualizes the coronary arteries on the surface of the heart.

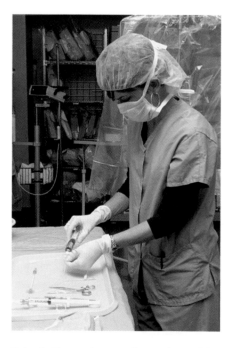

Prior to the angiogram, the equipment is prepared using sterile technique. Angiograms are usually performed in specialized areas called catheter labs or "cath labs."

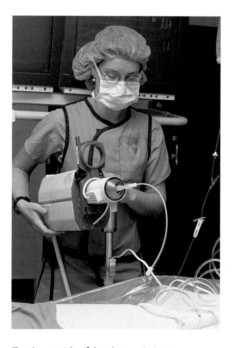

Equipment in this picture injects radiopaque contrast into the patient during the angiogram to enhance visualization of arteries. Contrast may be nephrotoxic and may cause an allergic reaction. If the patient has an iodine or shellfish allergy, the catheterization lab should be notified prior to the procedure.

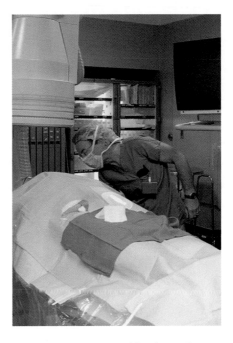

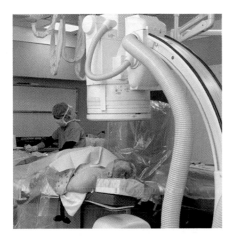

The patient is placed on a fluoroscopy table that allows X-ray images to be taken as the contrast is injected.

The patient receives mild sedation but is awake during the procedure. The health care members explain what they are doing during the procedure and ensure the patient's comfort.

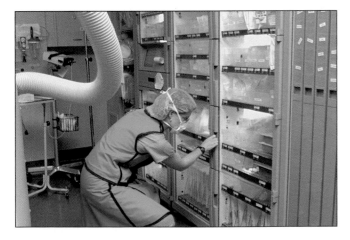

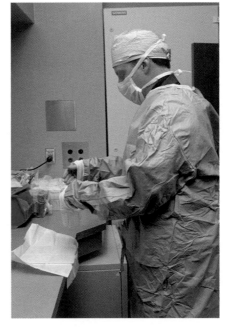

The patient is placed on a heart monitor during the procedure. Blood pressure and respiratory status is closely monitored as well.

Protective equipment is worn to protect the health care workers from body fluids and radiation emitted from the X-rays taken during the procedure.

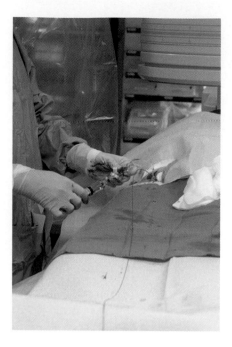

A small arterial puncture is performed and a guide wire is put in and the catheter is placed over the wire.

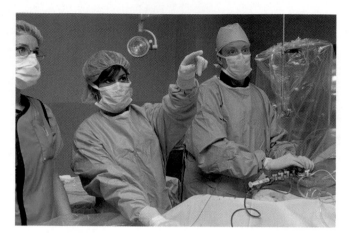

The radiopaque contrast is injected and the team observes the X-rays.

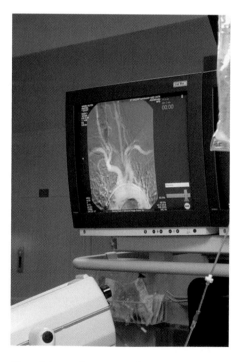

The pictures show up on large screens above the patient. Notice how the contrast enhances visualization of the arteries and blood flow.

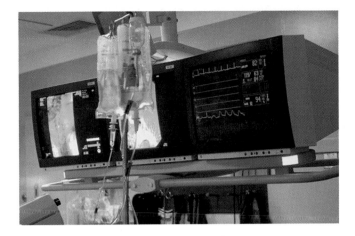

The patient received intravenous fluids during the procedure. Notice how the patient's heart rate and vital signs are displayed on a screen next to the X-rays so the patient can be closely monitored during the procedure.

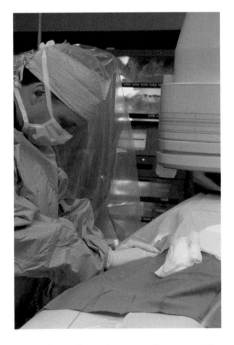

Once the catheter is removed, pressure is applied to the puncture site. Observing for hematoma formation, hemorrhage and for the presence of distal pulses are key nursing assessments post-procedure. To prevent bleeding, the patient will be instructed to not bend their leg or raise the head of bed.

BLADDER SCANNING

Bladder scanning is a procedure using ultrasonography to assess the amount of urine in the bladder. The non-invasive scan is performed at the bedside, and is painless and an accurate indicator of urinary retention. Once urinary retention is diagnosed, a urinary catheter insertion may be ordered to relieve symptoms and prevent urinary infection from residual urine in the bladder.

Assessment

- Medications that cause urinary retention (antihistamines, anticholinergics)
- Feeling of fullness in the lower abdomen
- Palpation of the bladder near the umbilicus
- Frequent urination
- History of benign prostatic hyperplasia
- History of spinal cord injury

Planning and Implementation

- Acute intake and output measurements
- Bladder scanning after urinating to determine the amount of post-void residual urine
- Retaining greater than 100 cc in adults and greater than 200 cc in the elderly is considered urinary retention
- Notify the physician if urinary retention is present

Evaluation and Outcomes

The patient will:

- Understand the bladder scanning purpose and technique
- Experience relief of symptoms of urinary retention

Nursing Considerations

- Inaccurate readings may occur in bladder scanning if the patient is extremely obese or has extensive surgical scarring.

- A consent is not required because the scan is noninvasive and does not have negative side effects.

- Ask the patient to attempt to void prior to scanning to obtain an accurate residual measurement.

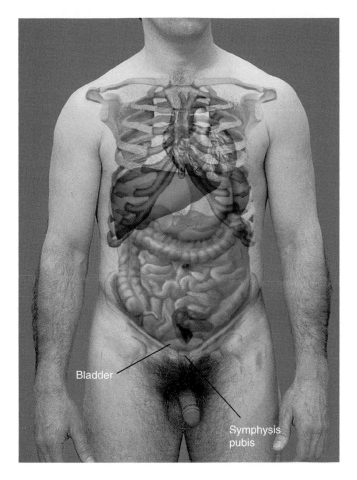

The bladder is located at approximately the symphysis pubis, the bony prominence above the pubic area as noted. As the bladder fills, the bladder may be palpated above the symphysis pubis.

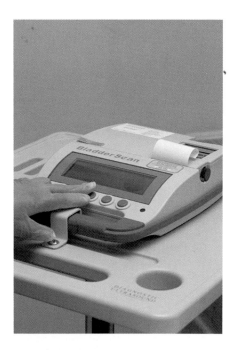

The microprocessor in the bladder scan unit calculates, displays the bladder volume in millimeters, and creates a printable reading. Once the procedure is complete, the ultrasound gel is removed from the patient, and the nurse uses the information to collaborate with the physician on further treatment.

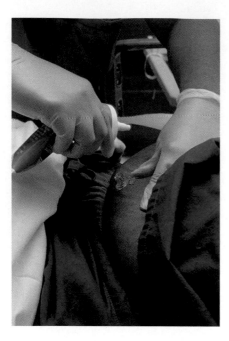

After explaining the procedure to the patient, the nurse locates the symphysis pubis and applies ultrasound gel to the area. An adequate amount of ultrasound gel is necessary for accurate readings.

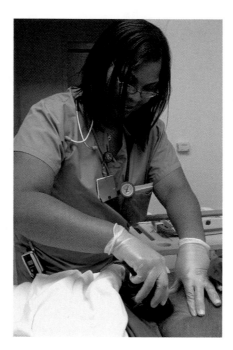

The nurse places the handheld ultrasound over the bladder. The ultrasound uses V-mode ultrasound technology to create a three-dimensional image of the bladder.

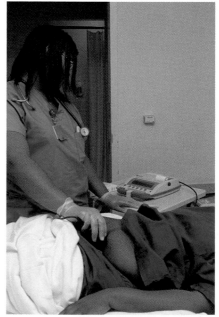

The nurse views the bladder scan screen to make certain the image is correct for certain volume measurements.

BRONCHOSCOPY

Bronchoscopy is the procedure in which a physician inserts a flexible tube through the patient's mouth, past the trachea and into the bronchus. The procedure allows direct visualization of lung tissue, allows biopsy of tissue, removal of obstruction and control of bleeding, if present. This procedure is performed using conscious sedation, and aids in the diagnosis and treatment of many pulmonary illnesses and diseases.

Assessment

- Nothing by mouth approximately 6 hours prior to the procedure
- History of any prior anesthesia reactions
- Bleeding history or anticoagulant use
- Empty bladder
- Removal of jewelry and dentures
- Obtain a written consent

Planning and Implementation

- Monitor pulse oximetry and respiratory status
- Monitor vital signs frequently
- Monitor sedation level

Evaluation and Outcomes

The patient will:

- Understand the bronchoscopy procedure
- Avoid respiratory complications from the procedure
- Experience the return of consciousness postprocedure
- Experience the return of gag and cough reflex postprocedure

Nursing Considerations

- If patient experiences large amounts of hemoptysis and severe shortness of breath after the procedure, administer oxygen and notify the physician immediately.

- Obtain a chest radiograph after the procedure to ensure no accidental lung damage occurred during the procedure.

- Do not allow the patient to eat or drink until the gag reflex has returned and the sedation effects have subsided.

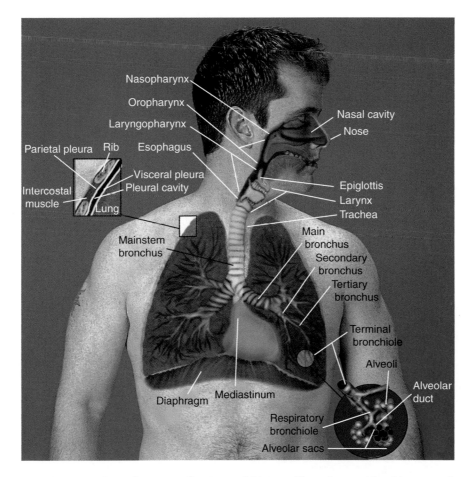

Nasopharynx

Oropharynx

Laryngopharynx

Nasal cavity

Nose

Parietal pleura   Rib   Esophagus

Visceral pleura

Pleural cavity

Intercostal
muscle

Lung

Epiglottis

Larynx

Trachea

Mainstem
bronchus

Main
bronchus

Secondary
bronchus

Tertiary
bronchus

Terminal
bronchiole

Alveoli

Alveolar
duct

Diaphragm   Mediastinum

Respiratory
bronchiole

Alveolar sacs

Bronchoscopy allows direct visualization and biopsy of lung tissue with tubing passed through the mouth through the trachea into the bronchi.

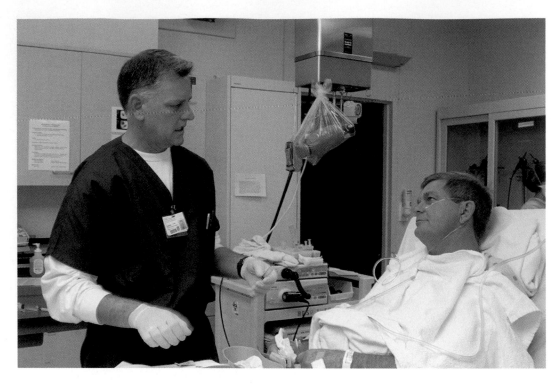

(A) Once the patient is in the procedure room, questions are answered, consent and preparation are verified before beginning the bronchoscopy.

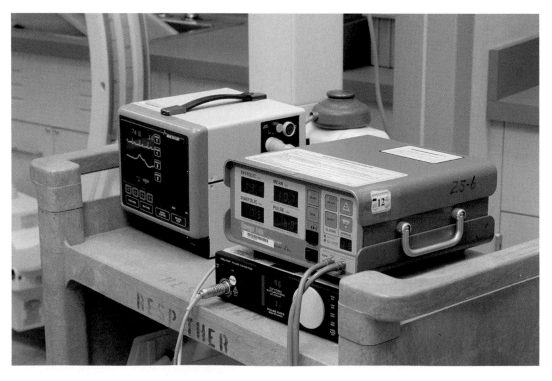

(B) Vital sign and pulse oximetry equipment is used to closely monitor the patient before, during, and after the procedure.

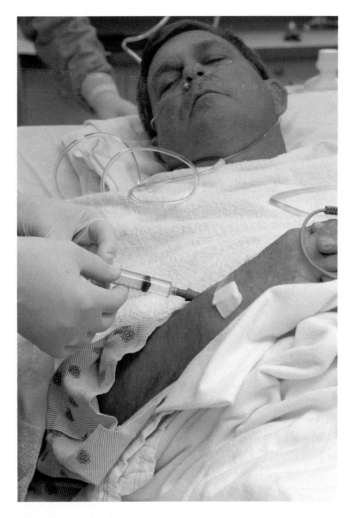

The patient receives conscious sedation during the procedure. Administration of conscious sedation is achieved with the use of intravenous sedation and relaxation agents. Close monitoring of sedation level allows the patient to maintain spontaneous respirations and comfort during the procedure.

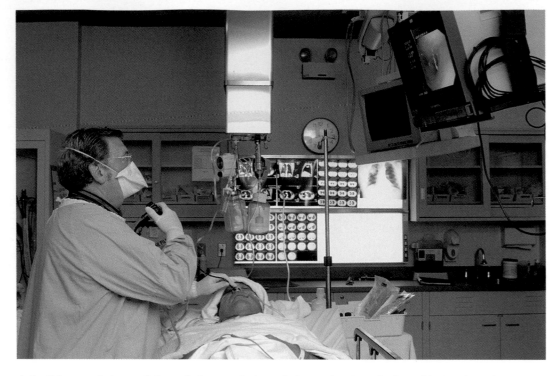

A flexible scope is inserted through the mouth through the trachea into the bronchi. Note how the screen in the upper right corner allows magnified, direct visualization of tissue, and it is watched as the tube is passed to the desired area.

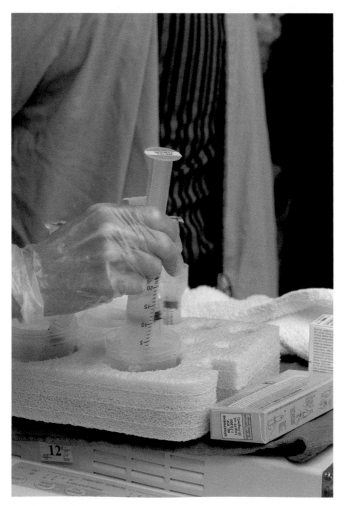

Bronchoscopy allows the tissue biopsy and sputum collection. Utilizing sterile technique, the samples are prepared, labeled, and sent to the laboratory for examination.

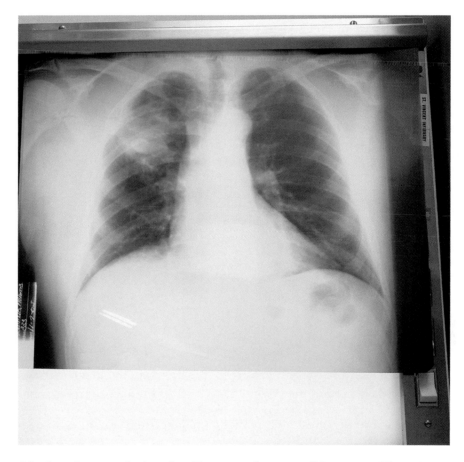

After bronchoscopy, obtain a chest X-ray to evaluate overall lung status. The patient is closely monitored until fully awake and the return of gag and cough reflexes.

CARDIAC SURGERY *

Cardiac surgery is a term covering any type of surgery of the heart. Common cardiac surgery procedures include coronary bypass, valve repair, valve replacement, and correction of cardiac structural defects. Patients undergoing cardiac surgery will experience general anesthesia and require postoperative care in an intensive care setting.

Assessment

- Preexisting conditions that may affect recovery (renal disease, diabetes mellitus, previous cardiac surgeries)
- Previous reaction or a family history of reaction to anesthesia
- Obtain written surgical and blood consents

Planning and Implementation

- Monitor respiratory and cardiac status
- Monitor wound for presence of infection
- Monitor and prevent common complications such as wound or pulmonary infection, cardiac arrythmias, or decreased cardiac output
- Monitor and treat pain

Evaluation and Outcomes

The patient will:

- Experience normal cardiac function
- Be free of complications
- Experience adequate pain control

Nursing Considerations

- Early discharge after cardiac surgery may lead to patients in the home setting unsure of medication and therapy regimes. Make certain the patient has a contact number for questions.

- Teach patients to splint the chest incision with a pillow when coughing, to decrease pain.

- If life-threatening cardiac arrhythmias such as ventricular tachycardia occur, treat immediately per protocol to prevent patient demise.

* Some of these images are from 3 different postoperative cardiac patients.

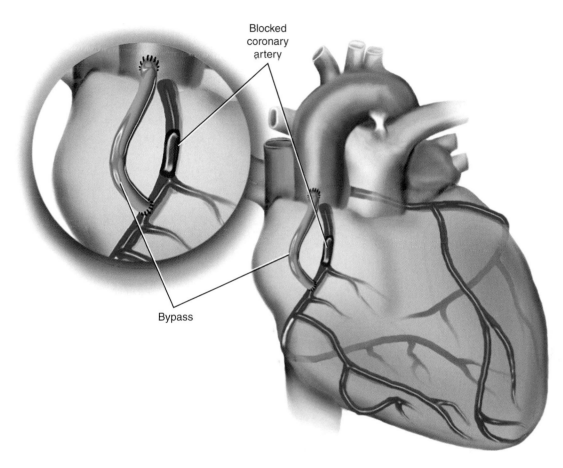

Blocked
coronary
artery

Bypass

Coronary bypass, the most common cardiac surgical procedure, is performed to bypass blockages in the coronary arteries. Note how the bypass begins from the aortic arch and connects to the vessel after the area of blockage.

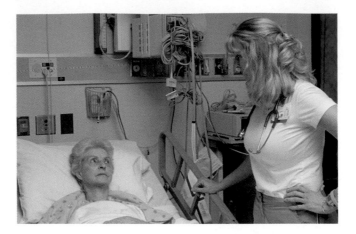

Preoperatively obtain consents, apply identification, allergy and blood bank bracelets. This patient is receiving teaching in the preoperative phase to prepare her for postoperative cardiac surgical care.

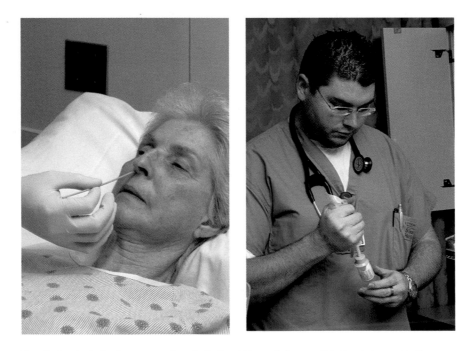

Prophylactic infection prevention includes (A) applying antibiotic ointment to the nares, and (B) administering intravenous antibiotics.

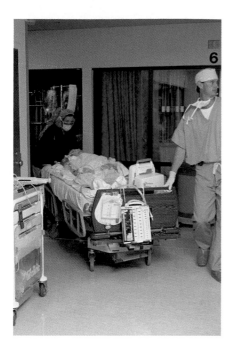

Upon completion of the surgery, anesthesiologist and surgeon transport the patient directly to the intensive care setting. The anesthesiologist oversees the patient via a transport monitor on the bed. Note the chest tube collection container and urinary catheter. Urine output should be at least 30 cc per hour and the chest output should not exceed 100cc per hour. If either output deviates, notify the cardiac surgeon.

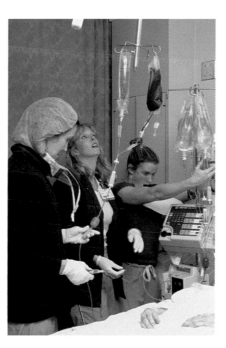

The anesthesiologist reports the patient's surgical course and status to the nurse. Multiple nurses admit the patient. Activities include applying a heart monitor, connecting the endotracheal tube to a ventilator, drawing blood for laboratory data, confirming intravenous medications, applying suction to the chest tube container, and leveling and zeroing hemodynamic lines.

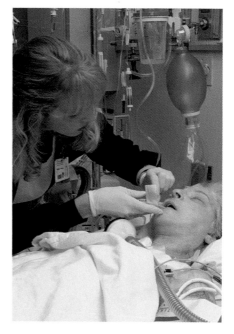

Initial and frequent patient assessments include monitoring the patient's airway, respiratory and cardiovascular status, chest tube and urinary output, pulse strength and level of consciousness. Note the effects of general anesthesia: the patient is unable to ventilate spontaneously and appears sedated. The patient will gradually become alert and able to breath spontaneously.

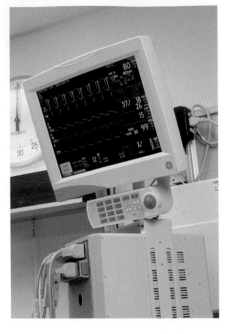

Hemodynamic monitoring includes heart rate and rhythm, arterial blood pressure, pulmonary artery pressure, central venous pressure, and pulse oximetry, as displayed from top to bottom. The patient has invasive lines to obtain these measures, including arterial and Swan-Ganz catheters. Hemodynamic monitoring reflects the patient's status and assists the nurse in guiding patient care. Patients often require multiple intravenous medications to support the hemodynamic status in the postoperative phase.

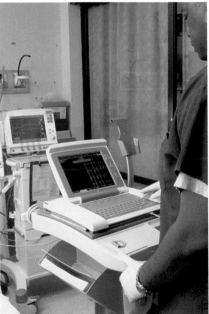

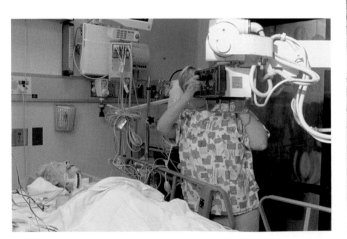

(A) Portable chest X-ray verifies endotracheal tube, chest tube, and central line placement. Additionally, lung status and cardiac silhouette are assessed. (B) 12-lead EKG confirms heart rate and rhythm, and identifies cardiac injury and ischemia.

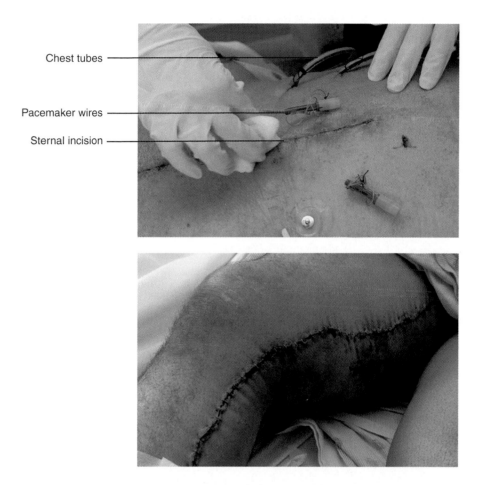

Chest tubes

Pacemaker wires

Sternal incision

Assess chest and leg incisions for infection, wound healing, and intactness. Provide wound care and dressings as ordered. In this postoperative patient the mediastinal incision is clean, intact, and well-approximated (A). Pacemaker wires allow emergent temporary pacing for life-threatening rhythms. Chest tubes allow excess blood to drain. Excessive blood drainage from chest tubes indicates hemorrhage and treatment is needed immediately. (B) Saphenous leg veins provide grafting material for patients receiving coronary bypass. Grafts may also be obtained from the radial artery and internal mammary artery.

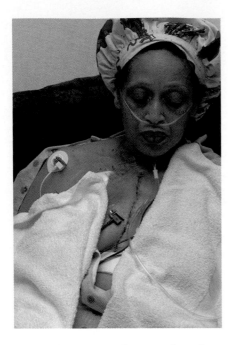

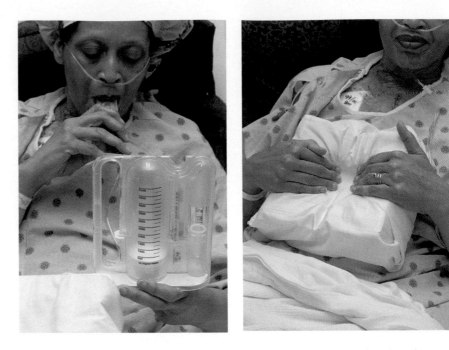

Appropriate personnel remove the endo-tracheal tube when the patient is alert with stable hemodynamic and respiratory status as per policy. This patient has oxygen per nasal cannula and requires continued respiratory status monitoring.

To prevent pulmonary complications such as pneumonia, encourage deep breathing and coughing. Incentive spirometer devices measure inspiratory volume and allow patients to visualize their progress. Splinting the sternal incision with a pillow lessens the pain caused by coughing. Maximize pulmonary efforts from the patient by maintaining adequate pain control.

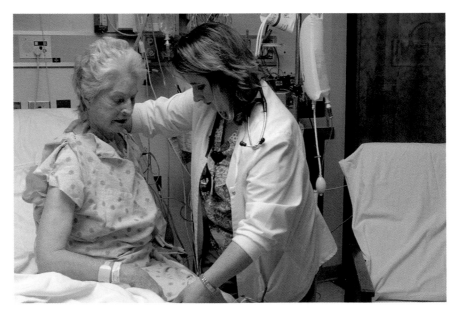

Assisting with early ambulation prevents complications associated with immobility (i.e., pneumonia, deep vein thrombosis). Protect all invasive lines and tubes when transferring to a chair. Cardiac rehabilitation starts during the hospital setting and continues after discharge. In addition to monitoring the patient during exercise, cardiac rehabilitation provides teaching and support concerning diet, exercise, medication, and home care considerations.

COMPUTERIZED TOMOGRAPHY (CT) SCAN

A CAT scan is a type of X-ray using computers to create a three-dimensional image from flat (i.e., two-dimensional) X-ray pictures. It may be performed with or without contrast. The scan generates pictures in "slices" from where the beginning of the area scanned to the end of the area scanned. This process allows health care providers to view anatomy in great detail.

Assessment

- Understanding of the procedure
- Remove jewelry or any metal objects that may interfere with x-ray results.

Planning and Implementation

- Instruct the patient on movement limitations
- Promote a comfortable environment

Evaluation and Outcomes

The patient will:

- Understand what a CAT scan is and its use in diagnosing.
- Avoid discomfort during the procedure.

Nursing Considerations

- Prior to the scan, female patients should be asked about the possibility of pregnancy. Do not perform CAT scans on pregnant women.

- Explain the intercom system in the CAT scan procedure room, so the patient is aware they can communicate during the procedure, if necessary.

- Do not infuse contrast in a patient with a history of contrast allergy.

- Infuse contrast via peripherally-inserted intravenous catheters.

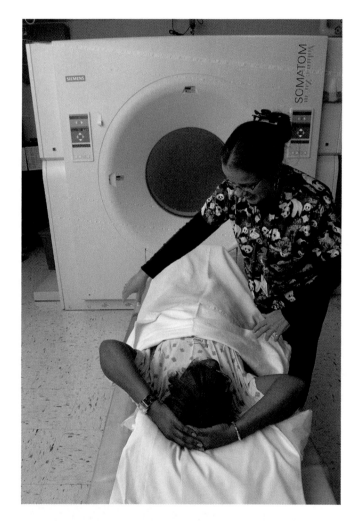

Once this patient is brought into the CAT scan room, the procedure is explained to the patient. At this time, verify the patient is not pregnant and all jewelry has been removed. As in the picture, if jewelry is still on, remove and place in a safe place labeled with patient information.

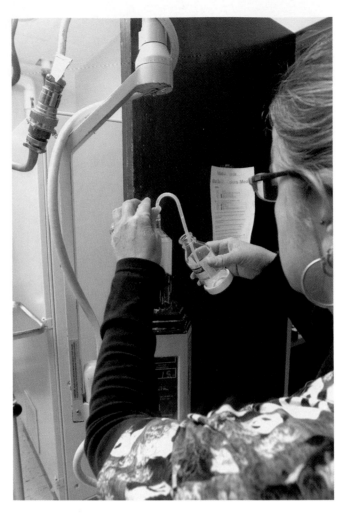

CAT scans may be performed with or without contrast. As pictured, contrast is readied for intravenous injection prior to the beginning of the exam.

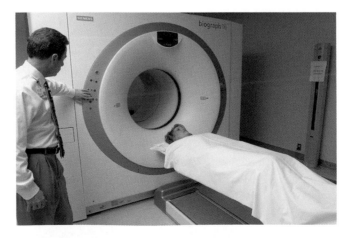

Once this patient is secure on the exam table and her comfort attended to, the exam is begun. Remind the patient to lie completely still until the exam is complete.

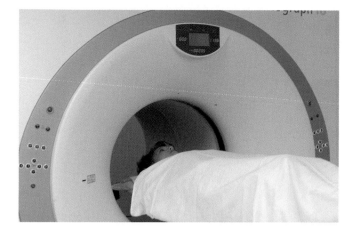

During the exam, the portion of the body to be examined is in the CAT scan machine. Claustrophobic patients may require sedation prior to the exam. Forewarn patients that loud knocking noises occur as the exam proceeds.

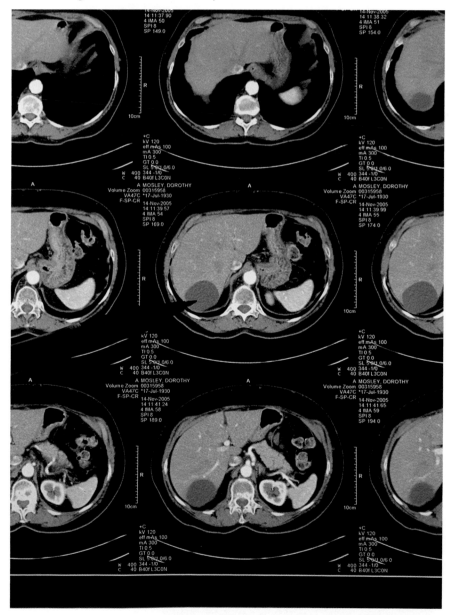

CAT scan results allow three-dimensional viewing of the examined area broken down into "slices" for viewing anatomy in impressive detail.

COLONOSCOPY

Colonoscopy is a procedure where flexible tubing is inserted through the anus allowing visual inspection, biopsy, and polyp removal in the colon, or large intestine. Colonoscopy is performed on an outpatient basis and is performed using conscious sedation. Colonoscopy is a screening tool for colorectal cancer and a diagnostic tool for conditions of the large intestine.

Assessment

- Bowel preparation is complete
- History of any cardiac or pulmonary problems
- History of medication allergy or previous reaction to anesthesia
- Obtain written consent

Planning and Implementation

- Monitor cardiac and respiratory status
- Monitor level of sedation
- Maintain patient safety during procedure

Evaluation and Outcomes

The patient will:

- Understand colonoscopy procedure
- Experience return of consciousness

Nursing Considerations

- Colon cancer is the second leading cause of cancer deaths in the United States, and most colorectal cancers are curable when diagnosed early.

- Monitor the patient's bowel movements priors to colonoscopy. Stool color should be clear and liquid.

- Arrange home transportation for the patient prior to the procedure.

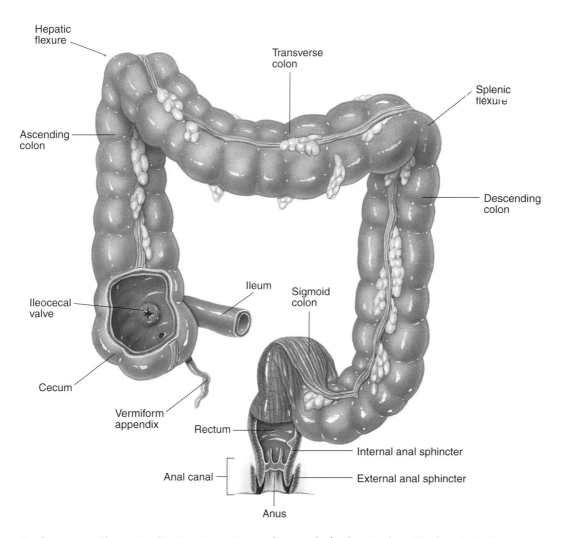

Hepatic flexure

Transverse colon

Splenic flexure

Ascending colon

Descending colon

Ileum

Sigmoid colon

Ileocecal valve

Cecum

Vermiform appendix

Rectum

Internal anal sphincter

Anal canal

External anal sphincter

Anus

A colonoscopy allows visualization, inspection, and removal of polyps in the entire large intestine or colon.

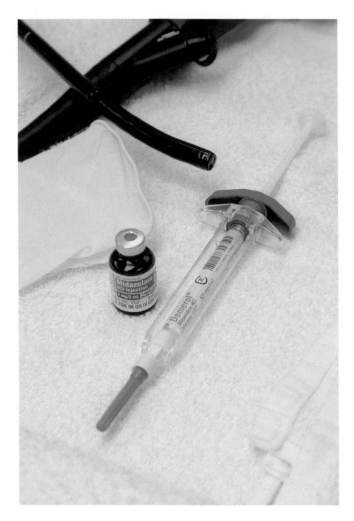

Patient preparation includes intravenous sedation to relax the patient and prevent discomfort while allowing spontaneous respirations. Bowel preparation is essential to clear the intestine of stool to allow adequate visualization during the procedure.

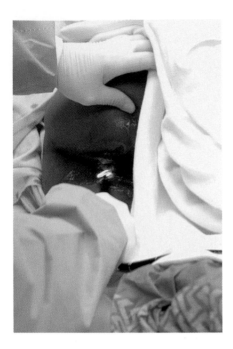

The patient is positioned on the side to allow access. Once sedated, lubrication is applied and the flexible tubing is inserted through the rectum.

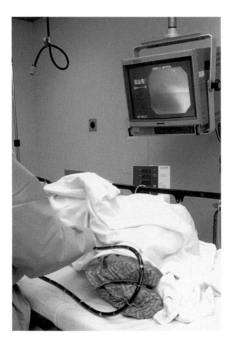

As the tube advances through the colon, simultaneous visualization occurs on the monitor. Notice below the monitor vital signs are displayed to observe the patient's status during the procedure.

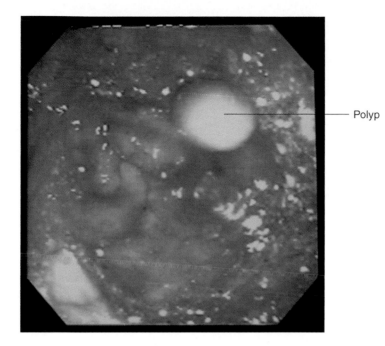

Polyp

Polyps are found, removed, and sent for biopsy during the colonoscopy procedure. Polyps are usually non-cancerous, but if left in the colon, may become cancerous over time.

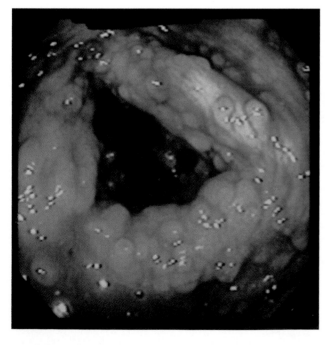

Colonoscopy may aid in the diagnosis of many conditions affecting the colon, including infection of polyps as pictured. Direct visualization aids in the prompt diagnoses and treatment.

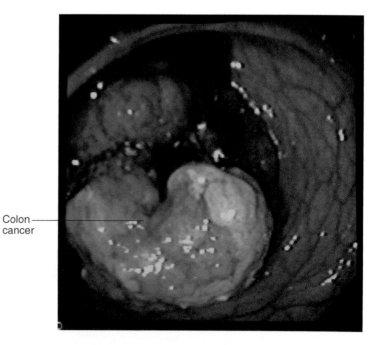

Colon cancer

Colon cancer is detected from colonoscopy. Colonoscopy is recommended every ten years after the age of fifty, to aid in the detection of colon cancer.

DIALYSIS

Hemodialysis is the process of removing fluid and waste from a patient that is experiencing reduced renal function. Blood is removed and returned to the patient and the wastes are drawn out through a semi-permeable membrane using the principle of diffusion. Dialysis may be performed on a temporary or long-term basis.

Assessment

- Signs of fluid overload (hypertension, shortness of breath, edema, weight gain)
- Creatinine levels
- Venous access device (arterial venous shunt)

Planning and Implementation

Vital signs

- Monitor access site for bleeding
- Monitor neurological status (dialysis disequilibrium)
- Monitor creatinine and electrolyte levels
- Monitor amount of fluid removed

Evaluation and Outcomes

The patient will:

- Experience normal vital signs
- Experience loss of fluid and waste
- Understand dialysis therapy

SpecialNursing Considerations

- Outpatient hemodialysis is usually performed three days a week, and is three to four hours in duration for each treatment. Discuss with the patient the considerable changes to lifestyle that take place when one requires life-long dialysis.

- Palpate the arterial venous shunt for a thrill and auscultate a bruit; both are caused by the turbulent blood flow with the mixing of venous and arterial blood. Document these findings every shift. A thrill and a bruit indicate the shunt is working correctly. If a bruit or thrill is not assessed, notify the physician immediately because this indicates the shunt is not working correctly.

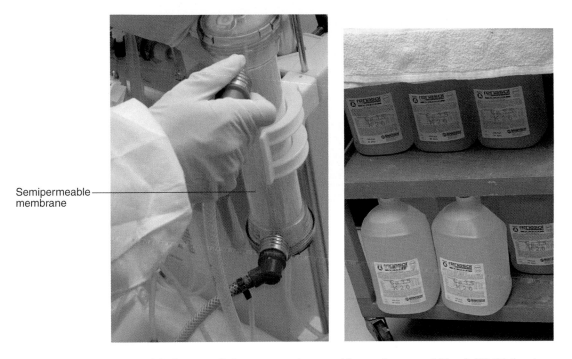

Semipermeable membrane

Three major components of dialysis are dialysate, a semi-permeable membrane, and blood. (A) Dialysate runs through a semi-permeable membrane using the principle of diffusion to draw out fluid and waste as the patient's blood flows inside the membrane. (B) Dialysate composition is patient-dependent, ordered by the physician, and it should be kept at room temperature.

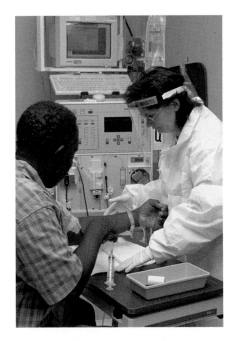

An arterial venous shunt is the surgical anastamosis of a vein and an artery; it is most commonly performed in the wrist area but may be created in the upper arm or thigh. When accessing a patient's arterial venous shunt, the nurse dons personal protective devices, including eye shield. Sterile procedure is followed to prevent blood contamination and subsequent infection.

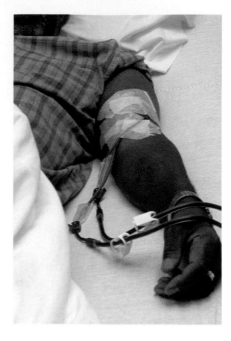

Venipuncture is performed in two sites and secured. The red marked tubing is considered arterial flow into the dialysis machine. The blue tubing is considered venous flow, and returns the blood from the machine into the patient.

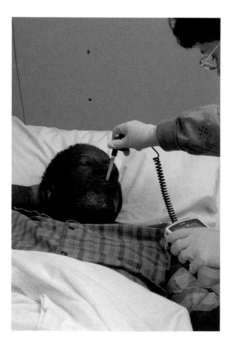

Vital signs and neurological status are closely monitored during and after dialysis. Fluid and waste loss may cause hypotension and changes in level of consciousness. If hypotension occurs, additional intravenous fluids may be ordered. If there is a change in the level of consciousness, provide a safe environment and notify the physician for further orders.

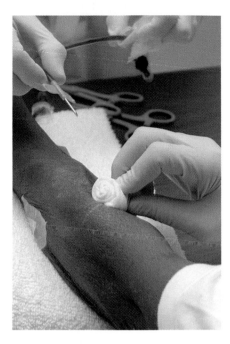

Once adequate fluid and waste are removed, the needles are removed and pressure is applied. The site is closely monitored for evidence of hemorrhage or hematoma formation. If either occurs, don protective equipment and hold pressure directly over the site

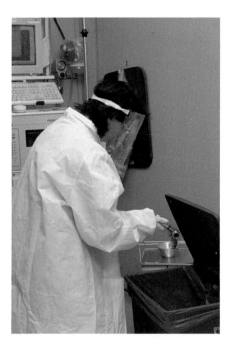

All equipment from dialysis is placed in a biohazard waste receptacle. Notice the personal protective equipment is not removed until proper disposal of all waste.

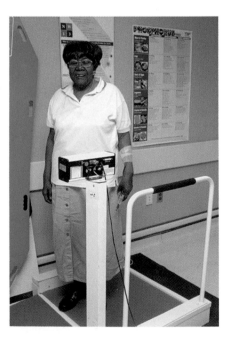

Record daily weights on all dialysis patients to monitor fluid balance. Obtain a "dry weight" or postdialysis weight to monitor fluid loss and to determine the patient's actual weight without excess fluid. Record the dry weight in the patient's record. This weight is used for medication calculations.

ESOPHAGOGASTRODUODENOSCOPY (EGD)

Esophagogastroduodenoscopy (EGD) is a procedure that allows the physician to directly visualize and biopsy the lining of the esophagus, stomach, and upper duodenum. A flexible scope with a camera and a light is inserted through the mouth. Patients undergoing EGD will require conscious sedation. EGD is an outpatient procedure that may aid in determining the cause of many gastrointestinal ailments.

Assessment

- Anticoagulation medications or a history of bleeding problems
- Nothing by mouth 6–8 hours prior to the procedure
- Remove dentures prior to the procedure
- Obtain written consent

Planning and Implementation

- Monitor vital signs
- Monitor respiratory status
- Monitor level of sedation

Evaluation and Outcomes

The patient will:

- Regain consciousness and gag and cough reflexes
- Maintain comfort during and after the procedure
- Understand the purpose and procedure for EGD

Nursing Considerations

- Nothing by mouth until the gag reflex has returned.

- If dentures are removed prior to the procedure, carefully label and store them.

- Arrangements for a driver to take the patient home after the procedure should be made prior to the procedure.

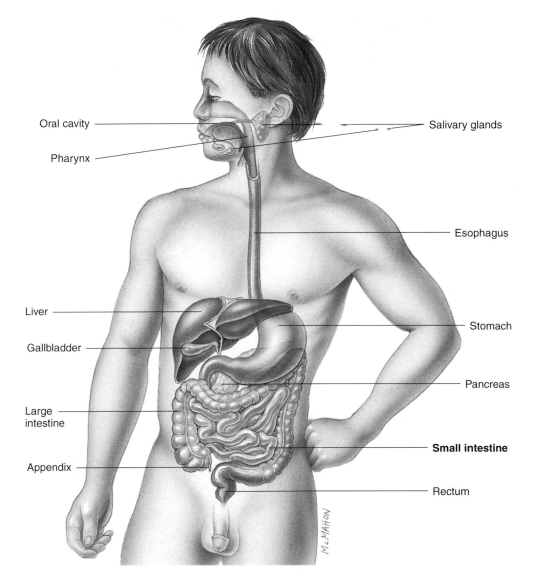

Oral cavity

Pharynx

Salivary glands

Esophagus

Liver

Gallbladder

Large intestine

Appendix

Stomach

Pancreas

Small intestine

Rectum

EGD (Esophagogastroduodenoscopy) allows direct visualization of the esophagus, stomach, and the duodenum portion of the small intestine. Biopsies may be taken during the procedure.

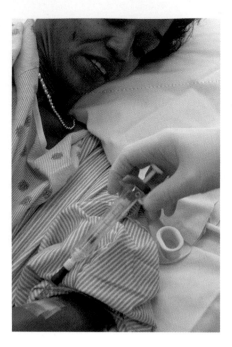

Patients receive intravenous conscious sedation during the EGD. The patient's level of sedation, vital signs, and oxygenation status are monitored throughout the procedure.

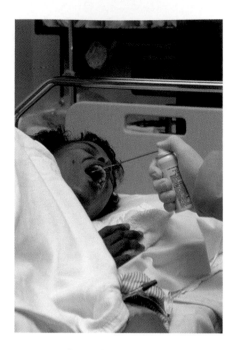

Spraying the oral cavity with a numbing medicine containing benzocaine lessens the gag reflex. Patients with known benzocaine sensitivity should not receive the spray. Depending on the severity of the allergy, another numbing medication may be given to lessen the gag reflex.

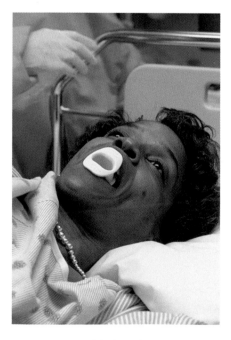

Inserting a bite block in the patient's mouth prevents accidental biting of the scope. The bite block remains in the mouth until the procedure is complete.

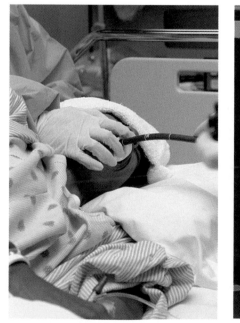

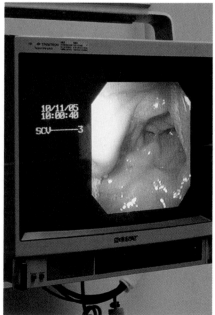

As the scope advances, a screen allows simultaneous viewing of the gastrointestinal lining. When viewing abnormalities, pictures are taken to document findings and biopsies may be performed. After the procedure, monitor the patient for wakening and the return of the gag reflex.

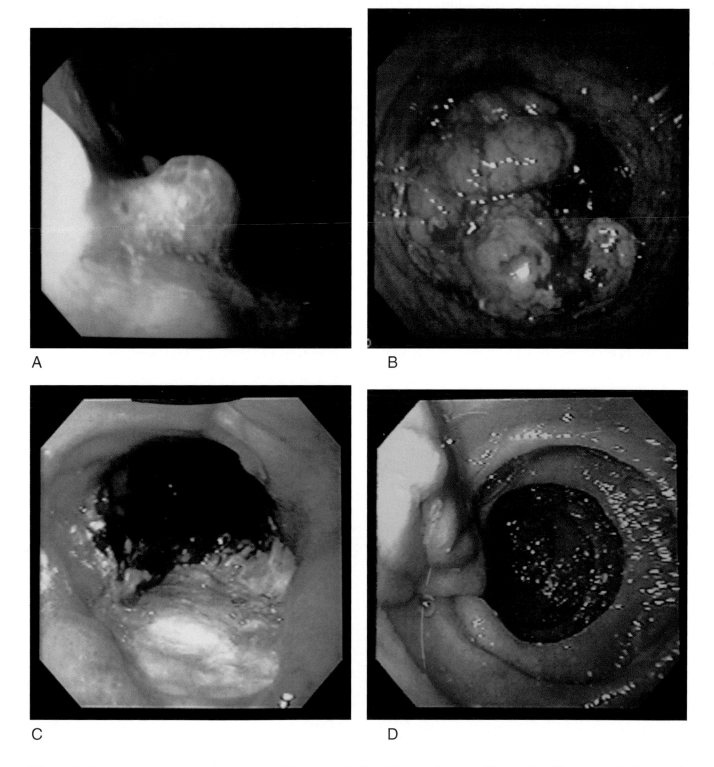

Diagnosis of many gastrointestinal conditions and diseases, including (A) stomach cancer, (B) gastritis, (C) esophageal ulcer, and (D) esophageal varices as shown in the pictures, occurs during the EGD procedure.

ENDOTRACHEAL INTUBATION

Endotracheal intubation is the insertion of an artificial airway into the trachea. Endotracheal intubation is required when a patient has general anesthesia and a variety of conditions that impair normal respirations and oxygenation (e.g., carbon monoxide poisoning, pneumonia, head injury).

Assessment

- Respirations, rate, and character
- Pulse oximetry
- Arterial blood gases
- Breath sounds

Planning and Implementation

- Insert large bore peripheral IV to administer sedation medications
- Monitor respiratory status including breath sounds, respirations, pulse oximetry, and arterial blood gases
- Maintain elevation of the head of bed
- Provide an alternate means of communication

Evaluation and Outcomes

The patient will:

- Be successfully intubated as evidenced by equal breath sounds, increase in oxygenation, presence of carbon dioxide with exhalation, and confirmation of endotracheal tube placement on X-ray.

Nursing Considerations

- Have emergency equipment available to support the patient's airway in case the endotracheal tube becomes dislodged.

- If the pulse oximetry reading does not increase with intubation, consider removing the endotracheal tube and reinserting, as this may indicate improper tube placement.

- Keep suction equipment available to remove oral secretions.

- Soft wrist restraints may need to be ordered and applied to protect the endotracheal tube.

- If the patient is sedated, correct body positioning should be maintained to prevent injury and skin breakdown.

- The endotracheal tube should be secured with a commercially available endotracheal tube holder.

- The level of the tube at the lip in centimeters should be documented to help confirm tube placement.

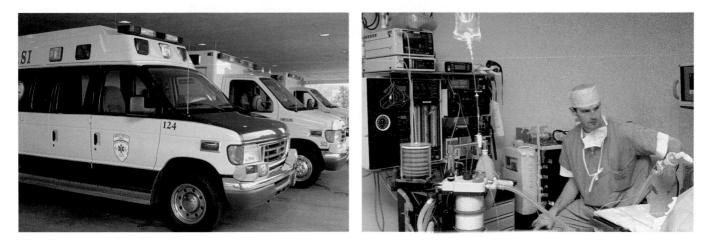

Patients require endotracheal intubation in a variety of settings, ranging from emergently outside of the hospital to the operating room for patients requiring general anesthesia. Regardless of setting, patients require endotracheal intubation when they are unable to spontaneously breathe (e.g., cervical spinal injuries, general anesthesia) or are unable to adequately oxygenate (e.g., severe pneumonia, smoke inhalation).

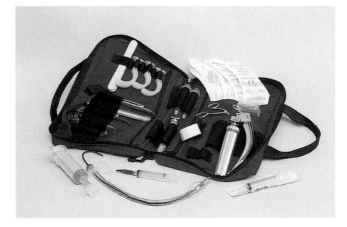

Equipment necessary to intubate includes a laryngeal scope and endotracheal tubes, and is found on most units in the hospital environment. Nurse anesthetists, respiratory therapists, paramedics, and anesthesiologists may perform endotracheal intubation, depending on the setting.

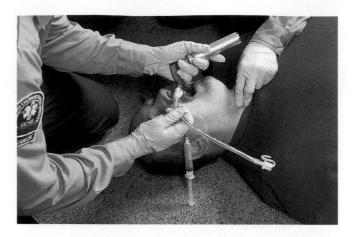

Rescue breathing, removing the headboard, moving the bed out, placing a roll behind the patient's shoulders to extend the neck, maintaining a patent intravenous line, monitoring vital signs and pulse oximetry, and ensuring there is supplemental oxygen and suction are functions of the nurse immediately prior and during the emergent endotracheal intubation process. Notice the person on the left intubating this patient; the person on the right is applying cricoid pressure to help visualize the vocal cords, a landmark used when intubating.

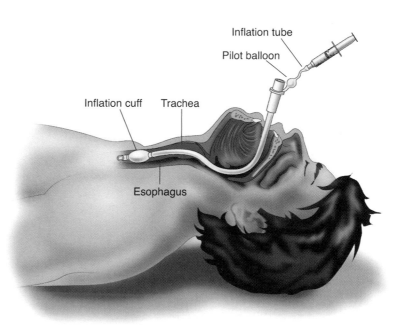

Proper endotracheal tube placement includes the tube being past the trachea above the carina. The tube has a cuff that is inflated to help prevent aspiration of oral contents into the lungs, a common cause of pneumonia. Notice the esophagus is posterior of the trachea, and the tube may be accidentally placed in the esophagus.

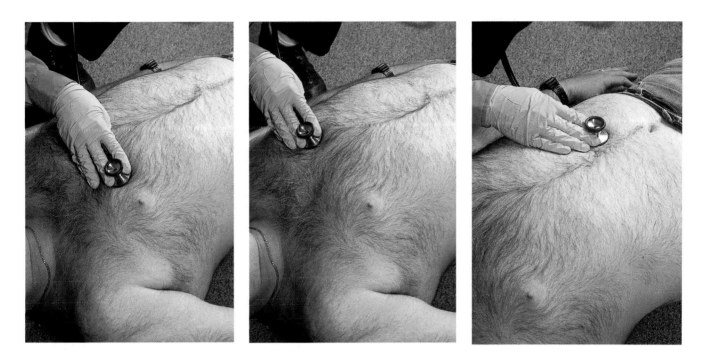

Verifying endotracheal tube placement is critical in this patient and all patients receiving an endotracheal tube. Auscultating bilateral breath sounds, observing equal chest movement, measuring for the presence of carbon dioxide with an end tidal CO_2 device, and improvement of patient's oxygenation status assist in verifying placement. Chest X-ray confirms placement. Air sounds over the epigastric area, lack of breath sounds, carbon dioxide and further patient deterioration indicate esophageal intubation. The tube should be removed immediately and rescue breathing resumed.

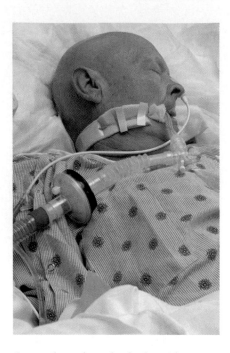

Secure the endotracheal tube with tape or commercially available devices to prevent dislodgement. Notice the nasogastric tube. Endotracheally intubated patients need a nasogastric tube for enteral feeding and oral medication administration, and require an alternate method of communication. The patient shown is in an intensive care setting and is sedated.

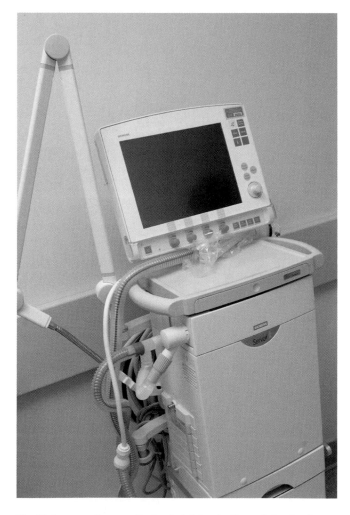

Ventilators, as shown, attach via tubing to the endotracheal tube. Ventilators have a variety of settings determined by the patient's ventilation and oxygenation needs. Alarms on ventilators require immediate attention when sounding.

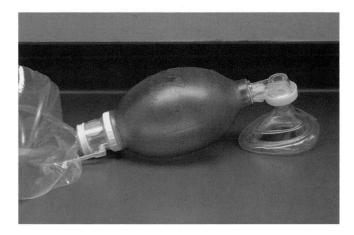

Intubated patients require that a bag valve mask resuscitator be in close proximity. Accidental dislodgement will require placing the mask portion over the patient's nose and mouth for rescue breathing. When the mask portion is removed from the resuscitator, the opening fits on the end of the endotracheal tube to perform rescue breathing for ventilator failure or when the patient requires transportation.

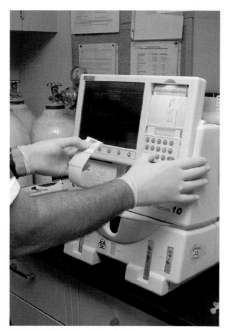

Arterial blood gas analyzer

Caring for endotracheally intubated patients requires monitoring of arterial blood gases, vital signs, chest X-ray results, and overall pulmonary status. Handwashing by all those in contact with the patient, frequent oral care, maintaining elevation of the head of bed, and suctioning using sterile technique reduce the chance of complication of ventilator-induced pneumonia.

HEMODYNAMIC MONITORING

Hemodynamic monitoring refers to measures that reflect many facets of the circulation of a patient's blood, and may be invasive or noninvasive consisting or one or more measures. The purpose of hemodynamic monitoring is early detection and prevention of life-threatening conditions, including cardiac failure, arrhythmias, shock, and hypoxia.

Assessment

- Blood pressure
- Arterial blood pressure
- Heart rhythm and rate
- Cardiac output
- Central venous pressure
- Pulmonary artery pressure
- Intracranial pressure
- Body temperature
- Pulse oximetry

Planning and Implementation

- Calibrate and monitor equipment
- Set alarm parameters
- Care of invasive lines per hospital protocol
- Close monitoring of hemodynamic status and report changes immediately

Evaluation and Outcomes

The patient will:

- Experience a stable hemodynamic status
- Encounter early detection of changes in hemodynamic status and with appropriate actions

Nursing Considerations

- Hemodynamic monitoring occurs with every patient in the hospital and clinic setting. Blood pressure, pulse rate, respirations, and temperature are baseline information required upon admission.

- Invasive hemodynamic monitoring occurs in specialty care areas, such as intensive care units, surgery, and the emergency room, and gives further information about the patient's status. For example, if a patient has cardiac surgery, invasive monitoring devices may include an arterial line (for continuous blood pressure measures and arterial blood gas sampling), a Swan-Ganz catheter (for central venous pressures, pulmonary artery pressures, cardiac output monitoring, and mixed venous blood sampling), continuous cardiac rhythm monitoring, and continuous pulse oximetry.

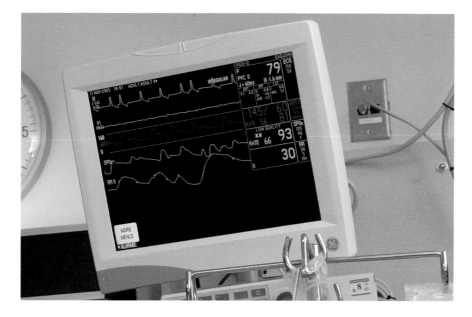

Hemodynamic monitoring provides crucial data reflecting a patient's cardiopulmonary status. Nurses determine and set alarm parameters and base them on the patient's condition. For example, if a patient were receiving medication to increase and minimally maintain a blood pressure of 100mm Hg systolic, the nurse would set the low alarm at 100mm Hg systolic and the high alarm at 130mm Hg systolic. By doing this, the nurse ensures the medication is maintaining the blood pressure and is not raising the blood pressure beyond a desired goal. Invasive lines require calibration and zeroing (eliminating the effects of atmospheric pressure on measured values) to maintain accurate readings. Changes in hemodynamic status are reported for prompt treatment and avoidance of patient demise.

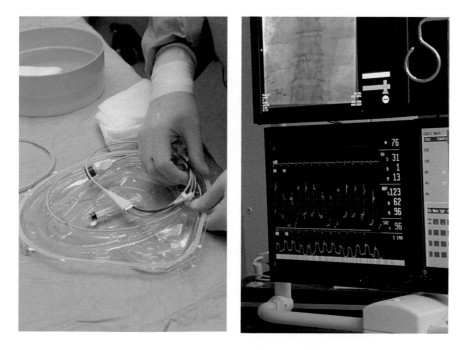

(A) Invasive lines to monitor hemodynamic statuses are inserted using sterile technique. Pulmonary artery catheters, as shown, require monitoring of the waveform and heart rhythm during insertion. The waveform reflects the position of the catheter as it advances through the heart. Additionally, during catheter insertion ventricular arrhythmias may occur due to mechanical irritation from the catheter. (B). Pulmonary artery catheters provide right and left heart pressures, cardiac output, and other cardiac determinants that aid in deciding treatment in critically ill patients. Treatment decisions may include using medications to increase or decrease the heart rate and blood pressure.

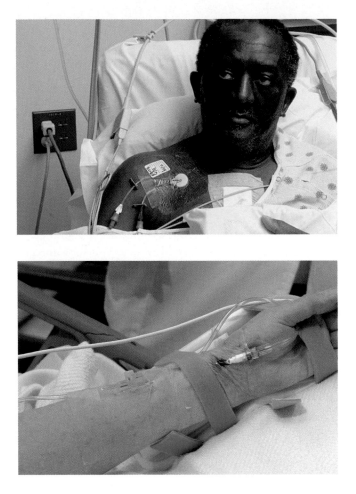

(A) Central venous catheters monitor central venous pressure (reflecting this patient's intravascular volume status), helping determine fluid volume deficit, overload, or euvolemia (adequate or normal intravascular volume status). (B) Another patient's radial arterial catheter provides a continuous blood pressure reading. All invasive catheters receive care according to the Centers for Disease Control guidelines to prevent catheter-related infections. Securing lines prevents accidental dislodging.

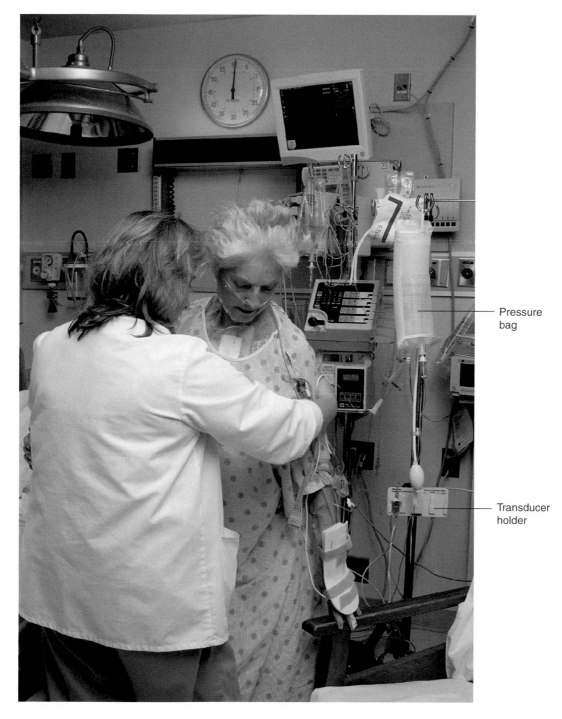

Pressure bag

Transducer holder

Connecting invasive hemodynamic lines to a pressure bag allows the pressure to be sensed and transmitted as a wave that displays on a monitor. Cardiac hemodynamic lines are leveled by maintaining the transducer in a holder level with the right atrium. As the patient's position changes, the transducer is moved to reflect positioning with the right atrium. In this picture, the nurse has placed the transducer holder so it will be level with the right atrium when the patient sits in the chair.

HYPERBARIC CHAMBER

Hyperbaric chamber therapy consists of placing a patient in a chamber where oxygen is administered at greater than normal pressure to the patient in order to treat specific medical indications. Indications include carbon monoxide poisoning, gas gangrene, chronic wound infections, and burns.

Assessment

- Medical condition requiring hyperbaric therapy
- Patient is free of flammable devices
- Loose, comfortable clothing
- History of anxiety or claustrophobia

Planning and Implementation

- Monitor patient during the procedure
- Observe for signs of anxiety

Evaluation and Outcomes

The patient will:

- Experience improvement of the medical condition requiring hyperbaric therapy
- Remain calm and anxiety-free
- Understand hyperbaric therapy and why it is being used

Nursing Considerations

- Short-term vision changes may occur in patients undergoing hyperbaric chamber therapy. Assess for visual changes and maintain safety.

- Patients with anxiety or claustrophobia may benefit from receiving an anti-anxiety agent prior to the procedure.

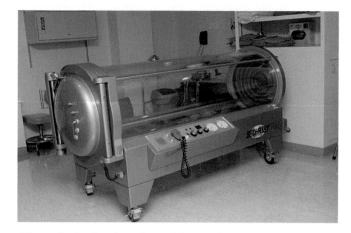

A hyperbaric chamber allows delivery of 100% oxygen at pressures greater than the atmosphere, allowing oxygen penetration not possible under normal pressure. The closed tube appearance may exacerbate feelings of claustrophobia for the patient. Monitor the patient for verbal and non-verbal signs of anxiety. Anti-anxiety agents may need to be ordered for the patient.

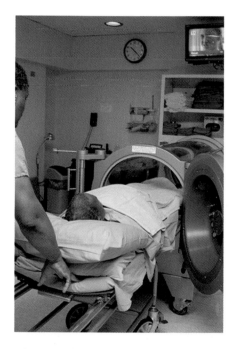

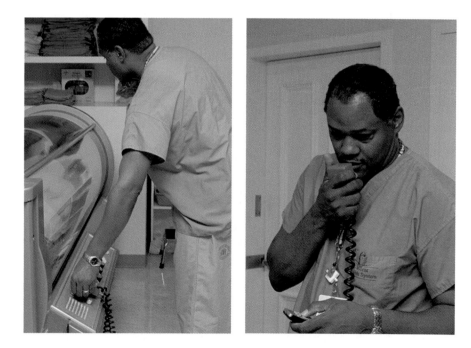

Obtain vital signs, ensure patient comfort, and place the patient within the chamber. Note the clock and television within the patient's view. Distractions help pass time while in the chamber. The amount of time the treatment takes, the number of treatments, and the pressure settings depend on the reason for the treatment. A typical length of time in the hyperbaric chamber is 90 minutes.

As the nurse increases the pressure, the patient is monitored for comfort, anxiety, and side effects of increased pressure, such as increased ear pressure or "popping." Having the patient open their mouth may help alleviate this. (B) Communicating with the patient in the chamber is reassuring to the patient and allows verbalization of feeling.

LAMINECTOMY

Laminectomy is a surgical procedure removing the bony arch, or lamina, of a vertebra for a variety of conditions, including spinal stenosis and herniated disc. A laminectomy is commonly performed when conservative treatment of back pain fails. Removal of the lamina relieves pressure on nerve roots, the cause of pain.

Assessment

- Back pain
- Loss of motor function
- Muscle atrophy on affected side

Planning and Implementation

- Vital signs
- Back pain
- Monitor for postoperative complications
- Monitor incision site for infection and cerebrospinal fluid leak

Evaluation and Outcomes

The patient will:

- Experience a decrease in back pain
- Avoid postoperative complications

Nursing Considerations

- Proper body mechanics should be reinforced in patients requiring laminectomy.

- The fourth and fifth lumbar vertebrae are the most common vertebrae requiring laminectomy.

- Observe the surgical dressing for the appearance of a "halo," a clear liquid with a yellowish ring around the edges. This may indicate the patient is experiencing a cerebrospinal fluid leak. If this occurs, leave the head of bed flat (to decrease the rate of leak) and notify the surgeon.

- If patients have been on long-term narcotic therapy for back pain, they may require higher doses of pain medication than those who have not been on long-term narcotic therapy.

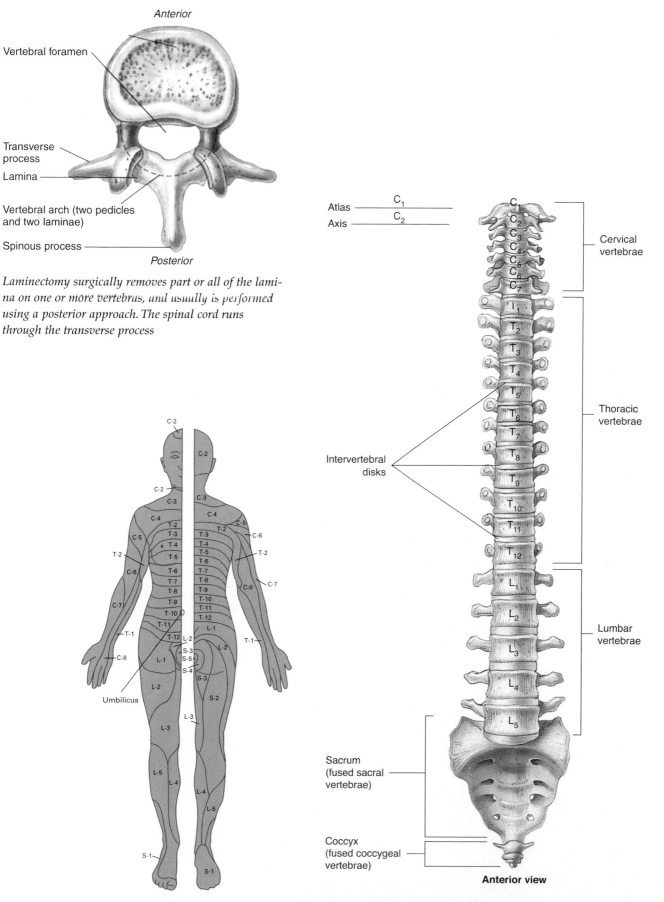

Anterior

Vertebral foramen

Transverse process

Lamina

Vertebral arch (two pedicles and two laminae)

Spinous process

Posterior

Laminectomy surgically removes part or all of the lamina on one or more vertebras, and usually is performed using a posterior approach. The spinal cord runs through the transverse process

Atlas — C₁
Axis — C₂

Cervical vertebrae

Thoracic vertebrae

Intervertebral disks

Lumbar vertebrae

Sacrum (fused sacral vertebrae)

Coccyx (fused coccygeal vertebrae)

Anterior view

Umbilicus

Laminectomy may be performed on any vertebra on the vertebral column (A). Spinal nerve roots innervate specific areas of skin, as noted in the dermatome (B). Compression of the specific nerve root causes pain along the vertebra's corresponding dermatome. Removing the lamina eliminates the pressure on the nerve and provides pain relief.

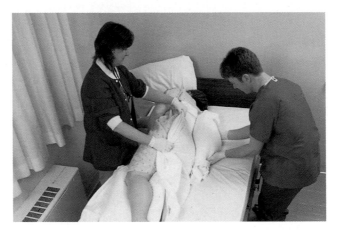

Logrolling prevents flexing of the spine in postsurgical patients, and allows the nurse to observe the surgical dressing. Cerebrospinal fluid leak is a post-operative complication noted by clear drainage with a ring around the edge (halo), and is usually coupled with a severe headache. Immediate treatment includes keeping the patient flat and notifying the surgeon. Epidural blood patches are often used to stop the leak. Assess distal pulses and color and the ability to move extremities. Compression stockings, encouraging early ambulation, use of incentive spirometry devices, and meticulous wound care prevent complications associated with surgery.

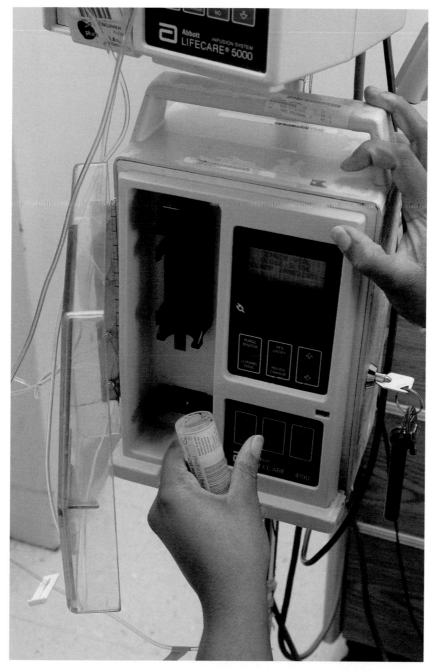

The nurse is preparing a PCA pump to control postoperative pain. Patient controlled analgesia (PCA) allows the patient to self-administer small doses of narcotics intravenously. The nurse monitors vital signs, oxygenation, pain, and sedation status. Keep narcan, a narcotic antagonist, available in case of signs of overdose, including respiratory depression and profound sedation.

MECHANICAL VENTILATION

Mechanical ventilation is artificial or mechanical assistance with ventilation. The assistance may include additional oxygen, volume, and pressure. The need for ventilation support occurs with a myriad of conditions, including neurological injury, general anesthesia, acute lung injury, and severe pneumonia. An artificial airway (endotracheal tube or tracheostomy) is attached to a ventilator to provide mechanical ventilation.

Assessment

- Pulse oximetry, arterial blood gases
- Breath sounds
- Spontaneous versus mechanical respirations
- Chest X-ray

Planning and Implementation

- Monitor respiratory status
- Provide means of communication
- Frequent oral care
- Keep emergency equipment at bedside in case of dislodgement of the airway

Evaluation and Outcomes

The patient will:

- Experience adequate respirations and oxygenation
- Maintain communication of needs
- Understand mechanical ventilation and why it is needed

Nursing Considerations

- A common complication of mechanical ventilation is ventilator-associated pneumonia. Handwashing by anyone in contact with the patient, frequent oral care, and keeping the head of the bed elevated 30 degrees reduce the incidence of this complication.

- High-pressure alarms signify increased pressure within the system, including increased pulmonary secretion, decreased lung compliance, or kinking of the tubing. If this occurs, assess the patient and if secretions are present, suction the patient.

- Low-pressure alarms signify a loss of pressure within the system, including a disconnection within the system, a leak in the endotracheal cuff, or accidental tube displacement. If this occurs, assess the patient and if disconnected, then reconnect; if the tube is displaced, remove and provide rescue breathing with a bag valve mask apparatus attached to oxygen.

- Collaborate with the respiratory therapist regarding the ventilator settings and the patient's condition. The respiratory therapist is responsible for the ventilator, but it is the nurse that is responsible for the patient.

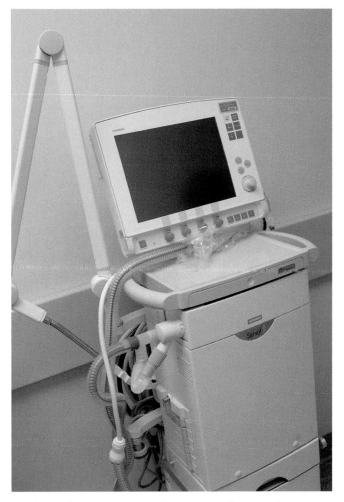

Mechanical ventilation provides oxygen, volume, and pressure through the use of a ventilator. Ventilator mode is chosen according to the patient condition, and may adjust as the patient condition changes. Ventilator alarms, set according to the patient and ventilator settings, may indicate changes in the patient's pulmonary status, dislodgement, or disconnection.

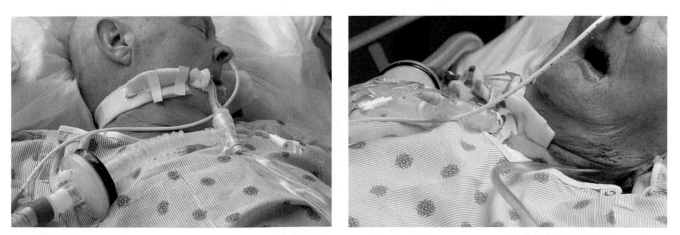

An artificial airway is necessary to provide mechanical ventilation. Endotracheal tubes, as seen on the left (A), and tracheostomy tubes, as seen on the right (B), are placed in the patient's trachea to afford a means to attach to a ventilator. Both types of artificial airways require care by the nurse. Notice how both are secured to prevent dislodgement. Frequent oral care and maintaining head of bed elevation lessen the incidence of pulmonary infections.

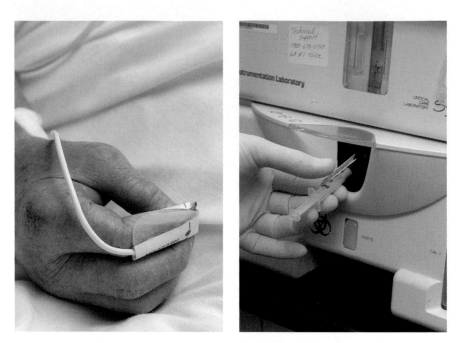

Continually watch the pulse oximetry, as shown on the index finger of the patient (A), to assess oxygenation status. Assess the patient's respiratory status frequently, including auscultating breath sounds, assessing respiration rate, depth, character, and effort. Monitor arterial blood gases to determine the effectiveness of mechanical ventilation, including oxygenation and acid-base balance(B). Chest X-ray confirms artificial airway placement and monitors pulmonary status.

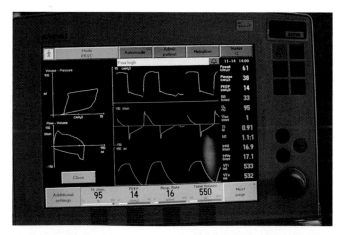

Ventilators give information about ventilation and lung status, including ventilation loops reflecting the pressure-volume relationship, tidal volume, respiratory rate, and airway pressures.

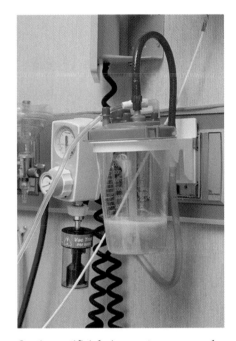

Suction artificial airways to remove pulmonary secretions. Keep suctioning equipment, a bag valve mask respirator with supplemental oxygen, and additional artificial airways available in case of dislodgement.

MAGNETIC RESONANCE IMAGING (MRI)

MRI is a noninvasive procedure using radio frequency waves and a strong magnetic field instead of X-rays to provide especially clear and detailed pictures of internal organs and structures. MRI is used to diagnose multiple medical conditions.

Assessments

- Remove all jewelry
- History of metal implants or shrapnel
- History of claustrophobia or extreme anxiety

Planning and Implementation

- Monitor patient during the procedure
- If the patient requires cardiac monitoring, ventilation, or infusion of intravenous fluids during the procedure, special non-metallic equipment will be required

Evaluation and Outcomes

The patient will:

- Understand the MRI
- Remain calm and anxiety-free during the procedure

Nursing Considerations

- Personnel assisting patients in and out of the MRI scanner may have magnetized cards (credit cards or identification cards) demagnetized by coming into contact with the machine.

- Consider requesting sedation orders for patients with extreme anxiety.

- Monitor the patient's pulse oximetry during MRI because when the patient is in the scanner, the nurse may be unable to directly observe respirations.

- Telemetry patients need to have the EGC adhesive patches removed before going to MRI. There are MRI compatible ECG adhesive patches available in the MRI suite

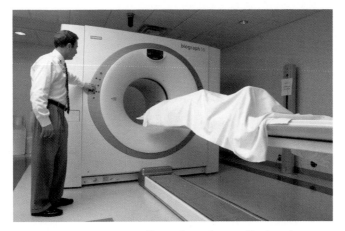

Have the patient remove all metal jewelry, medical equipment, and removable prostheses, because when the MRI is activated the machine will pull any metal towards the scanner. If the patient has a history of metal implants or shrapnel, MRI should be cancelled to prevent injury from the metal pulling out of the patient. Secure the patient and provide comfort and explanation prior to the procedure. During the procedure, personnel exit the room and monitor the patient.

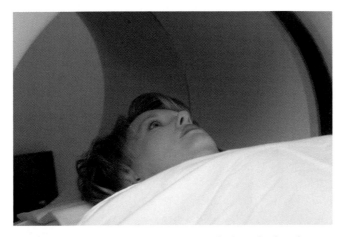

During the procedure, the patient is inside the cylindrical portion of the machine. Some patients experience feelings of claustrophobia. Reassure the patient and remain in verbal contact with them via the intercom system. Sedatives may be necessary.

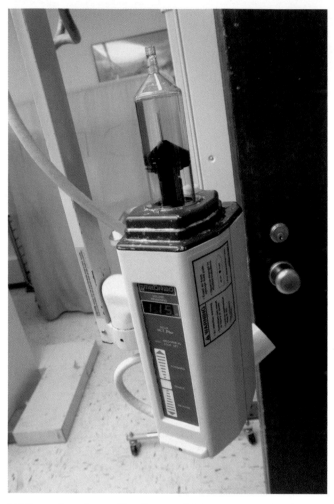

MRI may be enhanced by the use of intravenous contrast. Contrast helps differentiate between normal and abnormal tissue when diagnosing conditions such as tendonitis, multiple sclerosis, or infections. The contrast does not contain iodine and reactions are rare.

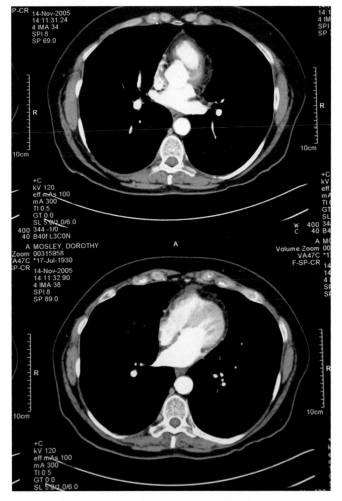

MRI pictures are shown in anatomical slices, provide great detail, and aid in diagnosing. These MRI films show slices of the chest showing the spinal cord, aorta, the heart, and the lungs.

OSTOMY CARE

Ostomy care is care to a surgically-created opening, or stoma, and the skin surrounding the site. The goal is to protect the skin surrounding the stoma, clean and remove waste products from the ostomy, and assess the stoma for viability. The care requires that the patient and family understand the need to continue the care once discharged from the hospital setting.

Assessment

- Stoma color
- Skin around the stoma
- Waste from the ostomy site

Planning and Implementation

- Monitor skin surrounding the stoma and the stoma itself
- Teach patients concerning foods that cause gas
- Return demonstration applying and removing appliances

Evaluation and Outcomes

The patient will:

- Demonstrate how to apply and change ostomy equipment
- Verbalize normal stoma color
- Understand foods that cause gas that may fill the ostomy bag

Nursing Considerations

- Often patients are uncomfortable looking at the stoma and with ostomy care. Encourage verbalization of thoughts and fears associated with ostomy care.

- Stomas should be pink and moist. If it becomes dark purple it may not be receiving adequate blood supply and the surgeon should be notified.

- If a patient with a stoma has an enema ordered, always clarify the route per the rectum or the stoma.

- Contact dietary to supply patients with lists of foods that produce little or no gas to prevent the ostomy bag from filling

- Ask patients if they have any questions about sexuality and their ostomy. Many patients are afraid to ask if there sexuality will be affected and need to understand the ostomy itself does not affect sexuality, but body image disturbances may.

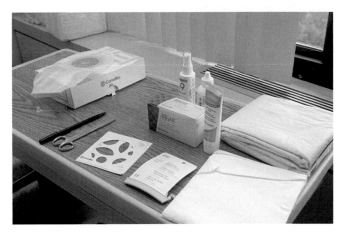

Ostomy care begins with explaining the procedure to the patient and gathering supplies, including ostomy care products, cleansing supplies. This time can be utilized for patient teaching and to answer any questions.

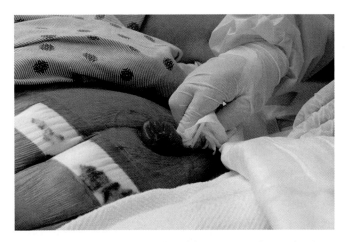

The existing pouch is removed and the stoma is cleansed. The stoma should be assessed for red color, moistness, and waste consistency. Purplish discoloration, dryness, or absence of output indicates problems and should be reported promptly. The surrounding skin is monitored for signs of irritation or breakdown.

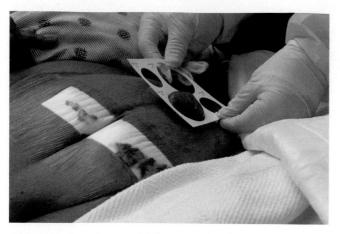

Sizing the stoma is essential for protecting the surrounding skin from contact with waste. Once the size is determined, the barrier will be cut to fit the stoma, ensuring no waste is in contact with skin.

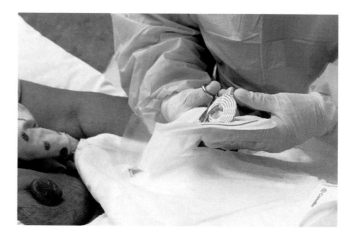

The pouch has two parts, the barrier and the pouch, and may be supplied in a one-piece system, as shown, or a two-piece system where the pouch attaches to the barrier. The barrier opening is cut to fit the patient's stoma.

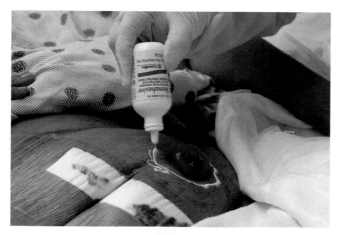

The skin surrounding the stoma is prepared with barrier wipes or barrier guard skin protectant as shown. The barrier wipes help adhere the barrier to the skin, and the skin protectant helps protect the skin from breakdown in case any waste comes into contact with the skin.

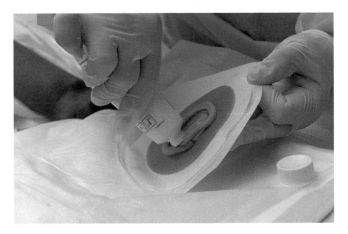

The barrier adhesive is applied and filler paste is added to the barrier portion of the pouch as shown. The paste ensures a complete seal.

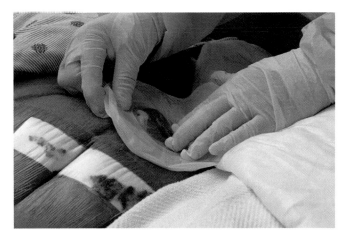

As the pouch is applied the nurse is able to observe that the barrier opening is the correct size and the seal is complete. Notice the pouch allows visualization of the stoma.

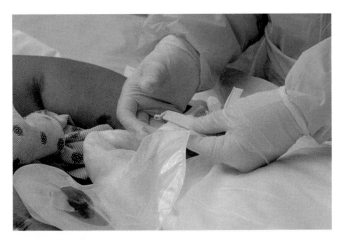

Clips on the bottom of a one-piece unit, as shown, allow drainage of waste material. Two-piece units disconnect from the barrier, allowing the pouch to be emptied and reconnected. Educate patients which foods create gas that fills the pouch and may cause an accidental popping off of the two-piece units. Odor controlling techniques, such as placing a couple of drops of vanilla in the pouch, should be discussed. How often the patient needs to empty and change the appliances depends on many factors, including the stoma placement and the consistency and amount of the waste created.

PNEUMONIA, TREATMENT OF *

The treatment of pneumonia, the inflammation and congestion of the lung tissue caused by bacteria or virus, depends on the specific cause and the severity. Goals of treatment include promoting oxygenation, clearing congestion, and eradicating the causative agent. Additionally, treating associated coughs, fever, and associated symptoms is included in the plan of care.

Assessment

- Breath sounds and respiratory status
- Color and quantity of sputum
- Vital signs including temperature and pulse oximetry

Planning and Implementation

- Monitor vital signs and respiratory status
- Administer antipyretics and antibiotics
- Administer oxygen therapy
- Respiratory treatments to promote expectoration of sputum
- Monitor chest X-rays

Evaluation and Outcomes

The patient will:

- Experience adequate oxygenation
- Understand pneumonia treatments
- Maintain adequate comfort

Nursing Considerations

- Pneumonia is a common respiratory complication in the hospital setting because of patient risk factors, including immobility and decreased immune systems from illnesses.

- The hospital environment, despite infection control measures, houses many drug-resistant infections, such as MRSA (methicillin-resistant Staphylococcus aureus).

- Encourage frequent oral care or provide it to the patient if they are unable. Bacteria in the oral cavity may be inadvertently aspirated in the lungs. Frequent oral care will reduce the bacteria in the mouth.

- Early ambulation provides exercise to the patient, helping with patient strengthening and adequate oxygenation.

- Excess sputum and atelectasis, a small area of the lung that collapses onto itself,

- increase the incidence of hospital-acquired pneumonia and should be avoided. Deep breathing and coughing promotes expectorating sputum, and prevents atelectasis.

*The pictures that follow are from different patients receiving pneumonia treatments.

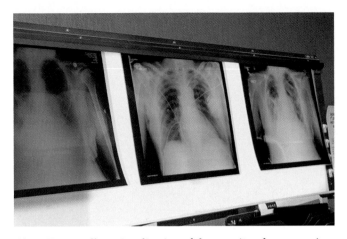

Chest X-rays allow visualization of the severity of pneumonia and aid in monitoring the effectiveness of therapies.

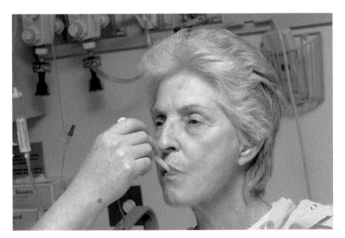

(A) Vital signs require monitoring, including pulse oximetry in patients with pneumonia. This patient is at risk for pneumonia because she is older and has had recent surgery. Fevers are treated with antipyretic medications. A drastic drop in blood pressure, tachycardia, or fever requires immediate intervention. It may indicate the patient is developing sepsis, a systemic infection that is a complication of pneumonia.

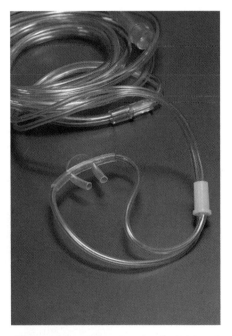

(B) Supplemental oxygen is administered for hypoxia indicated by pulse oximetry and patient reports of dyspnea. Depending on the severity of the pneumonia and the patient's pre-existing conditions, supplemental oxygenation delivery ranges from nasal cannula, as shown, to mechanical ventilation.

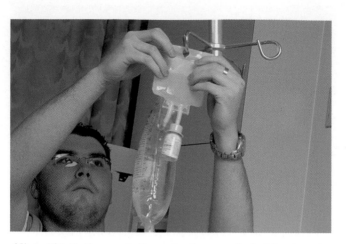

(C) Antibiotic therapy is the main pharmacological treatment for pneumonia. Administer antibiotics as ordered, orally or intravenously (as shown). Assess patient allergies before initiating antibiotic therapy.

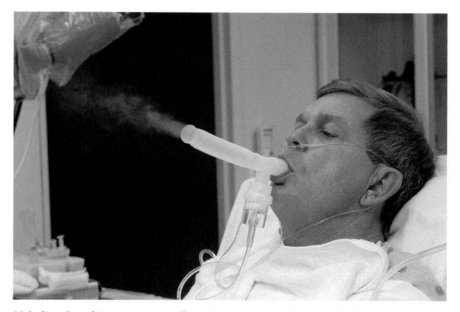

Nebulizer breathing treatments allow the inhalation of bronchodilating medication that promotes lung expansion and assists in loosening mucus to help expectoration. This patient is also receiving oxygen per nasal cannula in addition to the nebulizer treatment. Slight anxiety and tachycardia are common side effects of nebulizer treatments. Document quantity and color of mucus.

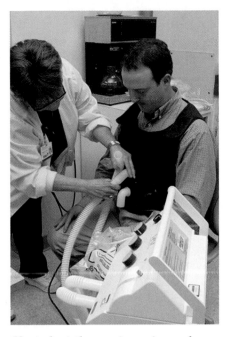

Chest physiotherapy is an airway clearance technique involving percussion of the chest wall, manually, with a hand-held mechanical percussor or a high frequency chest percussion device, as shown, for pneumonia. Chest physiotherapy loosens mucus and aids the patient in coughing up mucus.

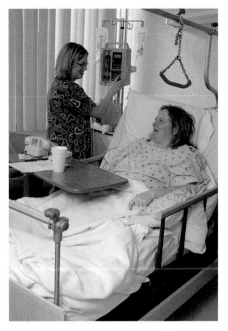

The head of bed is elevated for this patient and it facilitates easier breathing. Encourage deep breathing exercises, good oral hygiene and ambulation. Explaining the reason for activities involves the patient in the plan of care and increases compliance.

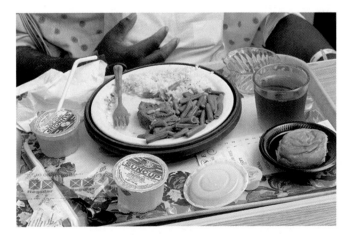

Adequate nutritional and fluid intake is important. Pneumonia increases caloric and fluid needs, the amount dependent on the patient and the severity of the pneumonia. The nurse should monitor intake and output, take daily weights, and record the amount of each meal the patient eats. If the patient is unable to meet nutritional and fluid demands, the use of intravenous therapy and enteral feedings may be necessary.

PRESSURE ULCERS, TREATMENT OF

The treatment of pressure ulcers depends on the stage of the pressure ulcer. Pressure ulcers rage in severity from stage 1, with intact skin, to stage 4, with involvement extending into deep muscle. The goal of the treatment of pressure ulcers is to heal and repair skin and underlying tissue, prevent infection, and prevent other pressure ulcers from forming.

Assessment

- Skin, especially bony prominences and coccyx area
- Determine stage of pressure ulcer
- Nutritional status

Planning and Implementation

- Treat pressure ulcer according to stage
- Change position every two hours
- Maintain adequate nutritional status

Evaluation and Outcomes

The patient will:

- Experience healing of pressure ulcer
- Maintain adequate nutrition
- Understand pressure ulcer treatment regime

Nursing Considerations

- Scales such as the Braden or Waterlow assist health care members in identifying patients at risk for developing pressure ulcers. Utilizing these scales will identify patients at risk for skin breakdown, and aggressive measures are used to prevent pressure ulcer formation, including skin care, frequent turning, and promoting good nutrition.

- Documenting skin care assessments on admission helps verify if a patient had skin breakdown on admission or if the breakdown occurred during the hospitalization.

- Collaborating with wound care nurses or wound care teams, help decide best treatment options for patients based on the breakdown type and location.

- Minimizing the use of incontinence pads or "chucks" reduces retained moisture from the patient and maximizes the effectiveness of therapy beds in preventing skin breakdown.

- Rectal tube pouches or tubes may reduce the incidence of skin breakdown in patients who are involuntary of prolonged diarrhea.

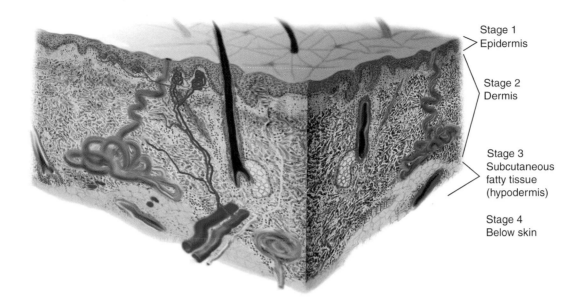

Stage 1
Epidermis

Stage 2
Dermis

Stage 3
Subcutaneous
fatty tissue
(hypodermis)

Stage 4
Below skin

Treatment of pressure ulcers depends on the stage. Stage 1 ulcers affect the epidermis and the skin is intact. The goal is to maintain the integrity of the skin and prevent further injury. Stage 2 involves the dermis, stage 3 extends into the subcutaneous layer, and stage 4 involves muscle and structures below the skin. In these more extensive ulcers, treatment goals include wound healing and infection prevention or care.

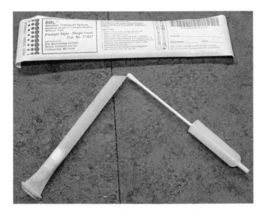

Wound cultures are obtained to verify infection status in Stages 2 through 4 pressure ulcers that are suspicious of infection (presence of drainage or odor). If infection is present, appropriate antibiotic therapy is initiated.

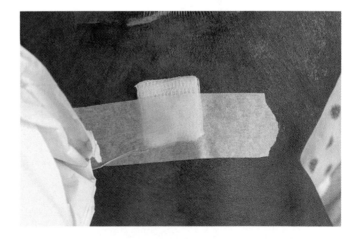

All pressure ulcer dressings begin with hand washing and donning appropriate personal protective devices. All wounds require cleansing prior to dressing. Stage 1 ulcers are treated with (as shown) occlusive dressings or protective ointment/creams. Frequent patient positioning, adequate hydration, and nutrition help the ulcer heal.

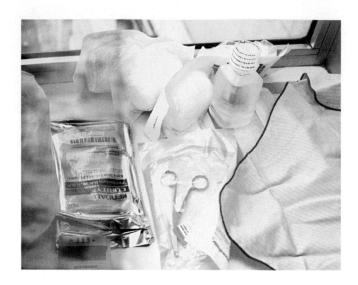

Application of moist dressings promotes granulation tissue by allowing drainage, maintaining a moist environment, promoting mechanical debridement, and obliterating dead space in Stage 2 or 3 pressure ulcers. Granulation tissue has a clean, bumpy appearance and is indicative of wound healing. Types of moist dressings include foam, gauze hydrocolloids, and hydrogels.

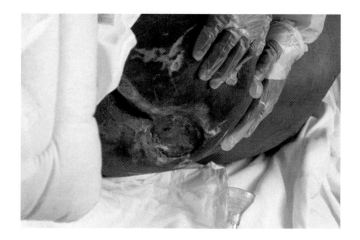

Surgical or enzyme debridement is commonly performed with Stage 3 and 4 pressure ulcer wounds to remove necrotic tissue and promote healing. Surgical debridement of the Stage 4 pressure ulcer pictured is evident by the clean regular wound edges.

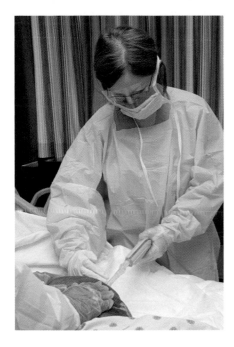

Pressure ulcer irrigation cleans the wound and provides mechanical debridement. Protective eye equipment is worn to reduce the risk of accidental splashing of the eyes.

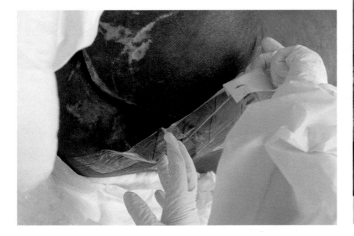

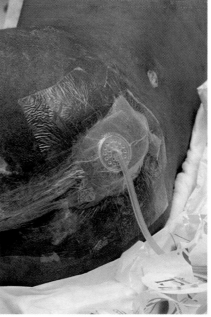

(A) A vacuum-assisted wound device uses a foam insert promoting granulation tissue, and applies gentle suction to remove wound exudates; its uses include Stage 3 or 4 pressure ulcers. The foam is cut to fit inside the wound and an occlusive dressing is applied. The dressing is usually changed every 48 hours or as ordered. (B) The suction tube is inserted into the foam and the wound is sealed. Suction is applied and note the foam flattens, which indicates the seal is adequate. Drainage collects in a container on the suction portion of the vacuum-assisted wound device.

SKIN GRAFT

A skin graft is a surgical procedure removing skin from one site and transplanting it to another site. Skin grafts are used for replacing skin lost from burns, injuries, infections, and for cosmetic purposes, and may be split-thickness (removing part of the dermis and the epidermis) or full-thickness (all skin layers). Skin grafts are obtained from the patient, cadaver, or from living bi-layer skin substitutes, such as Apligraf or Biobrane.

Assessment

- Skin graft color and temperature
- Presence of infection
- Wound healing

Planning and Implementation

- Meticulous skin care for donor and transplanted site
- Monitor for signs of adequate circulation
- Hand washing and infection prevention

Evaluation and Outcomes

The patient will:

- Be infection-free
- Experience wound healing to donor site
- Exhibit signs of skin graft healing

Nursing Considerations

- If a patient is unable to donate skin for skin grafts, cadaver, pig, and synthetic grafts are available.

- Adequate pain control is achieved with narcotics.

- Dressings maintain moisture with the skin grafts. If the graft becomes dry, it may dissect or pull away from the burn area.

- Fever, increased white blood cell count, poor healing, and wound drainage are indicative of infection and are reported to the physician.

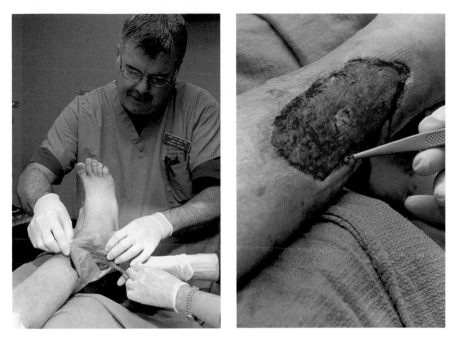

The dressing is removed and the skin graft site is prepared first by ensuring the area is infection-free and debrided (removal of dead or infected tissue) (A). Note how the healthy tissue bleeds once debrided (B).

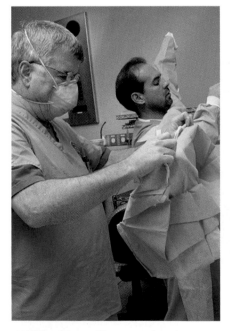

(A) The skin grafting procedure is performed using sterile technique.

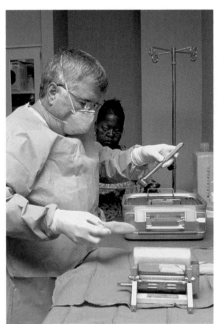

(B) The surgeon prepares equipment for the grafts, including a skin graft scapel that shaves skin for accurate thickness and a broad mesher to size the graft to fit the area to be grafted.

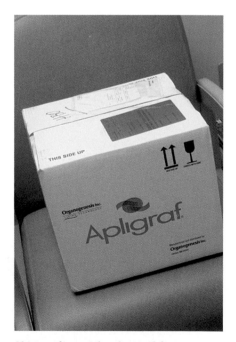

Skin grafts may be obtained from humans, xenografts, or living bi-layer skin substitutes such as Apligraf. The skin substitutes are living cells and structural proteins with bovine and human cells.

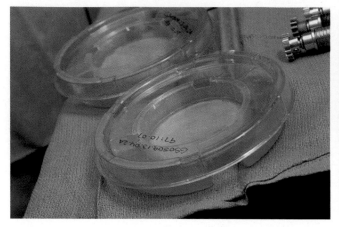

(A) The skin graft is prepared for the skin substitute skin graft. Skin substitutes, as shown, are living products.

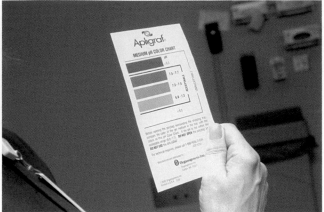

(B) The expiration date and the color chart (which makes certain the pH of the medium is in an acceptable range) are checked prior to applying to the patient. If the pH is not in an acceptable range or the expiration date is exceeded, the product is not used and is returned to the manufacturer.

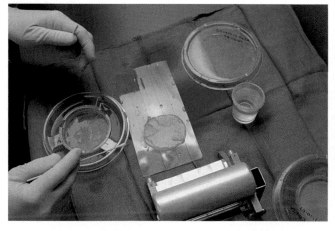

(A) The skin substitute or graft is removed from the medium (the pink round dish). The medium keeps the product viable and moist. The graft is expanded and fenestrated (tiny holes are placed) using the broad mesher (the silver tube-like piece of equipment).

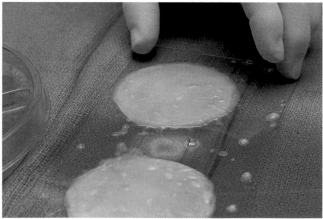

(B) The skin substitute is ready to apply to the patient.

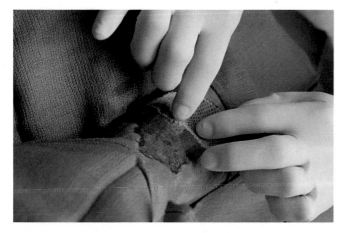

Using sterile technique, the graft is applied to the patient. Notice the fenestrations on the graft. The graft is set on the skin and may be stapled or sutured in place.

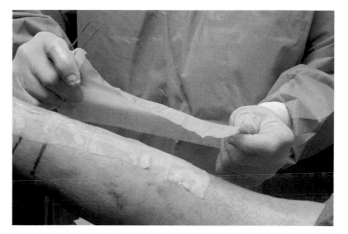

A non-adherent dressing such as Xeroform covers the skin graft. This dressing remains intact for 5 to 7 days to allow adequate time for healing.

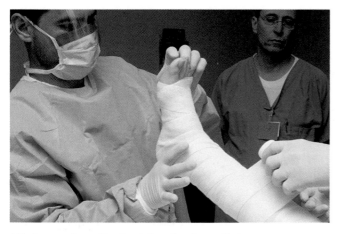

(A) A secondary absorbent dressing is applied.

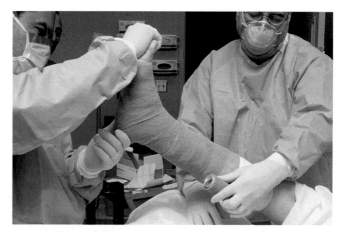

(B) Next, the dressing is covered with a compression bandage. Postoperatively, the affected site is elevated, and the patients level of consciousness, vital signs, distal extremity capillary refill, color, and pain levels are monitored.

TELEMETRY

Telemetry is the remote viewing of the electrical activity of the heart or the heart rhythm. Placing electrodes on a patient's chest and attaching them to a portable device allows physicians to monitor heart rate and rhythms. Telemetry is widely used in the hospital setting to monitor patients at risk for cardiac dysfunction.

Assessment

- Baseline heart rhythm
- Proper electrode placement
- Vital signs

Planning and Implementation

- Set monitor alarms
- Monitor heart rate and rhythm
- Notify the health care provider of changes in rhythm

Evaluation and Outcomes

The patient will:

- Understand the purpose for telemetry
- Experience normal heart rate and rhythm

Nursing Considerations

- Removing electrodes and leaving the area will interfere with monitoring. Teach patients to notify the nurse if either activity is required.

- Patient activity may appear as an arrhythmia, such as brushing teeth may appear as a ventricular arrhythmia or accidental removal of electrodes may appear as asystole. The patient's activity is noted and an assessment of the patient is performed before verifying any rhythm.

- When patients leave the unit for testing such as for a CAT scan, it is clarified with the physician if the patient will require cardiac monitoring during testing. If monitoring is required, a portable monitor is utilized.

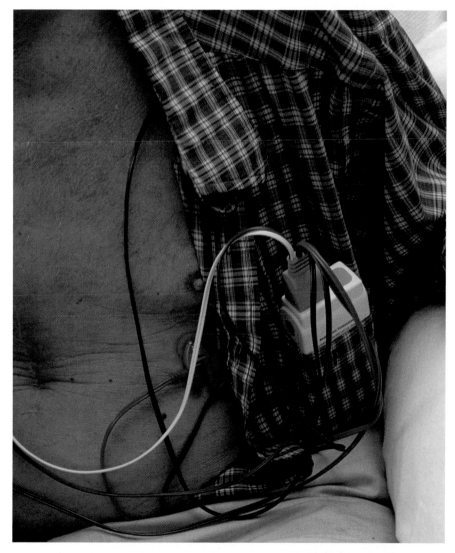

Telemetry units may be placed in the patient's pocket. Patients are instructed not to remove the device, wash with the unit intact, or leave the nursing unit. All said activities interfere with the ability to monitor the patient's heart rhythm. Electrode patches are applied daily and the battery in the telemetry unit is changed regularly.

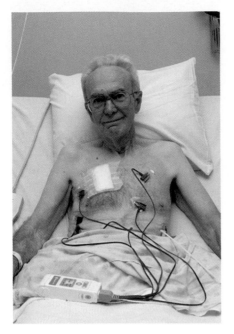

Electrodes are applied to the patient's chest avoiding hair and attached to the electrode wires and the telemetry units. Proper placement is important for receiving an accurate signal. Notice that the telemetry unit has a "road map" indicating proper electrode and wire placement.

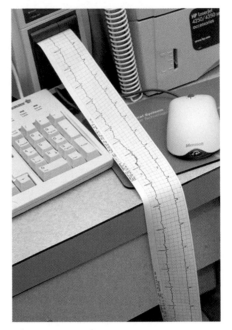

Telemetry permits the recording and documentation of the patient's heart rate and rhythm. Rhythm recordings are documented per unit protocol and when changes in the rhythm occur. PR, QRS, and QT interval size and interpretation of the recording is included in the documentation.

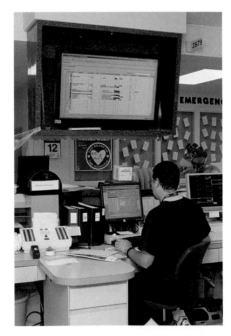

Telemetry allows the remote viewing of the patient's heart rate and rhythm. Alarms are based on patient's baseline heart rate and rhythm and set every shift. Note the monitor displays multiple patients' rhythms, allowing the nurse to monitor multiple patients simultaneously.

TOTAL HIP REPLACEMENT

Total hip replacement is the surgical replacement of the hip joint. Hip replacements are performed to relieve pain and improve function for patients experiencing osteoarthritis, rheumatoid arthritis, fractures, loss of blood supply to the hip, hip tumors, or deformities.

Assessment

- Pain
- Incision site
- Vital signs
- Distal pulse and extremity color

Planning and Implementation

- Encourage early ambulation with physical therapy
- Monitor vital signs
- Treat pain
- Wound care

Evaluation and Outcomes

The patient will:

- Improve mobility
- Maintain normal vital signs
- Experience pain control

Nursing Considerations

- Collaboration with the case manager or social worker explores home care considerations, such as stairs and living alone prior to surgery.

- Offer patients with scheduled hip replacements the option of banking their own blood prior to surgery.

- Teach patients to avoid flexing the operative hip beyond 90 degrees. Activities that flex the hip beyond 90 degrees include picking up objects off the floor, attempting to put on socks, sitting in low chairs, and bending forward in the bed to pull blankets up.

- Pain medications may cause constipation and any bowel difficulties are addressed promptly to avoid this problem.

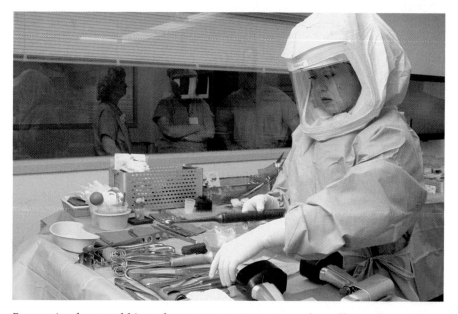

Preparation for a total hip replacement necessitates tremendous effort and expertise because of the amount of people involved, the equipment involved, and the procedure itself. (A) Surgical hoods protect against blood splashing and are commonly worn in orthopedic surgery.

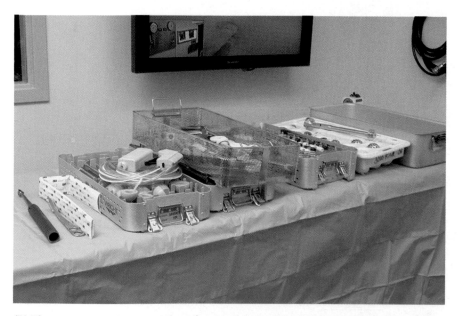

(B) The surgery requires a number of surgical instruments and equipment.

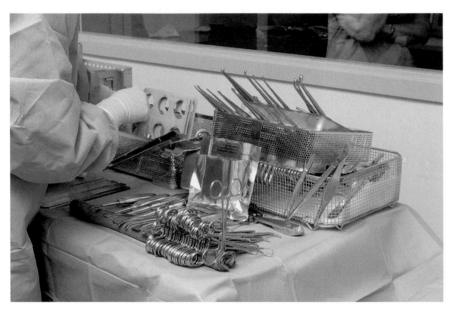

(C) Preoperatively, instruments are verified, counted, and set up by the nurse.

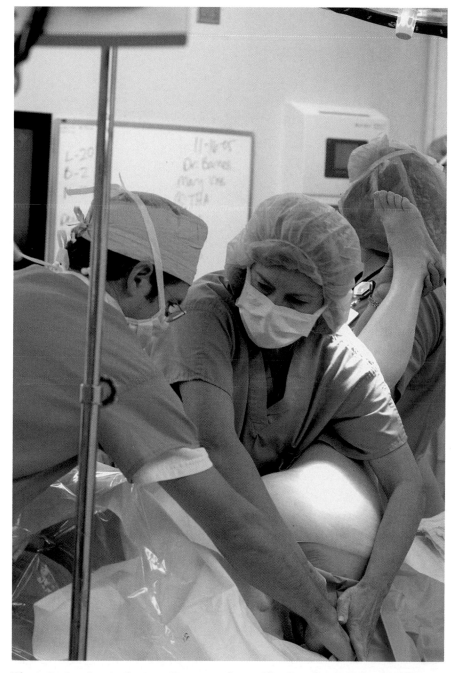

The patient arrives to the operating room after verification of patient identification and surgical site; surgical consents, laboratory reports, and allergies have been reviewed and verified. Careful patient positioning prevents complications and affords the surgeon better access to the surgical hip. The patient is positioned side-lying with the surgical hip exposed. Attention is made to pad pressure points and leave access to the patient's airway and intravenous lines.

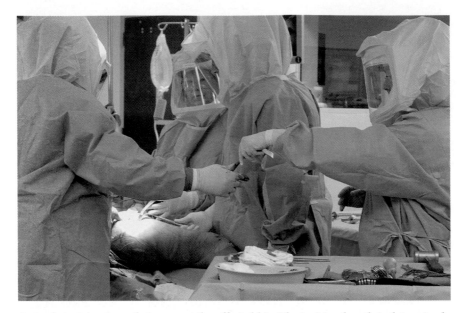

A single incision is made to expose the affected hip. The incision length is determined by the patient size and the exact nature of the surgery, and may be between 2 and 12 inches in length. Patients may opt to donate their own blood months prior to the surgery in case blood replacement is required.

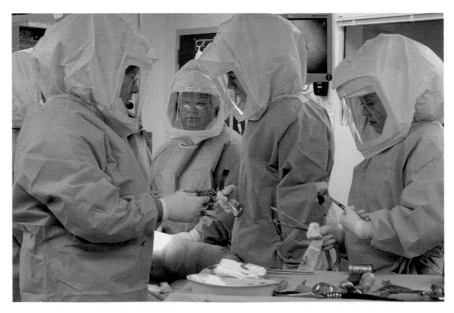

(A) Exposure of the hip joint allows removal of diseased bone.

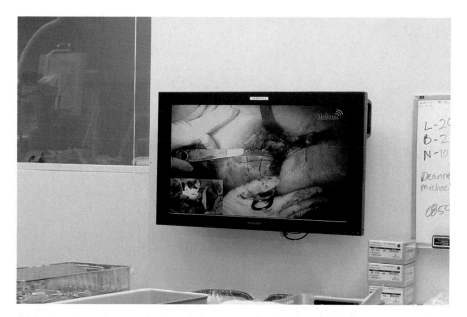

(B) TV screens allow monitoring of the surgery from outside the surgical suite. The metal retractors held by surgical team members pull the skin and muscle away from the hip area, allowing the bone removal and prosthetic implantation.

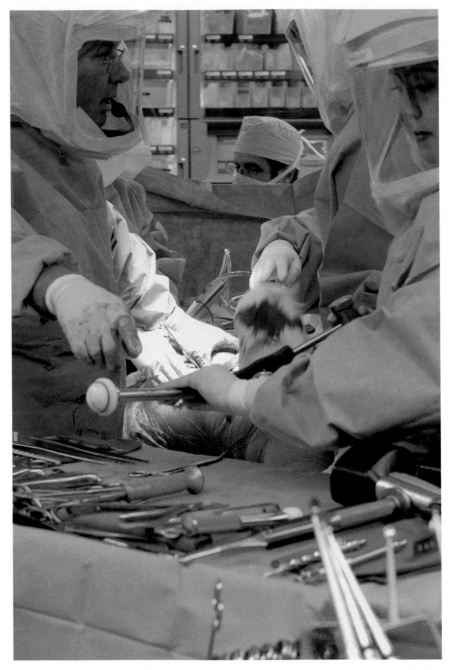

(A) Exposure of the area allows insertion of the prosthetic hip. Blood is removed with suction and sterile gauze during the procedure to help the surgeon visualize the hip.

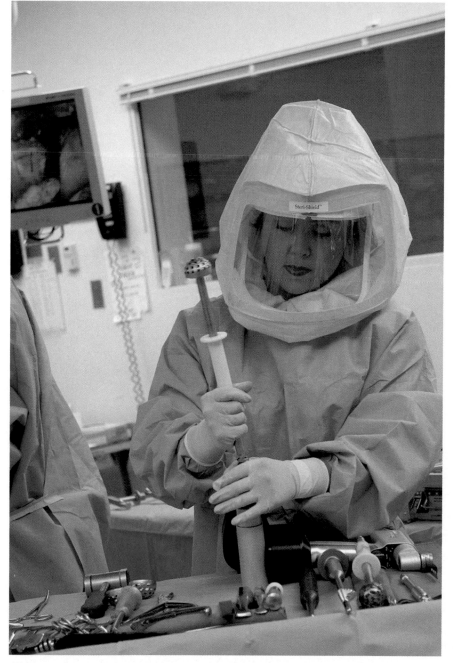

(B)Two main types of prosthetic hips, cemented and non-cemented, exist. The cemented type bonds the cup and the shaft of the prosthesis to the skeleton using a polymer compound. The non-cemented prosthesis is pushed into the skeleton and held by the elastic force of the skeleton. The surgeon and the patient preoperatively determine the type of prosthetic hip.

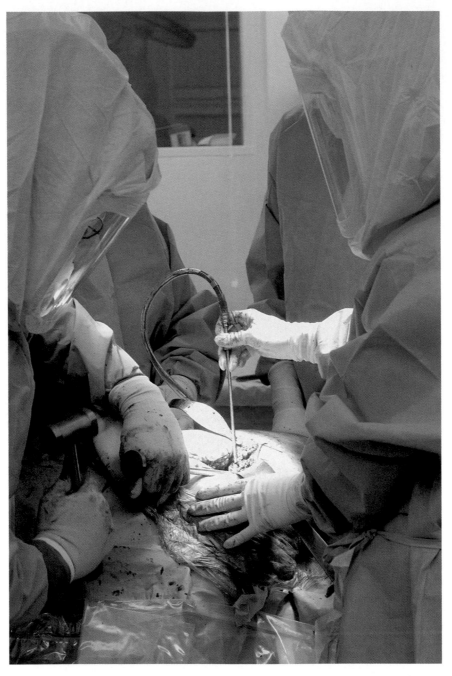

Closure of the incision begins and the surgeon may place drains at this time. The drains keep blood from pooling in the surgical hip.

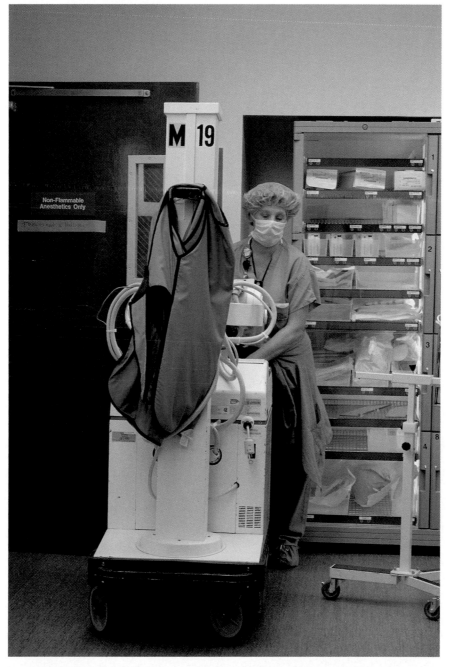

(A) A portable X-ray verifies proper placement of the total hip replacement.

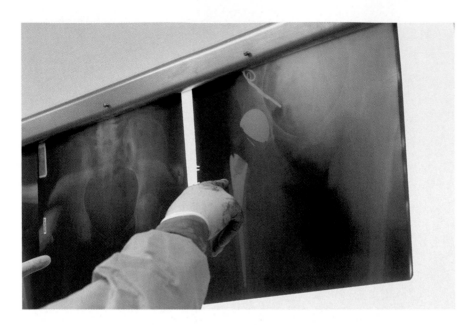

(B) The surgeon's finger points to the prosthesis. The acetabular shell (rounded edge) fits into the acetabulum and the hip implant extends into the femur.

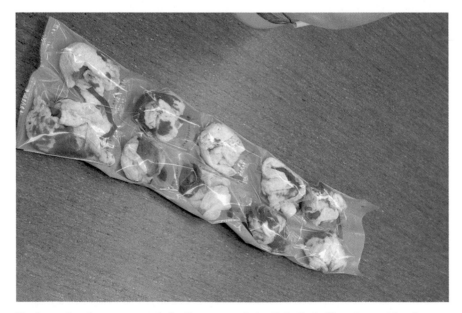

Equipment and sponge counts by the nurse substantiate that all equipment has been accounted for at the end of surgery. The recovery room monitors the patient as they regain consciousness. Once the patient is alert and stable, they are transported to the orthopedic unit.

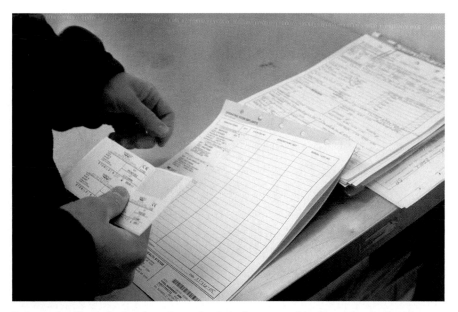

Information from the implanted prosthesis is documented in the patient's chart by the nurse. In case of future problems with the prosthesis, the exact serial number may be traced and the manufacturing company notified.

TRANSURETHRAL RESECTION OF PROSTATE (TURP)

Transurethral resection of the prostate (TURP) is a surgical procedure removing excess prostate tissue from benign prostate hyperplasia (BPH). BPH is common in men past the fifth decade of life, causing compression of the urethra and difficulty voiding. TURP relieves urinary symptoms of frequency, urine dripping, and urinary retention.

Assessment

- Urine color and quantity
- Pain
- Vital signs

Planning and Implementation

- Monitor urine output
- Maintain continuous bladder irrigation when ordered
- Call the physician for excessive bleeding or low urine output
- Treat pain

Evaluation and Outcomes

The patient will:

- Experience normal voiding
- Understand TURP and postoperative care

Nursing Considerations

- Administering alpha reductase inhibitors, adrenergic blockers, and prostate growth inhibitors may reduce the need for subsequent TURP procedures.

- Rarely, the bladder irrigation is absorbed, causing sodium and water imbalances, so therefore electrolytes are monitored.

- Foul-smelling urine may indicate a urinary tract infection.

- Teach patients that sexual activity may be resumed 6 to 8 weeks after the procedure.

- A low urine output during continuous bladder irrigation may indicate catheter obstruction from blood clots in the bladder and should be reported to the physician.

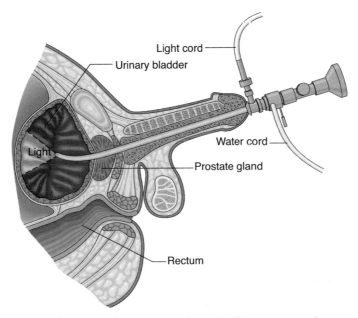

Light cord

Urinary bladder

Light

Water cord

Prostate gland

Rectum

Transurethral resection of prostate (TURP) allows access to the prostate via the urethra, eliminating the need for an abdominal approach to the surgery. Most TURPs are performed using spinal or epidural anesthesia. (Courtesy of the NCI, Terese Winslow)

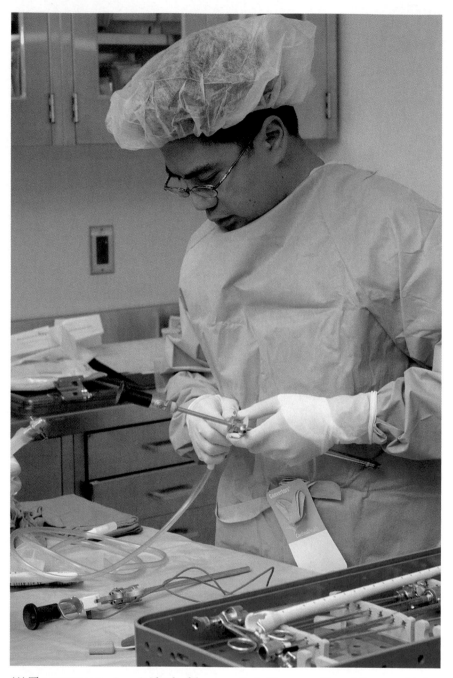

(A) The resectoscope is a rigid tube-like scope that allows resection of tissue and irrigation and cauterization (to control bleeding) of the prostate. A camera at the end of the tube allows direct visualization of the prostate during the procedure.

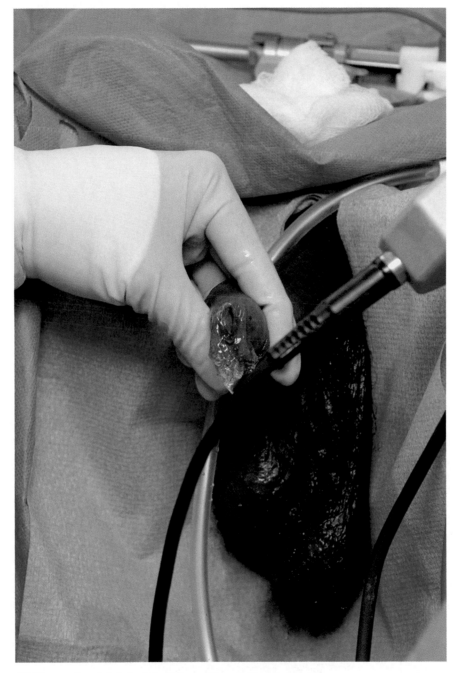

(B) The urethra is lubricated with a water-soluble lubricant.

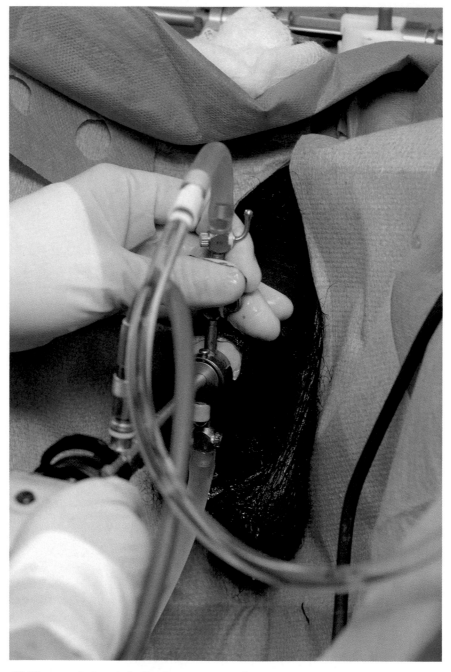

(C) The scope is inserted, allowing passage to the prostate.

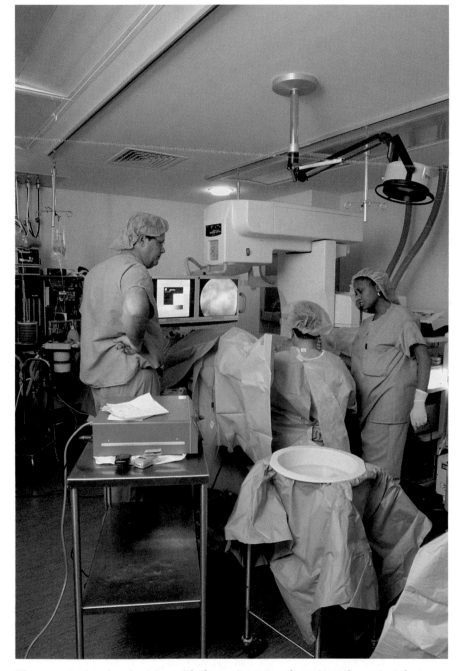

The nurse assists the physician with the equipment and monitors the patient during the procedure. The anesthesiologist monitors vital signs, oxygenation, and level of sedation during the procedure.

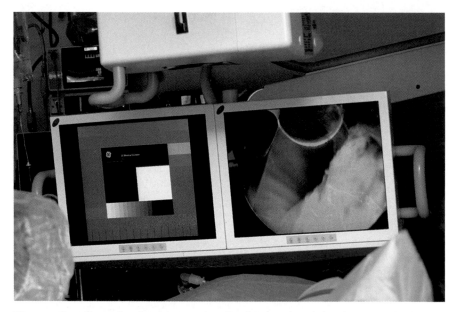

The monitor allows the physician to visualize landmarks while advancing the catheter. The scope is inserted at the penis and continues towards the bladder. The prostate is located before the bladder. The enlarged prostate tissue narrows the urethra, which is visualized on the screen.

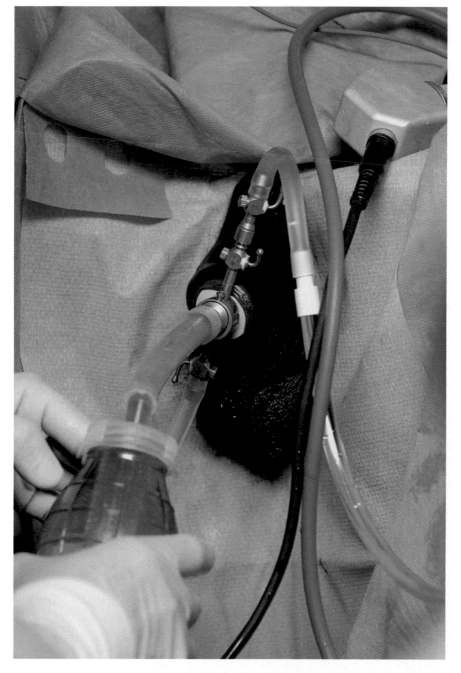

Resected tissue is collected from the prostate. The physician resects pieces of enlarged prostate with the scope until the urethra is enlarged and the prostate gland is within normal size. Tissue samples are sent to pathology for further analysis to rule out or confirm the diagnosis of prostate cancer.

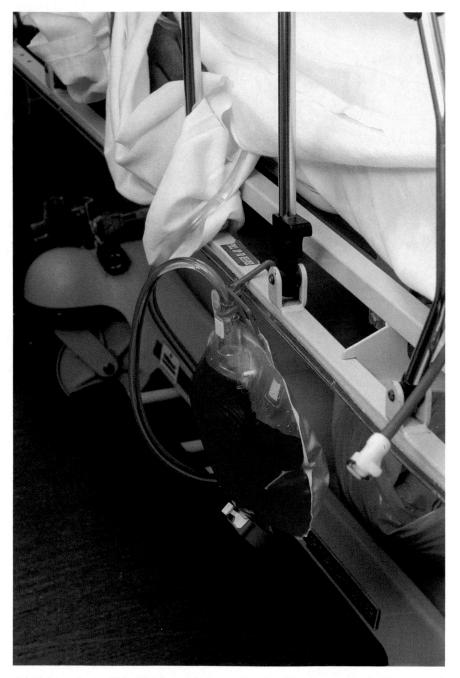

(A) Urine output will be bloody or "fruit-punch colored" post-operatively. The resected area of the prostate will have some bleeding after the procedure and that is normal. A urinary catheter is left in place that passes through the resected area and rests in the bladder. Irrigation is used to prevent clots from forming within the bladder.

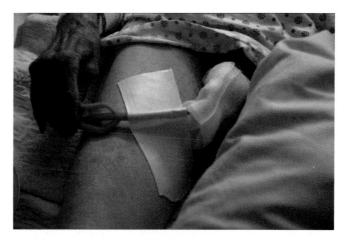

(B) Continuous bladder irrigation is performed with a three-lumen urinary catheter. One port allows irrigation to flow into the bladder, keeping blood clots from forming, and one allows urinary draining into a collection bag, while the third inflates a balloon to anchor the catheter inside the bladder. A low urine output and an increase in pain in the bladder, prostate, or rectum may indicate blood clots have formed and are obstructing the flow of urine and irrigant, and would be reported to the physician.

VENOUS STASIS ULCER DRESSING CHANGES

Ulcer dressing changes are a key treatment for the successful treatment of a venous stasis ulcer. The health care provider may request different types of dressing changes depending on the wound severity, size, and the response to treatment. Common dressings include the application of moist wound healing products and compression to the site using ointments, a gauze dressing, and with a vacuum assisted wound device. Other treatments include debridement (the removal of dead or infected tissue), skin grafting, and hyperbaric treatments.

Assessment

- Wound size, color, and depth
- Wound drainage
- Factors affecting skin healing (smoking, poor nutrition)

Planning and Implementation

- Dressing changes as ordered
- Document wound appearances
- Alert the physician or wound care nurse of changes in wound appearance
- Elevate affected extremity

Evaluation and Outcomes

The patient will:

- Experience wound healing
- Understand the dressing change purpose and procedure

Nursing Considerations

- Venous stasis ulcer dressing changes are commonly performed over a period of weeks to months. Patient understanding and compliance is paramount in the wound healing process.

- Healing may be affected in diabetic patients that have neuropathy or poor sensation in the extremities, causing unintentional injury to the ulcer site.

- Social isolation and self-esteem issues may arise because of the constant need to have the areas dressed, causing embarrassment when in public places.

- The type of dressing change ordered may change several times during the healing process.

- The patient's personal hygiene is performed close to dressing change times to avoid dressing contamination and additional dressing changes.

- Patients may not ambulate unless encouraged because they are fearful of the dressings falling off.

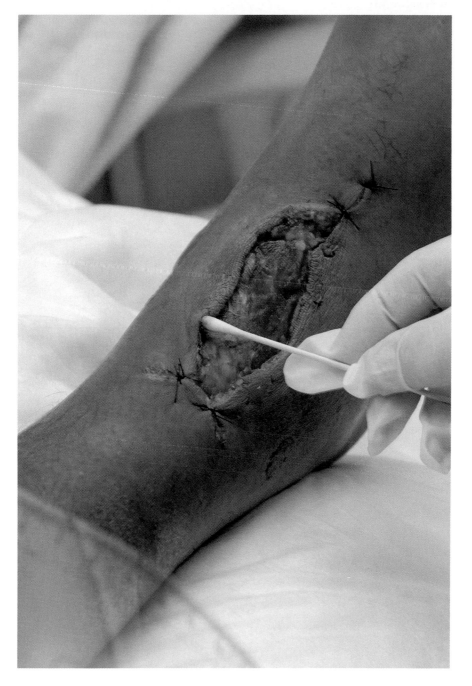

The goals of the dressing change are to keep the ulcer clean, free of infection and to promote healing. Types of dressings depend on the patient's mobility, the size of the ulcer, if it is infected and physician preference. (See Venous Ulcers)

Debridement is the removal of necrotic and infected tissue. This is performed to "clean the wound" and promote granulation or healing of the healthy tissue. This wound has been surgically debrided and the sutures help close the skin around the wound edges. Antibiotic ointment is applied to maintain the wound moisture and prevents bacterial growth. A gauze dressing is applied and the area is wrapped allowing mobility and security of the dressing. Compression of the dressing with a bandage or elastic stockings prevents edema, aiding in wound healing. The date, time, and initials are documented on the dressing. Wound appearance, size, and type of dressing are documented in the patient record. An example of documentation of an ulcer is: "Leg ulcer is located on the medial aspect of the left ankle and is 3cm by 4cm, the wound is clean with evidence of granulation tissue and is red in appearance. The wound edges are clean. Scant serosanguineous drainage is noted. The wound was cleaned using sterile saline and antibiotic ointment was applied. The wound was covered with a gauze wrap and then with an elastic wrap. The patient did not report any pain or discomfort during the procedure and it was tolerated well."

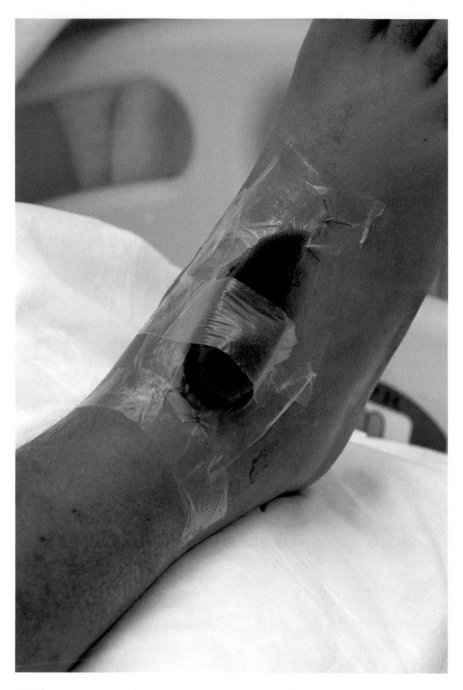

(A) This venous stasis ulcer dressing includes the use of a vacuum-assisted wound device using a foam type insert that promotes granulation and applies gentle suction to remove wound exudate. The wound is cleansed with sterile saline and the foam is cut to fit inside the wound, and an occlusive dressing is applied.

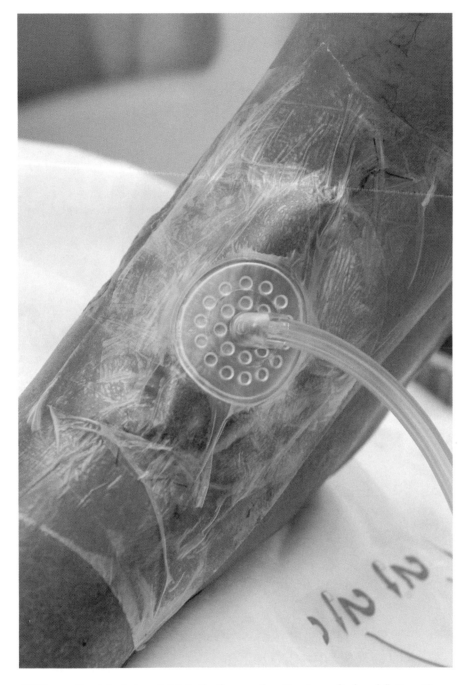

(B) The suction tube is inserted into the foam and suction is applied and flattens the foam, indicating the seal is adequate. If the seal is not adequate, the dressing must be reapplied. The suction maintains compression of the wound that aids in healing. (See Pressure Ulcers)

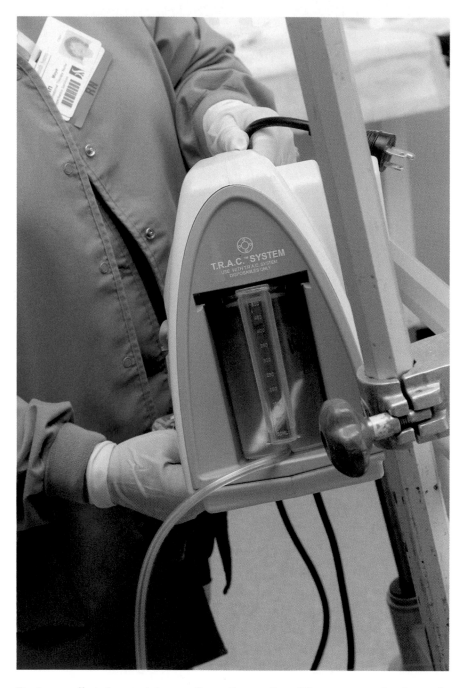

Drainage collects in a container on the suction portion of the vacuum-assisted wound device. The nurse notes the amount of output, the color, and the odor. The drainage is usually serosanguineous (pink-tinged), and not malodorous. Drainage that is tan, white, or yellow in color and malodorous may indicate the presence of an infection in the wound.

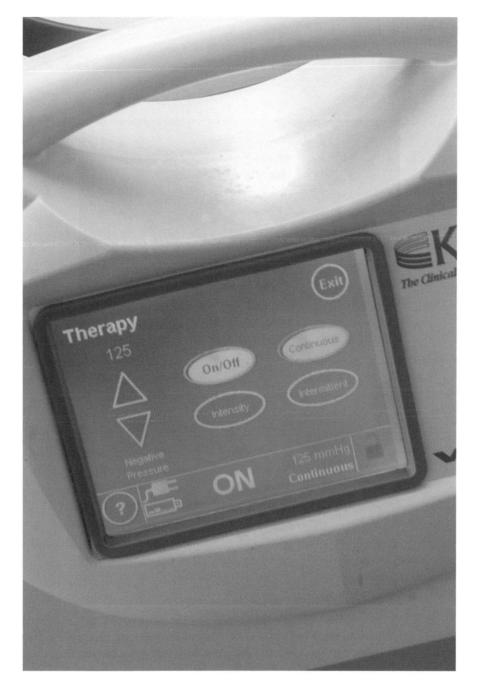

The wound vacuum device displays if negative pressure is present. It also shows the amount of pressure and if the prescribed amount of negative pressure is constant or intermittent. The settings are prescribed by the physician or wound care nurse. Negative pressure should be present at all times, except during dressing changes, to help remove drainage and promote healing. If it is not, it indicates there is an opening in the system, such as the dressing has become partially dislodged. The prescribed negative pressure is the amount of "vacuum" that aids in drawing out drainage. The amount and whether it is constant or intermittent depends on the wound size and the amount of drainage. For larger wounds with more drainage, the amount of negative pressure may be greater and constant compared to a small wound with minimal drainage that may have lower amounts of negative pressure and be intermittent.

12-lead electrocardiogram (ECG) A standardized recording of the electrical activity of the heart and may be used to detect heart irregularities, lack of oxygen to parts of the heart, and enlargement of the chambers.

A

A waves Plateau waves seen and related to severe intracranial hypertension. A waves have a range of 50 to 100 mm Hg.

abscess Collection or cavity of fluid, such as pus or cellular debris, which developed as result of an inflammatory response.

absolute hypovolemia Shock condition that occurs with the actual loss of fluid from the body including whole blood.

absorption A pharmacokinetic process that accounts for the movement of the drug from the site of administration into the bloodstream.

access Ability to obtain affordable health care when needed.

acculturation Process of learning the norms, beliefs, and behavioral expectations of a group.

acetylcholine A neurotransmitter in both the central and peripheral nervous system.

achalasia A motility disorder from failure of smooth muscle to relax or the absence of muscular contraction of the lower esophagus.

acidemia A decreased arterial pH, less than 7.35.

acne Results from thickening of the follicular opening, increased sebum production, the presence of bacteria, and the host's inflammatory response.

acquired immunity Refers to immunity that is not present at birth and develops as a result of exposure to pathogens; also called adaptive or specific immunity.

actin filaments The contractile part of a myofilament.

actinic keratoses Changes because of exposure to ultraviolet light

(sun) Considered as premalignant lesion.

active euthanasia Someone other than the patient performs an action that ends the patient's life.

acute abdomen Refers to a constellation of clinical signs and symptoms usually best treated by surgery. Abrupt onset of abdominal pain; a potential medical emergency involving one of the abdominal organs, i.e., appendicitis.

acute respiratory distress syndrome (ARDS) Classified as noncardiac pulmonary edema with disruption of the alveolar-capillary membrane due to injury to the pulmonary vasculature or the airways (formerly called adult respiratory distress syndrome).

Adams Bending Forward Test A test used to assess for scoliosis.

adaptation (adjustment) The ongoing process of modifying one's behavior in changed circumstances or in an altered environment to fulfill psychological, physiological, and social needs.

addiction A compulsive disorder in which an individual becomes preoccupied with obtaining and using a substance, the continued use of which results in a decreased quality of life.

adducts Free radicals that can bind closely with the patient's healthy tissues and create hybrid molecules.

adenoma A benign (not malignant) tumor made of epithelial cells, usually arranged like a gland.

adjuvant A remedy that enhances the effect of another therapy.

adjuvant therapy Treatment given after the primary treatment to increase the chances of a cure. Adjuvant therapy may include chemotherapy, radiation therapy, hormone therapy, or biological therapy.

adrenergic stress response The physical and psychological responses to threatening environmental stimuli and the rapid release of epinephrine (adrenalin) from the sympathetic nervous system.

adrenocorticotropic hormone (ACTH) Hormone released from the anterior pituitary that stimulates the secretion of corticosteroids by the adrenal cortex.

adult daycare Provides health, social, and recreational services to adults who require supervision during family absence.

advance directives Written documents that allow a person to state, in advance, specific decisions about how he or she wants his or her own health care managed if he or she becomes incapacitated and is unable to communicate.

adverse effects Negative response to a drug, can range from mild to life-threatening.

aerophagia Excessive amounts of air are swallowed.

affective domain Area of learning that involves attitudes, beliefs, and emotions.

afterload The load that the ventricular muscle exerts when it is pushing its contents into the aorta.

agency Capacity for intentional action.

Agency for Healthcare Research and Quality (AHRQ) A federally funded U.S. government agency established by Congress in 1989 to support research designed to improve the quality of health care, reduce its cost, improve patient safety, decrease medical errors, and broaden access to essential health care service.

ageusia Loss or impairment of taste.

agglutination Occurs when an antibody links to the same epitope on two different antigens; appears in the blood as clumping.

agranulocytosis Severe neutropenia, with less than 200 cells/μm.

airborne transmission Infectious material trapped in dust and carried on air currents.

airway pressure release ventilation (APRV) Two levels of pressures to ventilate the patient.

akinesia The loss of movement.

alaryngeal voice Alternative methods of speaking that do not include the larynx; method used by patients who have their larynx removed.

aldosterone   A mineral corticoid synthesized in the adrenal cortex; functions to maintain extracellular fluid volume.

alkalemia   An increased arterial pH, more than 7.45.

allele   One of two or more different genes containing specific inheritable characteristics that occupy corresponding positions on paired chromosomes.

allergen   A substance that induces an allergic reaction.

allogeneic   A remedy that replaces a patient's blood or bone marrow with blood or bone marrow from a donor.

allogeneic transplantation   Stem cells from a sibling or unrelated donor with matching human leukocyte antigens (HLA).

allograft   Skin graft.

allograft or homograft transplant   *See* allogenic transplantation.

allopathic   Mainstream, orthodox, conventional medical practice in the United States.

alopecia   The loss of hair.

alpha-fetoprotein (AFP)   A fetal protein produced in the yolk sac of the embryo for the first six weeks of gestation and then by the fetal liver.

altruism   Unselfish concern for the welfare of others.

amblyopia   A reduction in visual acuity caused by cerebral blockage of visual stimuli, which can develop in the eye affected by strabismus.

amenorrhea   Absence of menstruation most commonly caused by an underlying hypothalamic-pituitary-endocrine dysfunction or a congenital abnormality or acquired abnormalities of the reproductive tract.

amplification   The end result of the process in the formation of the erythrocyte whereby one rubriblast can form 14 to 16 erythrocytes.

amyloid   Extracellular protein-like substance.

anabolism   The constructive part of metabolism concerned especially with macromolecular synthesis.

analgesia   Insensitivity to pain.

anaphylaxis   Immediate, life-threatening hypersensitive allergic reaction.

anasarca   Generalized edema is associated with malnutrition, terminal illness, and metabolic fluid overload problems.

anastomosis   Surgical union of parts and especially hollow tubular parts.

androgens   The male sex hormones.

anesthesia   Absence of touch sensation.

anesthesia care provider   Anesthesiologist or nurse anesthetist who delivers anesthesia to patients in surgical settings.

aneuploid   A chromosome number that is not an exact multiple of the haploid number resulting in an extra or a missing chromosome.

aneurysm   A permanent bulging and stretching of an artery, in which the dilation is two times or greater the size of the artery.

angina pectoris   Pain in the chest.

angiogenesis   The establishment of blood supply through formation of new blood vessels.

angioneurotic edema   A condition associated with allergies and histamine release in which large welts develop below the surface of the skin, especially around the eyes and lips. The welts may also affect the hands, feet, and throat.

anion gap   The portion of negatively charged ions not measured with routine laboratory studies.

anions   Negatively charged particles.

ankle sprain   When the ankle is displaced or a sudden force is applied, the ligaments are stretched beyond their normal stretching capacity and a sprain of the ligament occurs.

annular   Ring-shaped (superficial fungal infections, such as ringworm, pityriasis rosea, seborrheic dermatitis, psoriasis, and others).

anosmia   Loss or impairment of smell.

anovulation   Failure to ovulate.

anthropophilic   Human source.

antibodies   Proteins produced by plasma cells that recognize and bind to a specific antigen.

anticipatory grieving   Intellectual and emotional responses and behaviors by which individuals work through the process of modifying self-concept based on the perception of potential loss.

anticipatory stress   A concern or worry about a potential problem or the uncertain outcome of a future event and the inability to control one's future.

anticoagulants   Pharmaceuticals that prevent further clot formation in the body.

antidiuretic hormone (ADH)   Hormone produced in the posterior pituitary and regulates the reabsorption of water in the kidneys, thereby regulating fluid volume.

antigen   A substance that stimulates an immune response.

antigen presenting cells (APCs)   Cells that ingest antigens, digest them, and display the epitope to stimulate immune response.

antineoplastic   A drug that prevents, kills, or blocks the growth and spread of cancer cells.

antiphagocytic   Something that destroys the function of the neutrophils and macrophages.

anuria   Less than 50 mL per 24 hours of urine.

aphakic vision   Absence of the crystalline lens of the eye.

aphasia   Impairment in the ability to speak or comprehend.

apheresis   Procedure that consists of withdrawal of blood from a donor, removal of one or more components (as plasma, blood platelets, or white blood cells) from the blood, and transfusion into patients with low platelet or white blood cell counts; the remaining blood is transfused back into the donor.

aphonia   Loss of voice.

aphthous stomatitis   Ulcerative conditions of the gums and mucous membranes; are labeled mouth ulcers.

apneustic breathing   A pattern of respirations characterized by a prolonged inspiratory phase, followed by expiration apnea (the rate of apneustic breathing is usually 1:5 cycles per minute).

apoptosis   An intact regulation of physiological cell death, which protects the organism from the development of a cancerous tumor.

approximated   Wound edges also called borders, or margins, that are well connected without gaps.

arcus senilis   Lipid deposition on the periphery of the cornea.

aromatherapy   The therapeutic use of concentrated essences or essential oils that have been extracted from plants and flowers to stimulate, uplift, relax, or soothe by promoting balance between the sympathetic and parasympathetic nervous systems.

arrhythmias   Deviations from normal cardiac rhythm.

arteriosclerosis   Hardening of the arteries and defined as a thickening and solidifying of the endothelial lining of the walls in small arteries and arterioles.

arthroscopy   A diagnostic test performed in the knee joint; an arthroscopy is an endoscopic procedure used to diagnose and repair meniscal, patellar, extrasynovial, and synovial diseases.

articulation   Where a bone meets another bone to form a joint.

ASA scale   Evaluation method used by anesthesiologists to determine risk of patients undergoing surgical procedures.

ascending cholangitis   An infection in the gallbladder that moves in the direction of the liver.

ascites   The accumulation of fluid in the peritoneal cavity.

asepsis   Practice of ensuring that bacteria are excluded from open sites during surgery, wound dressing, blood sampling, and other medical procedures.

assessment   The first step in the nursing process that involves the systematic collection, verification, organization, interpretation, and documentation of data for use by health care professionals.

assisted living   Provides personal, social and health care, plus 24-hour supervision.

assisted suicide   Similar to active euthanasia; often associated with a health care provider assisting another to end his or her own life.

astereognosis   Lack of ability to identify objects by touch.

astigmatism   Occurs when there is an unequal curve of the cornea and the light rays are bent unevenly.

ataxia   A lack of muscle coordination.

atherogenesis   Developmental process of the atherosclerotic lesion.

atherosclerosis   Atherosclerosis begins as fatty streaks of the arterial wall in adolescence, progressing to hard fatty plaques that narrow and "harden" the arteries lumen in adulthood.

atopic dermatitis (AD)   A hereditary and chronic skin disorder; also called eczema.

atopy   A personal or familial tendency to become sensitized and produce immunoglobulin E (IgE) antibodies in response to ordinary exposure to allergens.

atresia   Absence or closure of a natural passage of the body.

atypia   Deviation from the standard cell form.

auditory   Pertaining to the sense of hearing.

auditory learners   Style of learning in which an individual learns by hearing.

aura   Sensation that occurs immediately before a disorder, such as a migraine headache or a seizure.

auricle (pinna)   The external ear.

auscultation   Listening to sounds produced by the body, which are created by movement of air or fluid.

autoantibody   An antibody that reacts against a person's own tissue.

autograft   A permanent graft where a piece of skin from a remote unburned area of the body and transplants it to cover the burn wound.

autoimmunity   The loss of tolerance (self-tolerance) of the body's antigenic markers on cells.

autologous   The collection and storage of blood or blood components from a patient for subsequent transfusion to that same person.

autologous donation   Occurs when a patient's own blood or blood products are donated 72 hours or more prior to surgery in anticipation of the need for blood or blood product replacement during surgery.

autologous transplantation   Transplant of the patient's own stem cells.

autolytic debridement   Uses moist wound dressings maintain a natural level of moisture, facilitating a normal inflammatory response.

automaticity   When a group of cardiac cells have the ability to generate an electrical impulse spontaneously.

autonomic dysreflexia   Disordered discharge of autonomic responses, which results in massive discharge of sympathetic responses.

autonomously   Independent provision of primary health care.

autonomy   Self-rule that is free from controlling influence by others and from limitation, such as inadequate understanding.

autosomes   Any chromosome other than the sex chromosomes.

axis   The imaginary line drawn between two electrodes.

ayurveda   A healing system based on Hindu philosophy, which embraces the concept of an energy force in the body that seeks to maintain balance or harmony.

azoospermia   Absence of spermatozoa in the semen.

azotemia   A build up of nitrogenous waste products.

B

B waves   Waves seen with intracranial pressures of 20 to 50 mm Hg.

balanitis   Inflammation of the glans penis.

balanoposthitis   A condition in which posthitis occurs concurrently with balanitis.

bariatric therapy   Specialization dealing with patients who are overweight or obese.

barium   An oral preparation that allows roentgenographic visualization of the internal structures of the digestive tract.

barium enema   A rectal infusion of barium sulfate.

baroreceptors   Pressure sensitive receptors located primarily in the arch of the aorta, which sense the pressure generated in the arteries by the pumping action of the heart.

barotrauma   An injury to the lungs as a result of increased air pressure in the lungs.

basic human needs   Need that must be met for survival.

basophils   Granulocytes that attack fungi.

beneficence   Requires that actions are of benefit to others.

bereaved People mourning a loss.

bioavailability Percentage of the drug that is available to achieve its intended effect in the body.

biofeedback A mechanism of providing feedback of physiological process to help patients learn how to manipulate those responses through mental activity.

biotechnology Use of data and techniques of engineering to solve problems related to natural organisms.

Biot's (ataxic) breathing The presence of an abnormal pattern of breathing, which is characterized by totally irregular rate and depth of respirations with periods of apnea.

blepharitis Inflammation of the hair follicles (cilia) and glands along the edges of the eyelids.

blood pressure Force exerted by the blood against the walls of the blood vessel to maintain tissue perfusion during rest and activity.

body mass index (BMI) Formula using weight and height to determine the percentage of total body fat.

bone marrow aspiration and biopsy A diagnostic test used to examine the bone marrow for abnormal tissue growth or to monitor the progress of bone marrow disease.

bone scan A diagnostic nuclear scan used to detect early bone disease, bone metastasis, and bone response to therapeutic regimens.

borborygmi sounds Loud, hyperactive bowel tones.

borborygmus Hyperactive bowel sounds.

Bouchard's nodes In rheumatoid arthritis, bony enlargements of the proximal interphalangeal joints.

brachytherapy The treatment with radioactive sources placed into or near the tumor or affected area.

bradykinesia Slowness in performing spontaneous movements.

bradypnea An abnormally slow rate of breathing.

brain dead Loss of consciousness, brainstem reflexes, and respiration with essentially flat electroencephalograms.

brash water Occurs when the mouth suddenly fills with saliva; secondary to reflex salivary secretion stimulated by acid back flow into the esophagus.

breakthrough pain Acute flares of pain when medication or therapy does not relieve all of the pain.

breast augmentation Surgical enlargement of the breasts.

bronchophony The presence of distinct, clear, and relatively loud sounds heard over areas of the lung in which the normal alveoli are filled with fluid or replaced by solid tissue.

bruit An adventitious sound of venous or arterial origin heard during auscultation.

Buerger's disease An occlusive disease mostly located in small to medium-sized arteries and occasionally in veins. Though commonly found in the upper and lower distal extremities, it is associated with clot formation and fibrosis of the vessel wall. In prolonged cases, large extremities vessels may be affected.

buffy coat An area that is light-colored and contains the mostly white blood cells seen in a test tube that is centrifuged or allowed to stand.

bullae Enlarged airspaces that do not contribute to ventilation but occupy space in the chest.

bullous myringitis The presence of an infectious vesicle and inflammation of the tympanic membrane caused by the organism *Mycoplasma pneumoniae.*

burn shock Massive fluid shifts of plasma, electrolytes, and proteins into the burn wound causing the inability of the circulatory system to meet the needs of cells, tissues, and vital organs.

burrows Linear lesions produced by tunneling of animal parasite, such as in scabies.

bursae Synovial fluid-filled sacs near a joint.

C

C waves Small waves seen with pressures less than 20 mm Hg.

cachexia A breakdown of muscle mass resulting from rapid weight loss or a general wasting due to illness or stress.

calcitonin A hormone produced by the thyroid gland when circulating calcium levels are elevated.

calculi A substance of abnormal concretion composed of mineral salts commonly produced within the renal system.

cancellous Found in the ends of the long bones and in smaller amounts in some of the flat bones.

carbuncles Aggregates of infected follicles originating deep in the dermis and subcutaneous tissue.

cardiac index The patient's cardiac output divided by the patient's body surface area.

cardiac output (CO) Total blood flow through the systemic or pulmonary circulation per minute.

cardiogenic shock Shock that occurs when inadequate oxygen and nutrients are supplied to the tissues because of severe left ventricular failure.

carditis Inflammation of the heart.

caregiver role strain Caregiver's felt difficulty in performing the family caregiver role.

carrier An individual who is heterozygous for a normal gene and an abnormal gene.

casts Accumulation of materials in a space that fills the contours of the space.

catabolism Destructive metabolism involving the release of energy and resulting in the breakdown of complex materials within the organism.

cations Positively charged particles.

cell-mediated immunity Refers to immunity that is mediated by T lymphocytes.

cellular components The parts of the blood that are derived from the stem cell. These include erythrocytes, granulocytes, platelets, B lymphocytes, and T lymphocytes.

cellulitis Generalized inflammation of the deeper connective tissue.

centering Bringing body, mind, and emotions to a quiet, focused state of consciousness; being still and nonjudgmental.

centrifugal Extends outward away from the center.

cephalalgia Headache.

cerebral perfusion pressure The pressure at which cerebral tissue is perfused. It is calculated by subtracting the intracranial pressure from the mean arterial pressure.

cerebrovascular accident ([CVA] stroke) Damage to the brain due to lack of blood flow.

cerumen A thick, wax-like substance secreted by the sweat glands within the ear canal.

chakra A concentrated area of energy of which there are seven primary centers in the physical body according to Hindu belief.

cheilosis Small fissures at the corners of the mouth.

chemoembolization An embolizing drug impregnated with chemotherapy drugs to deliver a concentrated dose directly to the area close to the tumor.

chemokines Chemicals that attract other cells, particularly leukocytes.

chemotaxis Response to a chemical stimulant to attract white blood cells to a specific site.

Cheyne-Stokes breathing The presence of an abnormal pattern of breathing, characterized by alternating periods of crescendo-decrescendo depth of breathing with periods of apnea.

cholangitis Inflammation of the bile duct.

cholecystitis Inflammation of the gallbladder.

cholelithiasis Gallstones.

cholestasis Any condition that impedes bile flowing freely through the bile ducts.

cholesteatoma A cyst that contains an accumulation of squamous epithelium, keratin, and other debris.

chondrosarcoma A cartilaginous sarcoma.

chorea Abnormal and excessive involuntary movements.

chromosomes Thread-like structures within the nucleus of a cell that carry the genes.

chyme The contents of the stomach, which are semiliquid.

climacteric The perimenopausal period.

clinical decisions Decisions that promote the optimal clinical response in a patient.

clinical ethics Ethical issues that impact patient care.

clinical practice guidelines (CPGs) Systematically developed statements to assist clinicians and patients in making decisions about appropriate health care for specific clinical circumstances.

clonus A slight involuntary pushing against the foot.

closed reduction External manipulation of a fracture, which forces it into alignment.

clubbing An abnormal enlargement of the distal phalanges.

coagulopathies Disorders that lead to abnormal clotting of the blood.

Cochrane Collaboration Global nonprofit and independent collaborative founded in 1993 in the United Kingdom that disseminates evidence summaries for use by clinicians, health policy makers, and consumers of health care.

Cochrane library Subscription service repository of full text reports and abstracts of evidence summaries.

code of ethics Principles that guide professional practice.

cognitive domain Learning by understanding the material that is presented with the mind.

colectomy Surgical operation to remove all or part of the colon.

collective bargaining Process where employer and worker representatives negotiate conditions of employment.

coma depasse Irreversible coma.

comedones Plugged secretions of horny material retain within a pilo-sebaceous follicle.

compartment syndrome Swelling in the soft tissues and muscles that in turn cause compromised circulation to that area.

competence Individual's demonstrated command of a body of knowledge or skills and the ability to consistently perform to a standard and achieve a desired outcome.

complement A cascade of proteins in serum that, when activated, attract more leukocytes to the site of activation, encourage phagocytosis, and lyse pathogen cell membranes.

complementary and alternative medicine (CAM) Therapy that has a focus beyond specific symptom management.

complementary therapy Otherwise known as alternative therapy; methods of medicine that are not Western based but that offer alternative ways to accomplish health care goals. Examples include massage therapy and hypnosis.

compliance The distensibility or elasticity of the lung that decreases as lung tissue becomes stiffer.

concept map A special form or diagram used for exploring knowledge and gathering and sharing information.

concussion Mild form of brain injury.

conductivity The ability of the cardiac cells to transmit an impulse.

condyloma Genital warts caused by the human papillomavirus (HPV).

conscious sedation A drug-induced depression of consciousness during which patients respond purposefully to verbal commands, either alone or accompanied by light tactile stimulation.

consensual response Pupillary constriction on the opposite pupil.

constipation Straining at stool with the production of hard stools, decreased frequency, and a feeling of not completely evacuating the colon.

contact dermatitis An acute or chronic skin inflammation triggered in the epidermis by contact with a specific antigen or irritant.

contextual features Social, economic, and cultural factors that make each person a unique individual.

continuing care Provides ongoing care for disabilities, chronic diseases, or permanent changes in functional capacity.

continuous mandatory ventilation (CMV) Breaths are delivered at preset intervals, regardless of patient effort. This mode is used most often in the paralyzed or apneic patient because it can increase the work of breathing if respiratory effort is present.

continuous positive airway pressure (CPAP) Pressure that adds to the functional residual capacity in patients who are spontaneously breathing.

continuous quality improvement (CQI) Application of scientific process analysis methods to improve quality and productivity.

contractility The capability of muscle fibers to shrink.

contracture Shortening of a muscle.

conventional medicine The common medical practice in the United States by medical doctors, doctors of osteopathy, and their adjunct practitioners: nurses, physical therapists, and social workers.

convulsion   The abnormal motor response or jerking movements that occur during a seizure.

coping   Conscious or unconscious methods used to deal with, and attempt to overcome, problems and difficulties such as stressful events, violence, and illness.

coping efficacy   Perceived effectiveness of the coping effort to manage a stressful event.

cor pulmonale   Hypertrophy or failure of the right ventricle resulting from disorders of the lungs, pulmonary vessels, or chest wall.

corneal reflex   Stimulation of the trigeminal nerve (cranial nerve V) causes this protective blink.

coronary artery bypass grafting (CABG)   A surgery where veins and arteries are used as conduit to bypass the coronary artery stenosis.

coronavirus   A virus that normally only leads to upper respiratory infection.

cortical or compact (bone)   The hard outer layer of bone surfaces.

corticosteroids   Any of the hormones, except androgen, synthesized by the adrenal cortex.

cortisol   A major glucocorticoid that functions in the regulation of blood glucose levels.

cough   To expel air from the lungs suddenly and noisily to keep the respiratory passages free from irritating material.

counterpulsation   The synchronization of the intra-aortic balloon pump to assist the heart according to the cardiac cycle.

crash cart   Mobile cart with defibrillator, resuscitation equipment, and medications used when patients go into cardiac arrest.

crepitus   A crinkly, crackling, or grating feeling or sound in the joints, skin, or lungs.

critical access hospital (CAH)   Provides outpatient, emergency, and inpatient services in a rural area.

critical incident   A patient or event that causes a stress reaction in the health care worker.

cryopexy   Freezing of the retinal tear area.

cryotherapy   The use of ice or cold water over an injury site to decrease inflammation.

cultural assimilation   Individuals from a minority group are absorbed by the dominant culture and take on the characteristics of the dominant culture.

cultural awareness   A conscious learning process in which people become appreciative of and sensitive to the cultures of others.

cultural competence   The complex integration of knowledge, attitudes, and skills that enable the nurse to provide culturally appropriate health care.

cultural context   Environment or situation that is relevant to the care, beliefs, values, and practices of the culture under study.

cultural diversity   The difference among people that results from ethnic, racial, and cultural variables.

cultural encounter   The process that encourages individuals to engage directly in cross-cultural interactions with people from culturally diverse backgrounds.

cultural knowledge   The process of understanding the vital aspects of a groups' culture as it relates to health and health care practices.

cultural skill   The ability to collect relevant cultural data regarding health histories and performing culturally specific assessments.

culture   The knowledge, values, beliefs, art, morals, law, customs, and habits of the members of a society.

culture for caring   Ideas, customs, skills, and arts of a work group that are transferred, communicated, or passed along to succeeding generations of health care workers.

Cushing response   A late sign of increasing intracranial pressure with signs of slowing respirations, slowing heart rate, and increasing blood pressure.

cystectomy   Removal of the bladder.

cytokines   Chemicals that affect the way other cells behave.

cytotoxic (killer) T cells   Lymphocytes that lyse host cells infected with a virus; also called CD8 T cells.

D

dactylitis   An inflammatory affection of the fingers.

dead space   That portion of ventilation that does not participate in gas exchange.

debridement   A mechanical method of eliminating necrotic tissue.

deep partial-thickness burn   Also called second-degree burn; a burn that involves the entire epidermis and the lower two thirds of the dermis.

deep sedation/analgesia   A drug-induced depression of consciousness during which patients cannot be easily aroused but respond purposefully following repeated or painful stimulation.

deep vein thrombosis (DVT)   A blood clot in a deep vein that accompanies an artery.

defibrillation   Delivering an electrical shock to the heart so that it completely depolarizes the cardiac cells in an effort to terminate ventricular fibrillation.

dehiscence   The separation of a wound or scar. A rupture or splitting open, as of a surgical wound or of an organ or structure to discharge its contents as splitting open.

deletion   The loss of varying amounts of genetic material that is detectable at the DNA or chromosomal level.

demargination   A process whereby the granulocytes can suddenly leave the peripheral tissues.

dendritic cells   Large phagocytic antigen presenting cells that activate T cells.

deontology   Philosophy concerned with the moral duty and obligation of an action rather than the action's outcome.

deoxyribonucleic acid (DNA)   The molecular basis of heredity, consisting of purine and pyrimidine nucleotides arranged in two long strands, twisted about each other to form a double helix.

depolarization   Electrical changing in the interior of an excitable cell from negative to positive, which results in an action potential.

dermatomal   Localized into a dermatome supplied by one or more dorsal ganglia (herpes zoster and segmental vitiligo).

dermatome   The body region supplied by a pair of a dorsal root ganglia.

detumescence   The process that occurs following orgasm where the blood flow decreases and the vasocongestion is relieved.

diabetes mellitus   A chronic metabolic disorder characterized by hyperglycemia (elevated blood sugar levels) related to a lack of insulin, lack of effects of insulin, or a combination.

diapedesis   Cells squeeze through pores in capillary wall.

diaphoresis   Profuse sweating.

diarrhea   An increase in the liquid state of the stool.

diastolic blood pressure   Phase in the cardiac cycle when the heart is at rest.

didelphic   Duplication; usually refers to two uteri, two cervices, and two vaginas.

differentiation   A process involving constant turnover of new cells of the epidermis.

diffusion   The movement of solutes from an area of high concentration to an area of low concentration.

dimorphic   Existing in two shapes or forms.

diploid   Two complete sets of chromosomes, double the number present in gametes (ova or sperm cells). In humans, the diploid number is 46.

diplopia   Double vision.

direct calorimetry   A measurement of energy expended by measuring temperature changes in a closed structure.

direct contact transmission   Body surface to body surface contact.

direct response   Pupillary constriction on the pupil being tested.

directed or controlled coughing   Cough technique to expectorate sputum and avoid fatigue associated with undirected, forceful coughing that consists of slow, maximal inspiration followed by breath holding for several seconds and then two or three coughs.

disaccharides   A class of sugars, which yields two monosaccharide molecules through hydrolysis.

disease prevention or health protection   Behavior motivated by a desire to actively avoid illness, detect it early, or maintain functioning within the constraints of an illness.

disequilibrium   An imbalance in solute concentration across the blood brain barrier.

displaced fracture   A fracture in which the bones have gone out of natural alignment.

disseminated   Spread over a large area of the body, tissue, or organ.

disseminated intravascular coagulation (DIC)   Clotting and bleeding disorder that results from the generation of tissue factor activity within the blood. This trigger of the coagulation cascade quickly leads to significant thrombin production, which perpetuates its own formation and results in bleeding.

distress   Stressor that is perceived as negative or stress that produces a negative response; a certain level of negative stress is needed for growth and development.

distribution   The movement of the drug, after absorption into the bloodstream, to the site of intended action.

diverticula   Sac-like outpouches of mucosa through the muscular layer of the bowel.

diverticulosis   When there are multiple infected diverticula that result in pathology.

do not resuscitate (DNR)   A health care provider's order that there be no attempt to restart a failed heartbeat or apply cardiopulmonary resuscitation.

domains of nursing   The four main areas of nurses' practice, which includes clinical practice, education, administrative practice, and research.

dominant culture   Group whose values prevail within a society.

double effect   Palliative therapy, itself, hastens death.

drawer test   An assessment technique used to diagnose rupture of cruciate ligaments.

Dressler's syndrome   Inflammation of the pericardium that can occur 2 to 10 weeks after a myocardial infarction.

droplet transmission   Particles propelled through the air.

dual energy X-ray absorptiometry (DEXA) scans   Diagnostic tests that assist with the early diagnosis of osteoporosis.

Durable Power of Attorney for Health Care (DPAHC)   Advance directive that appoints an agent or proxy decision maker to make health care decisions for a person who has lost decisional capacity.

dysarthria   Difficulty in oral movement to form words.

dyscrasia   Nonspecific term for blood disease.

dysdiadochokinesia   The inability to perform rapidly alternating movements.

dysesthesia   Burning or tingling.

dysfunctional uterine bleeding (DUB)   Abnormal uterine bleeding not caused by malignancy, inflammation, or pregnancy.

dysgeusia   Disturbed sense of taste.

dysmenorrhea   Pain associated with menstruation.

dysmetria   Impaired judgment of distance, range, speed, and force of movement.

dyspareunia   Painful intercourse.

dyspepsia   An uncomfortable feeling in the upper abdominal region.

dysphagia   Difficulty swallowing.

dyspnea   Difficulty breathing.

dysrhythmia   A disturbance in rhythm.

dyssynergy   A lack of coordinated muscle movement.

dysthymia   A low-level depression that can last at least two years, and if left untreated, can lead to more severe depression.

dysuria   Painful urination.

E

echocardiogram   A noninvasive test in which ultrasound is used to reflect cardiac structures. It can be performed at rest or in conjunction with a stress test.

ectopy   Heartbeat arising from a location other than the sinoatrial node on a monitor screen.

ectropion   When the lower eyelid is turned away from the globe of the eye.

eczematoid   Lesion suggesting inflammation with tendency to thickening, oozing, vesiculation, or crusting (related to eczema).

edema   An abnormal collection of fluid in the interstitial spaces between cells resulting in a lifting and separating of the layers of the skin.

effluent   Waste materials.

egophony   The presence of loud, nasal, and "bleating" sounds when auscultating the lungs.

ejection fraction (EF)   An index that estimates contractile function of the left ventricle. The expected ejection fraction is 60 to 70 percent.

electrolytes   Charged particles found in body fluids.

emboli   A blood clot or other particle (plaque) that break loose and block blood vessels.

embolization   Introduction of an angio catheter to visualize the internal spermatic vein, to correct dysfunction of the spermatic vein.

emmetropia   In normal vision the light falls onto the retina without any distortion or abnormal bending of the light.

empowerment   To assist or encourage a person to be involved in decision making and development of the plan of care; the ability to assume self-care management.

endemic   Restricted to a particular region, community, or group of people.

endocarditis   Inflammation of the endocardium.

endocardium   The membrane that lines the cavities of the heart and forms part of the heart valves.

endocrine glands   Those glands that produce hormones that are secreted into the bloodstream and travel to their target organs or tissues.

endogenous   Produced or originating from within a cell or organism.

endometriosis   Ectopic growth of functioning endometrial tissue.

endorphins   Peptides secreted in the brain that boost mood and help fight depression and pain.

endothelium   The layer that lines the blood and lymphatic vessels, the heart, and various other body cavities is a prominent contributor to the activation of the inflammatory immune response. Cells produce several compounds that affect the vascular lumen and platelets.

endotracheal intubation   The passage of tube into the trachea through either the mouth or nares to maintain an open airway or facilitate mechanical ventilation.

enterokinase   An enzyme that hastens effective digestion.

enterprises   Organized systems of any size in any location that provide any type of health care for compensation.

enthesitis   Traumatic disease occurring at the insertion of muscles where recurring concentration of muscle stress provokes inflammation with a tendency toward fibrosis and calcification.

entropia   An eye that deviates inward.

entropion   When the lower eyelid is turned in toward the globe of the eye.

enucleation   Surgical removal of an eye.

environmental control   Relationships between people and nature and a person's perceived ability to control activities of nature.

enzymatic debridement   Accomplished using a chemical debriding agent.

eosinophil   A granulocyte that helps to control the inflammatory process.

epidemiological investigation   Study looking at a specific disease, its distribution, and initial source.

epididymitis   Infection of the epididymis.

epilepsy   Chronic recurrent pattern of seizures.

epiphyses   The widened ends of the long bone.

epispadias   The urinary meatus is located along the superior (upper) aspect of the penis.

equianalgesia   The provision of equal analgesic effects in changing from one drug and/or delivery method to another or choosing a different delivery method.

ergonomics   Science that seeks to adapt work or working conditions to suit the worker.

erythromelalgia   A burning sensation in the digits of the extremities.

erythropoietic   Relating to the formation of red blood cells.

erythropoietin (EPO)   A hormone produced by the kidney in response to low oxygen states or a low hematocrit, which stimulates red blood cell production in the bone marrow.

eschar   Burned skin that is dead and must be removed before healing can occur.

escharotomy   Incision through full-thickness circumferential burn tissue

to restore and maintain circulation or chest expansion.

esotropia   Convergent strabismus.

ethics   The study of philosophical ideals of right and wrong behavior.

ethics of care   Belief that health care professionals have a moral obligation and duty to provide care to those in need.

ethnicity   A cultural group's perception of themselves (group identity). This self-perception influences how the group's members are perceived by others.

ethnocentrism   Belief that one's own culture is superior to all others.

eugenics   The selection and recombination of genes already existing in the gene pool.

euglycemia   A normal concentration of glucose in the blood.

euploidy   A term referring to the correct number of chromosomes in a cell.

eupnea   The presence of normal respirations, or normal rate and depth of breathing.

eustachian tube   A tube that connects the middle ear to the nasopharynx.

eustress   A certain level of positive stress that is needed for growth and survival.

euthanasia   Practice in which a person other than the patient directly administers medication that causes the death of a patient.

euthenics (euphenics)   The techniques for correcting defects in individuals after they have been born.

euthyroid   Having a normal functioning thyroid gland.

evidence-based practice (EBP)   Process through which scientific evidence is identified, appraised, and applied in health care interventions.

evidence summary   Report of the state of scientifically produced knowledge that is developed using rigorous methods to synthesize knowledge across a number of research studies so that study variations and contradictory study results can be understood in a single conclusion statement.

Ewing's sarcoma   A diffuse endothelioma or endothelial myeloma forming a fusiform swelling on a long bone.

exacerbation A sudden increase in the seriousness of the disease with greater intensity in signs and symptoms, which lasts from minutes to hours or days.

exanthema Breaking out in a rash.

excitability The capacity for that cell to depolarize in response to an electrical impulse.

exocrine glands Those glands that secrete substances into ducts that empty into a body cavity or onto a body surface.

exogenous Originating outside an organ.

exotropia (wall eyes) An eye that deviates outward.

expiratory reserve volume (ERV) The maximal amount of gas that can be expired at the end of a normal exhalation.

expressive aphasia (Broca's aphasia) A condition in which a patient cannot express what he or she wants to say.

extracellular fluid (ECF) The fluid located between cells and includes interstitial and intravascular fluid.

extravasation The inadvertent administration of vesicant into the surrounding tissues.

extrinsic distortion Occurs when the interpreter is improperly prepared.

exudate Accumulated fluid in a vity.

F

fascia An inelastic connective tissue that covers and separates muscles, tendons, and ligaments.

fasciotomy Incision through a fibrous layer that separates muscles.

fast pain (rapid pain) Pain that originates in the free endings of the large myelinated nerve fibers of the skin; such pain respond to strong pressure and high temperature, thus eliciting the withdrawal reflex.

fecalith Hard mass of fecal material.

fibroadenomas Benign fibrous growths or tumors of the glandular epithelium in breast tissue.

fibromyalgia A disorder characterized by muscle pain, stiffness, and easy fatigability.

first pass effect After absorption, oral drugs are transported via hepatic portal circulation to the liver, where they are metabolized (broken down) before they can pass into the general circulation.

flatulence Gas formed within the gastrointestinal tract and expelled via the rectum.

foam cell Engorged lipid-laden macrophages that are the major component of the fatty streak.

focused assessment An assessment that is limited in scope to focus on a particular need or health care problem or potential health care risk.

folliculitis Acute inflammation of the hair follicle caused by physical irritation, infection, or chemical irritation.

fracture A break in a bone.

fremitus The feeling of vibration, which will be increased or decreased in certain conditions.

fulguration Destruction of tissue using high-frequency electric sparks.

full-thickness burn Also called third-degree burn; involves the entire epidermis and dermis that extends to subcutaneous tissue and possibly muscle and bone.

furuncles (boils) Localized bacterial infections that can manifest as painful, indurated, or fluctuant, fluid-filled masses.

G

galactorrhea Excessive secretion of milk.

gametes A mature male or female reproductive cell.

gender identity The biological sex of male, female, or intersexed.

gender role The masculine or feminine role adopted by a person, which is often culturally and socially determined.

gene A segment of a DNA molecule that is the heredity unit that occupies a fixed chromosomal locus.

gene therapy The process of treating or curing a genetic disorder by providing the affected individual with an intact, functional copy of the gene in question.

general inhibition syndrome (GIS) "Possum" response to stress because of overstimulation of the parasympathetic nervous system (PNS) as a means of survival or a paralyzing or numbing effect when facing a life-threatening event; a state of panic or freezing.

genetic counseling The interaction between health care provider and patient to manage the human problems associated with the occurrence, or risk of occurrence, of a genetic disorder in a family.

genetic engineering Changing a particular molecule in the structure of the gene, either to eliminate a certain bad trait or to improve the genotype.

genetic screening Population screening for a genetic variation or mutation, for example, PKU screening at birth.

genetic testing Testing of an individual at significant risk because of family history or because of presentation of symptoms, for example chromosome abnormalities.

genogram A family tree related to health history.

genomics The study of genome composition, structure, and function in combination with environmental factors that has led to the discovery of numerous health care products.

genotype The genetic constitution or blueprint of an individual, the gene pairs that are inherited from the parents.

global aphasia A condition in which a patient has both expressive and receptive aphasia.

globalization Organized or established worldwide.

glossitis An inflammation of the tongue.

glucagon A hormone released from the pancreas in response to low levels of blood glucose and is a counterregulatory hormone.

gluconeogenesis The process of the liver converting predominant amino acids to glucose in the fasting state.

glycogen hydrolysis Conversion of stored glycogen into usable glucose to meet the immediate energy needs of the body.

glycogen synthesis Conversion of glucose to glycogen that can be stored in preparation of times of fasting.

glycogenolysis The physiological process of the breakdown of stored glucose to raise blood sugar levels.

grading The degree of malignancy or cell differentiation of the tumor cells.

granulocytes Class of leukocytes with prominent granules.

granuloma A mass of inflamed granulation tissue.

graphesthesia Identify letters, numbers, or shapes drawn on hand.

grief resolution An adjustment to actual or impending loss.

gross domestic product (GDP) Total value of final goods and services produced in a year within the United States.

growth hormone (GH) Hormone that affects all tissues of the body, is secreted from anterior pituitary, and is one of the counterregulatory hormones.

gynecomastia Breast enlargement in men.

H

half-life The time required for the body, tissue, or organ to metabolize or make inactive half the amount of a substance taken in.

haploid One complete set of chromosomes. The haploid number in humans is 23.

haptens An antigen that does not cause an immune response unless bound to a carrier molecule.

harvesting A procedure to collect tissue such as the spongy bone marrow from inside bones containing stem cells.

healing touch (HT) An energy-based therapeutic therapy that alters the energy field through the use of touch.

health A state and a process of being and becoming an integrated and whole person.

health care Care related to all states of health from severe illness and injury to supreme good health; diagnosis and treatment of disease and strategies that maintain and improve health.

health care system Network of individuals, technologies, and processes that provide and support health care.

health insurance Insurance policy that provides payment for benefits of a covered sickness or injury. Included under this definition are various types of insurances, such as accident insurance, disability insurance, medical expense insurance, and accidental death insurance.

health maintenance Behavior directed toward maintaining a current level of health.

health maintenance activities The activities or behaviors an individual performs to maintain or improve a current level of health.

health maintenance organizations (HMOs) Type of managed care plan where access to care is controlled by a primary care provider and coverage is limited to the approved medical services, administered by a network of health care providers, hospitals, skilled nursing facilities, and other providers included in the plan. Emphasis is on prevention.

health promotion Process undertaken to increase levels of wellness in individuals, families, and communities.

heartburn (pyrosis) A substernal burning sensation often radiating to the neck that is experienced within one hour of eating or one to two hours after reclining.

Heberden's nodes Hard nodules or enlargements of the tubercles of the last phalanges of the fingers.

Heinz bodies Degraded hemoglobin.

helper T cells Lymphocytes that orchestrate the immune response; also called CD4 T cells. There are two subclasses TH1 and TH2.

hemarthrosis Untreated bleeding into the joint.

hematochezia Stools containing red blood rather than tarry stools.

hematoma Excessive bleeding that occurs around a wound site as a result of broken blood vessels from trauma or surgery.

hematomas A swelling noted in tissue, caused by extravasated blood.

hematopoiesis The ability to maintain the body's blood supply and its components.

hematopoietic Pertaining to the formation of blood or blood.

hematuria Blood in the urine.

hemiparesis Weakness on one side of the body.

hemiplegia Inability to move of one side of the body.

hemoglobinuria Hemoglobin in the urine.

hemolysis Destruction of red blood cells.

hemoptysis Indicates either the presence of frank blood or blood-streaked sputum.

hemorrhagic stroke When a blood vessel bursts leaking blood into brain tissue or surrounding spaces.

hemosiderosis A condition in which iron is toxic to the cells.

hemovac A type of surgical drain with a piece that connects to a mechanical suction device.

hepatomegaly Enlarged liver, palpated below the level of the ribs.

hereditary angioedema (HAE) An inherited abnormality of the immune system that causes swelling, particularly of the face, and abdominal cramping.

heterograft (xenograft) A graft of skin obtained from another species.

high-density lipoprotein (HDL) The substance that transports plasma cholesterol away from atherosclerotic plaques and to the liver for metabolism and excretion and is considered "good" cholesterol because increased levels decrease the tendency to CAD.

high efficiency particulate air (HEPA) filter Filter used to remove submicron particulate matter from the air.

hirsutism Condition characterized by the excessive growth of hair or the presence of hair in abnormal places.

histamine A chemical released by the immune system during allergic reactions.

histocompatibility leukocyte antigens (HLA) A complex set of proteins on the surface membrane of human nucleated cells, tissues, and blood cells (except red blood cells).

holism The concept that the whole is greater than the sum of its parts. Holism encompasses consideration of the physiological, psychological, sociocultural, intellectual, and spiritual aspects of each individual.

Homans' sign Dorsiflexing the foot, causing pain in the calf.

homeopathy Treatment of disease with minute drug doses to activate an illness that then stimulates the body's normal defense system to eliminate illness.

homeostasis Physiological and psychological equilibrium or balance.

homograft A graft of skin obtained from a cadaver 6 to 24 hours after death that is used as a temporary graft.

homonymous hemianopsia Inability to see out of one half of both eyes, and the visual field cut.

hope A feeling expressed as future-oriented, which allows the person to set goals, devise strategies for achieving the desired goals, and a sense of being in control.

hormones The chemicals produced and stored by the endocrine system that help regulate metabolism and energy, cardiac output and blood pressure, reproduction, and growth and development.

hospice Provides end-of-life care for patients and their families.

hospice care Coordinated program of palliative care services with a goal of attaining the highest possible quality of life for patients and their families at the end of life and continuing through the bereavement period.

human leukocyte antigen (HLA) MHC class I.

humectants Substances that promote moisture in skin.

humoral-mediated immunity Refers to immunity that is mediated by B lymphocytes, plasma cells, and antibodies.

hyaline Cartilage that covers the end of each bone to reduce friction and distribute weight-bearing forces.

hydronephrosis Dilation of the renal pelvis because of an obstruction of urine flow or from ureteral reflux.

hypalgesia Diminished sensitivity to pain.

hyperalgesia (allodynia) A state of neural supersensitivity where a slight painful stimulus can be interpreted as very painful.

hypercapnia An accumulation of $PaCO_2$ in the blood, indicating hypoventilation.

hypercholesterolemia High serum cholesterol.

hyperesthesia Increased sensitivity of the skin.

hypergesia Increased sensitivity to pain.

hyperglycemia An elevated blood sugar level.

hyperlipidemia Elevated blood cholesterol levels.

hyperopia (farsightedness) Occurs when the light passing through the eye is focused behind the retina when looking a close objects.

hyperplasia Increase in number.

hypersensitive response An extreme physical response to an allergen, in which large amounts of IgE are produced.

hypertension Sustained elevation of blood pressure.

hypertonic A solution with a concentration higher than that of blood.

hypertrophic Increase in size of an organ or structure secondary to inflammation or overgrowth of cells not related to tumor formation.

hypertrophy Abnormal enlargement, increase in size and mass, of a body part or organ.

hyperuricemia An abnormal amount of uric acid in the urine.

hypervolemia Excess intravascular fluid.

hypesthesia Diminished sense of touch.

hypoalbuminemia Decrease in albumin in the blood.

hypocapnia Less than normal $PaCO_2$ in the blood, indicating hyperventilation.

hypogeusia Diminished taste sensitivity.

hypokyphosis Less than normal curvature in the thoracic spine.

hypospadias The urinary meatus is located along the inferior (lower) aspect of the penis.

hypotany Low intraocular pressure.

hypotension Blood pressure lower than needed for adequate tissue perfusion and oxygenation.

hypothermia Condition where the body temperature falls to less than 36° C (96.8° F). It is classified as mild, if not less than 32° C (89.6° F).

hypotonic A solution with a concentration less than that of blood.

hypovolemia Insufficient intravascular fluid.

hypoxemia A decrease in PaO_2 below 80 mm Hg.

hypoxia A general term for decrease in tissue oxygenation.

I

icterus Yellow coloration in the sclera of the eye.

idiopathic A disease state that arises from an unknown cause.

idiopathic pain Spontaneous or unpredictable breakthrough pain.

ileus Refers to intestinal obstruction because of a partial or complete arrest of intestinal peristalsis; also known as paralytic or adynamic ileus.

illness care Care aimed at relieving the discomfort of disease.

imagery The use of one's sense to create an image in one's mind.

immune response A body response to an antigen that occurs when lymphocytes identify the antigenic molecule as foreign and induce the formation of antibodies and lymphocytes capable of reacting with it and rendering it harmless.

immunity The quality or state of being immune; a condition of being able to resist a particular disease through preventing development of a pathogenic microorganism or by counteracting the effects of its products.

immunodeficiency Inability to produce a normal complement of antibodies or immunologically sensitized T cells especially in response to specific antigens.

immunogen A particle that can cause an immune response.

immunoglobulins (IG) The class of proteins that antibodies belong to. Body manufactures five isotopes: IgM, IgD, IgG, IgA, and IgE.

immunotherapy The process of introducing allergens to the body by injection for the purpose of increasing immunity.

imperforate hymen Congenital malformation of the hymenal ring resulting in lack of a vaginal opening.

inborn error of metabolism A condition in which the metabolism of an organism is abnormal because of the presence of one, or a pair of, abnormal alleles.

incentive spirometer A machine used to allow patients a quantifiable aid in deep breathing postoperatively.

incidence The number of new cases of a condition, symptom, death, or injury that arise during a specific period of time such as a month or a year.

indirect calorimetry A method for estimating energy expenditure by measuring oxygen consumption and carbon dioxide production.

indirect contact transmission Inanimate object involved in transfer.

infertility The inability to conceive within one year when a couple is engaging in unprotected sexual intercourse at the appropriate times in the female's menstrual cycle.

infiltration Inadvertent administration of a solution into the surrounding tissues.

inflammation A nonspecific response to any foreign invader involving the immune system.

inflammatory immune response (IIR) A response that is composed of several body systems that are constantly on alert to detect nonself and harmful intruders from the normal cells and proteins in the body.

informed consent A patient's authorization for care based on full disclosure of risks, benefits, alternatives, and consequences of refusal.

innate immunity Immunity that is inherent within a species and develops regardless of exposure.

inspection Careful, systematic visual observation.

inspiratory reserve volume (IRV) The maximal amount of gas that can be inspired at the end of a normal inspiration.

insulin Hormone produced by the beta cells of the pancreas to lower blood glucose levels.

integrated care delivery system Network of organizations that provides a coordinated continuum of services to a defined population and that is willing to be held clinically and fiscally accountable for the outcomes and health status of the population served.

integrative review Alternative term for an evidence summary.

integrative therapy Therapy that combines conventional medical therapies with complementary alternative medicine (CAM) therapies for which there is some high-quality scientific evidence of safety and effectiveness.

interdisciplinary team Clearly defined group of members of specific disciplines who work collaboratively to develop a coordinated plan of care.

interferons (IFNs) Proteins formed when cells are exposed to invaders such as viruses that are able to activate other components of the immune system.

interleukins (IL) Generic name for cytokines released by leukocytes.

interstitial fluid The fluid located between cells.

interstitial space The area surrounding the nephron loops and the peritubular capillaries, which has a high osmotic pressure due to extremely high levels of sodium. The renal interstitial space facilitates the massive volume water reabsorption required to maintain fluid balance.

intra-aortic balloon pump A catheter with an oblong balloon on the end that eases the workload on the patient's heart by decreasing afterload and coronary perfusion.

intracellular fluid (ICF) The fluid located inside each cell.

intracranial pressure (ICP) The amount of pressure placed on the structures within the brain.

intractable pain Pain that is refractory or resistant to some or all forms of treatment.

intradermal route An injection into the skin.

intraductal papilloma Small benign tumor that grows within the terminal portion of a solitary milk duct of the breast.

intraoperative The operative period from entry into the operating suite through departure from the post-anesthesia care unit (PACU).

intrarenal Occurring within the kidney.

intrathecal Within the spinal canal, the space between the double-layered covering or lining of the brain and spinal cord.

intravascular fluid The fluid located inside the blood vessels, excluding the fluid inside the cells in the blood vessels.

intrinsic distortion Occurs when information is passed on from one person to another through an interpreter.

intussusception Invagination, or telescoping, of one part of the intestine into itself.

inverse ratio ventilation Ventilating the patient with a longer inspiratory time as compared to the expiratory time.

inversion stress test A physical examination test used to assess for ankle joint laxity. It is performed by bracing the heel with left hand, inverting the foot with right hand, and comparing to the opposite side.

ischemic stroke Damage to the brain due to a clogged artery.

isokinetic Exercise involving resistance through full range of movement.

isotonic Solution that has the same osmotic pressure as the referent solution (e.g., plasma).

J

jaundice Yellow pigmentation of the skin and sclera.

joint aspiration A procedure performed to examine the synovial fluid in the joint cavity and to relieve pain in the joint resulting from edema and effusion.

Joint Commission on Accreditation of Hospitals (JCAHO) An independent, not-for-profit organization that sets standards for measuring health care quality. Accredited hospitals receive an on-site review every three years.

justice Requires that like cases are treated in like fashion.

K

karyotype A photomicrograph of the chromosomes of an individual that have been arranged in the standard classifications system by group and size.

keratinization A process that is used by epidermal tissue to replenish itself.

keratitis Inflammation of the cornea.

keratometry Measurement of the cornea.

kernicterus Yellow discoloration and degenerative lesions in the central nervous system causing brain damage.

kinesthesia The ability to perceive the movement of one's body.

kinesthetic learners Learning style in which a person processes information by experiencing the information or by touching and feeling.

knowledge transformation Five sequential steps that convert primary research knowledge to evidence that a specific health care intervention achieves positive clinical outcomes.

Kupffer cells Specialized reticulo-endothelial cells of the liver, which belong to the monocyte-macrophage system.

Kussmaul breathing The presence of abnormally deep and rapid respirations, with the presence of a fruity odor to the breath.

kyphoscoliosis A combination of kyphosis and scoliosis.

kyphosis An exaggeration of thoracic spine convexity.

L

labyrinth A complex, closed, fluid-filled system of interconnecting tubes in the inner ear.

lacunae Reservoirs in which the mature bone cells are embedded.

lamellar bone The thin layer of mature bone tissue.

laminar airflow Filtered air circulating in parallel-flowing planes.

lancinating Stabbing or piercing.

laparoscopic cholecystectomy A surgical procedure using a laparoscope to remove the gallbladder.

laparoscopy A diagnostic procedure where the peritoneal cavity (pelvis and abdomen) are examined.

laparotomy Surgical incision made in the wall of the abdomen.

lateral epicondylitis Pain over the lateral epicondyle of the humerus or head of the radius. Also called tennis elbow.

latex allergy An immediate type of hypersensitive reaction to latex exposure.

lavage The irrigation (wash out) of the stomach contents.

learning Process of assimilating information with a resultant change in behavior.

learning plateaus Peaks in effectiveness of teaching and depth of learning.

learning style Way in which an individual incorporates new information.

leiomyomata Benign smooth muscle tumors of the uterus commonly called fibroids.

length of stay (LOS) Length of time a patient remains hospitalized, an outcome variable that refers to the efficiency of a health care delivery system.

lentigines Flat brown spots seen on aged exposed skin.

lesions Circumscribed altered area of tissue that should be treated as abnormal finding.

leukapheresis The removal of blood to collect specific blood cells; the remaining blood is returned to the body.

leukocytes General name for all white blood cells.

leukopenia A decrease in the total circulating white blood cells.

Levine's sign Clenched fist over the chest is the universal sign for angina.

liberty Independent from coercion.

lichenification Thickening of the epidermis.

ligaments Strong bands of connective tissue that attach bone to bone or bone to cartilage.

lipodystrophy A localized complication of insulin administration characterized by changes in the subcutaneous fat at the site of the injection.

liver lobule The functional unit of the liver.

liver sweats The movement of plasma from the lymphatic system into this potential space in the abdomen.

living will (LW) Advance directive that allows a person to document specifically what medical treatment they wish, or do not wish, to have.

locus The position of a gene on a chromosome.

long-term care Extended assistance for the chronically ill, mentally ill, or disabled.

low-density lipoprotein (LDL) The main lipid component of the atherosclerotic plaque and is considered "bad" cholesterol because increased levels reflect increased tendency to CAD.

lower motor neuron Motor pathway that originates in the spinal cord and

continues on as spinal nerves sending impulses to the peripheral areas of the body.

lumpectomy Wide local excision or partial mastectomy that involves excision of all cancerous tissue to microscopically clean margins.

lymphadenopathy Painless lymph node enlargements from obstruction and pressure.

lymphocytes Primary cells in the immune response.

M

macronutrients Carbohydrate, protein, and lipids.

macrophages Phagocytic cells found in tissues.

macules Flat circumscribed changes of the skin (flat nevi, café au lait spots, vitiligo, telangiectases or capillary hemangiomas).

macular rash A rash with flat red spots.

major surgery Operations that involve risk to life in some way, such as those involving multiple systems, or that require long periods of time in the operating suite.

malaise Body discomfort and fatigue.

malignant Cells that invade and destroy nearby tissues and spread to other parts of the body.

malignant hyperthermia (MH) Life-threatening, acute pharmacogenic disorder, developing during or after a general anesthesia.

malrotation Failure during embryonic development of normal rotation of all or part of an organ or system.

mammary duct ectasia Noncancerous condition of the breast in which the milk ducts beneath the nipple become dilated and sometimes inflamed.

mammoplasty Surgical procedure to increase or decrease the size or shape of the breast.

managed care organizations (MCOs) Groups implementing health care using managed care concepts including pre-authorization of treatment, utilization review, and a fixed network of care providers.

mandatory minute ventilation (MMV) A mode of ventilation that allows the ventilator to adjust its breaths based on the patient's minute ventilation.

mass casualty incident (MCI) An influx of patients that overwhelms a hospital and affects its capability to care for patients.

mastalgia Breast pain.

mastitis Inflammation or infection of the breast.

mastodynia Breast pain.

mastoidectomy An incision of the mastoid sinuses.

mastoiditis Infectious process of the mastoid sinuses.

mechanical debridement Uses gauze dressings to remove necrotic or devitalized tissue from wounds.

mechanical ventilation A means of providing ventilatory assistance by a mechanical device.

mechanism of injury The manner in which an injury occurs.

Medicaid Program that pays for medical assistance for certain individuals with low income and resources. It is jointly funded by federal and state governments.

medical futility When a particular therapy offers no medical benefit.

Medicare National health insurance program for people age 65 years and older, people under aged 65 with disabilities, and people with end-stage renal disease. Medicare provides coverage to approximately 40 million Americans.

Medicare Hospice Benefit Reimbursement benefit provided by the federal government for hospice services.

meditation A mind-body technique by which an individual can consciously quiet the mind by focusing one's attention in order to control some functions of the sympathetic nervous system.

meiosis A series of two specialized divisions of diploid germ cells to produce four gametes containing the haploid number of chromosomes.

menarche Initial menstrual period, normally occurring between 9 and 17 years of age.

menopause Permanent cessation of menstrual activity, usually occurring between 35 and 55 years of age.

menorrhagia Cyclic menstrual bleeding that is abnormally long or heavy.

menstrual cycle Periodically recurring series of changes associated with uterine endometrial growth in preparation for fertilization and shedding of endometrium when fertilization has not occurred.

meta analysis Statistical procedure used to summarize the results of research across multiple research reports.

metabolic syndrome Diagnosed when three or more factors such as high blood pressure, abdominal obesity, high triglyceride levels, low high-density lipoprotein (HDL) cholesterol and high fasting blood glucose levels are present.

metabolism or biotransformation Biotransformation process in which the drug is broken down by enzymes to a form that can be excreted from the body. The primary organ of metabolism is the liver. The chemical changes in living cells by which energy is provided for vital processes and activities, and new material is assimilated.

metastasis Spread of cancerous tumor to other distant locations.

metrorrhagia Bleeding at times other than normal menstrual cycle.

microtrauma Trauma to muscles, tendons, ligaments, and bones on a microscopic level.

minimal sedation (anxiolysis) Drug-induced state during which patients respond normally to verbal commands. Although cognitive function and coordination may be impaired, ventilatory and cardiovascular functions are unaffected.

minor surgery Operations that do not involve risk to life in some way, such as those that involve one system that can be done in a short period of time or can be performed in a health care provider's office.

minority group Ethnic, racial, or religious group that constitutes less than a numerical majority of the total population.

mitigation Activities a hospital undertakes to help lessen the severity and impact of potential emergencies that may affect operations or services provided by a hospital.

mitosis Somatic cell division resulting in the formation of two cells, each

with the same chromosome complement as the parent cell.

mitral facies A florid appearance with cyanosed cheeks.

mixed venous oxygen saturation (SvO$_2$) A measurement of the amount of hemoglobin saturated with oxygen compared to the total amount of hemoglobin in the pulmonary artery.

modulation Alteration in the level of pain intensity (by either increasing or inhibiting it), including the processing of incoming impulses from the sensory nerve to the dorsal horn of the spinal cord; modulation also occurs via descending messages originating in the midbrain and sent to the dorsal horn.

monoclonal antibodies Genetically engineered immunosuppressive agents that are used in combination with other drugs to prevent graft rejection.

monocytes Phagocytic cells found in the blood.

monosaccharides Simple sugar molecules not decomposable by hydrolysis.

moral distress Occurs in response to awareness of the right and moral action, coupled with inability to carry out that action.

morals Customs or habits that are ethically correct.

morbidity The number of ill persons in relationship to a specific population.

mortality The ratio of the number of deaths in a given population.

mosaicism Tissue composed of cells of two different genotypes or karyotypes.

motivation The internal drive or externally arising stimulus to action or thought.

mucositis An inflammation and ulceration of the lining of the mouth, throat, or gastrointestinal (GI) tract most commonly associated with chemotherapy or radiotherapy for cancer.

Müllerian dysgenesis Malformation of the embryonic duct that becomes the fallopian tubes, uterus, and vagina.

multiple organ dysfunction syndrome (MODS) Evidence of a progressive inflammatory response has caused more than one of the body's organs to fail. The presence of altered organ function in an acutely ill patient such that homeostasis cannot be maintained without intervention.

Murphy's sign Pain on deep inspiration when an inflamed gallbladder is palpated by pressing the fingers under the rib cage.

music-thanatology A holistic and palliative method for using music to help dissipate obstacles to patients' peaceful transition to death.

mutation A permanent change in genetic material.

myalgia Pain in the muscles.

myectomy Excision of a portion of the muscle.

myelogram A diagnostic test used to determine defects in and around the spinal column.

myelosuppression A decrease in the production of red blood cells, platelets, and some white blood cells by the bone marrow. Also, inhibition of the production of blood cells, a bone marrow function.

myocardial infarction (MI) Prolonged ischemia, 20 minutes or more, that results in myocardial cellular death.

myocarditis An inflammation of the myocardium.

myoclonus Twitching or clonic spasms of a muscle or group of muscles.

myomectomy Surgical removal of fibroid tumors in the wall of the uterus.

myopia (nearsightedness) Occurs when the light passing through the eye is overbent or overrefracted.

myosin The protein that compose the thick filaments of a myofibril.

myotonia Tonic spasm of a muscle or temporary rigidity.

myringoplasty Plastic surgery of the tympanic membrane.

myringotomy Incision into the tympanic membrane.

N

nadir The period of time following chemotherapy, usually 7 to 10 days after chemotherapy, when blood counts drop, thereby increasing susceptibility to infection or bleeding.

narrative review Less rigorous form of summary process used in nursing.

nasal airway A soft, flexible tube that is inserted into the nasal passage to maintain an open airway.

National Guideline Clearinghouse Searchable database of nearly 1,500 clinical practice guidelines.

native kidney One's own kidney as opposed to a transplant graft.

negative feedback Response of a gland by increasing or decreasing the secretion of a hormone.

neoadjuvant Adjunctive or adjuvant therapy given prior to the primary (main) therapy.

neoangiogenesis Development of new blood vessels.

neoplasm An abnormal mass of cells, can be benign or malignant.

nephrectomy Surgical removal of the kidney.

nephritis Infection contained to the kidney.

nephrolithiasis Kidney stone disease.

nephropathy Disease of the kidneys.

nephrotoxic Having the ability to harm the kidney.

neuralgia Pain associated with peripheral nerves, which follows the course of nerves.

neuropathies Dysfunctions of the peripheral nervous system.

neuropeptides Amino acids produced in the brain and other sites in the body that act as chemical communicators.

neurotransmitters Chemical substances produced by the body that facilitate nerve impulse transmission.

neutropenia A decreased number of circulating neutrophils, usually less than 1,500 cells/μm.

neutrophils Chief phagocytic cell of early inflammatory response.

nociceptive pain Pain that occurs when there is normal processing of the pain impulse.

nociceptor A free nerve endings that is a receptor for painful (noxious) stimuli. Nociceptors are found in almost all types of tissue.

nocturia Urination at night.

nodules Circumscribed elevated, usually solid lesions (fibromas, neuro-fibromas, xanthomas, erythema nodosum, and various benign or malignant growths).

nonmaleficence Use of ability, judgment, or skill to help someone else without intent to cause injury or harm.

normovolemia State of normal blood volume.

nosocomial Infection acquired in a health care facility.

nuchal A stiff painful neck due to irritated meninges.

nutraceuticals Any natural substance found in plant or animal foods that acts as a protective or healing agent.

nystagmus An involuntary rhythmic movement of the eyes in a back and forth or cyclical movement.

O

objective data Data that are observable and measurable.

occult fracture A fracture that does not show up on plain radiographic films until the healing process begins and calcification is seen.

odynophagia Pain that is experienced when a person swallows.

oligomenorrhea Menstrual cycles occurring farther apart than usual.

oligospermic Having low sperm motility with a low semen volume.

oliguria Low urine output.

oncogenes Cancer susceptibility genes. When altered or mutated proto-oncogenes promote tumor formation or growth.

oncotic pressure Osmotic pressure because of proteins.

onycholysis The loosening of the nails starting at the border.

oocytes The early or primitive ovum before it has developed completely.

opportunistic Organism causing disease in a host whose resistance to fight infection is diminished.

oppression Rules, modes, and ideals of one group are imposed on another group.

opsonization A process that coats a foreign substance and makes it more susceptible to phagocytosis.

oral airway A stiff plastic tube that prevents the tongue from sliding back into the pharynx and blocking the airway.

orchitis Acute inflammation of the testes.

orthostatic hypotension Hypotension occurring when changing position from supine to upright.

osmolality   The number of solutes per kilogram of fluid.

osmolarity   The number of solutes per liter of fluid.

osmosis   The movement of water from an area of low concentration of solutes (low osmolality) to an area of high concentration of solutes (high osmolality).

osmotic pressure   The ability of a solution to draw fluid across a semipermeable membrane.

ossicles   Three tiny bones (in the middle ear) that play a crucial role in the transmission of sound.

osteoarthritis (OA)   Noninflammatory degenerative joint disease characterized by degeneration of the articular cartilage, hypertrophy of bone at the margins, and changes in the synovial membrane.

osteogenesis   The process of bone formation and remodeling.

osteomalacia   A condition marked by softening of the bones with pain, tenderness, muscular weakness, anorexia, and loss of weight, resulting from deficiency of vitamin D and calcium.

osteomyelitis   Inflammation of the bone caused by a pyogenic organism.

osteopenia   A significant amount of decrease in bone mineral density.

osteoporosis   A reduction in the amount of bone mass, leading to fractures after minimal trauma.

osteosarcoma   Malignant tumor of bone.

ostomy   A surgically created opening made between the intestine and the abdominal wall.

otalgia   Ear pain.

otitis media   An inflammation of the middle ear.

otorrhea   Liquid discharge or drainage from the ear.

otosclerosis   A progressive hearing loss of predominately low tones.

ototoxic   A substance that damages the acoustic nerve or hearing mechanism.

outcome variables   Consequences of care delivery categorized as humanistic, financial, and clinical.

overuse syndrome   An injury to musculoskeletal tissues affecting the upper extremity or cervical spine, resulting from repeated movement, temperature extremes, overuse, incorrect posture, or sustained force or vibration. Also called repetitive motion injuries or cumulative trauma disorders.

ovulation   Periodic maturation and release of an ovum from a follicle on the ovary.

oxyhemoglobin dissociation curve   A relationship between the partial pressure of oxygen in the blood and the saturation of hemoglobin with oxygen.

P

P wave   Graphic representation of atrial depolarization.

Paget's mammary disease   Uncommon skin cancer characterized by a chronic eczema-like rash of the nipple and adjacent areolar skin.

pain   An unpleasant sensory and emotional experience arising from actual or potential tissue damage or described in terms of such damage.

pain scales   scales used to quantify patient's pain so that consistent relief measures can be taken.

pain threshold   The lowest intensity of a painful stimulus perceived by the individual as pain.

pain tolerance   The degree of pain that an individual is willing to endure.

palliation   The process of easing symptoms and maximizing quality of life when cure or control is not possible.

palliative care   Active total care of patients whose disease is not responsive to curative treatment.

palpation   The use of the sense of touch to assess texture, temperature, moisture, organ location and size, vibrations and pulsations, swelling, masses, and tenderness.

palpebrae   Eyelids that cover and protect the eyes by covering the anterior aspect of the eyes.

panhypopituitarism   Defective or absence of function of the entire pituitary gland.

papillary reflex   Stimulation of cranial nerve II that causes direct and consensual reactions to light.

papilledema   A swelling of the optic disc.

papules   Elevated circumscribed lesions (elevated nevi, verrucae, molluscum contagiosum, and individual lesions of lichen planus).

paracentesis   The aspiration of fluid from the abdominal cavity.

paraphimosis   The entrapment of the retracted foreskin behind the glans penis of an uncircumcised male.

paraplegia   Paralysis involving the lower extremities.

parathyroid hormone (PTH)   Hormone that is secreted by the parathyroids and is not controlled by the pituitary and hypothalamus but by negative feedback.

parenchyma   Functional elements of an organ.

paresthesia   Numbness, tingling, or prickling sensation.

parity   The number of viable births.

passive euthanasia   Omission of an action, thereby allowing death to occur.

patient controlled analgesia (PCA)   Devices that can be used by the patient to deliver pain medications (usually via intravenous [IV] route) as needed.

peak drug level   Time it takes for the drug to reach its highest concentration in the blood.

pediculosis   Infection by human lice.

pediculosis pubis   Infection in pubic area by lice.

pedigrees   Diagrammatic representations of a family history indicating the affected individuals and their relationship to proband or index case.

percent solution   A measure of parts per hundred.

perception   A person's sense and understanding of the world.

percussion   Short tapping strokes on the surface of the skin to create vibrations of underlying organs.

percutaneous coronary interventions (PCI)   Category of procedures performed during the cardiac angiography using catheters, balloons, and devices to treat atherosclerotic lesions (e.g., percutaneous transluminal coronary angioplasty [PTCA]).

perfusion   The exchange of oxygen and carbon dioxide at the alveolar-capillary level.

pericarditis   An inflammation of the pericardium.

pericardium A double-layered serous membrane that surrounds the heart.

periductal mastitis Inflammation of the breast that can occur in nonlactating older women.

perimenopause Five- to 10-year period before menopause.

perinephric Surrounding the kidney.

perioperative Inclusive term to denote preoperative, intraoperative, and postoperative periods.

periosteum The outer portion of the cortical bone that supplies nutrients and a blood supply to the bone.

peripheral vascular resistance (PVR) The pressure against the flow of blood to or from the arteries or veins outside the chest.

peristalsis Successive waves of involuntary contraction passing along the walls of a hollow muscular structure (as the esophagus or intestine) and forcing the contents onward.

petechiae Small, pinpoint hemorrhages.

phagocytosis Process by which foreign substances are ingested and destroyed.

Phalen's maneuver A physical test involving flexion of the fully extended hand at the wrist to aid in the diagnosis of carpal tunnel syndrome.

phantom limb sensation When the patient has the perception of a limb that is no longer there. If the patient feels pain it is known as phantom limb pain.

pharmaceutic Phase that an oral drug disintegrates and dissolves into a form that can be used by the body.

pharmacodynamics Phase that describes the biochemical and physiological effects the drug has on the body.

pharmacogenomics The study of how an individual's genetic inheritance affects the body's response to drugs.

pharmacokinetics Phase that describes how drugs are acted on in the body from ingestion to elimination, includes the processes of absorption, distribution, metabolism (biotransformation), and excretion.

pharmacology The scientific study of drugs and their origins, actions on, and interactions with, living things through chemical processes.

phenotype The physical, biochemical, and physiological nature of an individual as determined by the genotype and the environment. It is the outward expression of the individual's genes.

philosophy Statement of beliefs that is the foundation for one's thoughts and actions.

phimosis The inability of the foreskin to be stretched and retracted over the glans of the penis.

phlebitis Inflammation of a vein.

phlebostatic axis Location at the midpoint of the anterior and posterior chest at the fourth intercostal space. This is the point at which transducers should be leveled for hemodynamic parameters.

photoaging Degenerative changes in connective tissue caused by chronic exposure to ultraviolet A (UVA).

photoallergic Sensitivity to light that causes allergic reactions.

photochemotherapy UVA therapy combined with oral or topical 8-methoxypsoralen.

phototherapy The treatment of certain dermatological conditions with artificially produced, nonionizing UV light.

phototoxic Rapidly developing non-immunologic skin reaction when exposed to light.

physical dependence Body is dependent on a substance and abrupt cessation or reduction in the dose may result in withdrawal symptoms.

physician-assisted suicide Medical hastening of death by a physician in consultation with a terminally ill patient.

phytonutrients Chemicals found in plants that act as protective or healing agents.

pica Craving for substances other than food, such as dirt, clay, starch, or ice cubes.

pigmentation Color of the skin (produced by melanocytes in the epidermis).

plaques Elevated disc-shaped lesions (psoriasis, lichen simplex or chronicus neurodermatitis).

plasma The liquid portion of the circulation system.

plasma half-life (t $_{1/2}$) The time required to eliminate one half of the ingested medication after administration.

plasmapheresis (plasma exchange) Plasma is removed from the patient and replaced with the fresh frozen plasma.

pleuritic chest pain Discomfort detected on expiration or inspiration caused by an inflammation of the lining of the lungs.

pneumothorax A collection of air in the pleural cavity may occur as a result of trauma, tuberculosis, or chronic respiratory diseases. This collection of air leads to a collapse of all or part of a lung.

polycystic cysts Cysts with closed sacs that develop abnormally within an organ and have a distinct enclosing membrane.

polycythemia An abnormal increase in the number of red blood cells.

polypharmacy Situation in which multiple drugs are prescribed to treat a variety of conditions.

positive end expiratory pressure (PEEP) A ventilator setting that adds pressure at the end of expiration to keep alveoli open and enable gas exchange.

posthitis Inflammation of the foreskin.

postoperative Takes the patient from the time of departing from the surgical suite through the length of their hospital stay and beyond.

postrenal Occurring after the kidney.

posttraumatic stress disorder (PTSD) A psychological reaction that occurs after experiencing a highly stressing event, such as wartime combat, physical violence, or a natural disaster.

Power of Attorney for Health Care Legal document that allows the patient to choose a person called a health care proxy or agent to make decisions about the patient's medical care when the patient is unable to do so for himself or herself.

PR interval An estimate of the amount of time it takes the impulse to travel from the SA node through the AV node, the bundle of His, and the main part of the left bundle branch.

prana The life force of the Indian culture that is believed to fill the body with a vital energy.

preferred provider organization (PPO) Type of managed care plan in which members receive more coverage if they choose health care providers approved by or affiliated with the plan.

preload The amount the myocardial fibers are stretched at the end of diastole. This stretch reflects the amount of pressure and volume in the ventricle immediately preceding systole.

preoperative Prior to the intraoperative period or events leading up to entry into the surgical suite.

preparedness Activities that build the hospital's capacity to manage the effects of an emergency or disaster.

prerenal Occurring prior to the kidney.

presbyopia A loss of near acuity (near vision) as the lens loses its elasticity and accommodation of the lens fails.

presbyphagia Dysphagia in the elderly.

prevalence The number of current cases of a disease in a specific population at a given time period.

preventive care Focuses on health promotion, including educational and preventive programs designed to promote healthy lifestyles.

priapism The presence of a prolonged, often painful, penile erection.

primary amenorrhea Failure of the menstrual cycles to begin.

primary anorgasmia Never having achieved orgasm.

primary brain tumor The growth originated in the brain or central nervous system.

primary care Basic, routine health care.

primary immune response Occurs when an antigen is initially introduced into the system. It involves both mast cell degranulation and activation of plasma proteins, i.e., complement, clotting factors, and kinin (polypeptides that increase blood flow and permeability of small blood capillaries).

primary intention Utilizes normal repair processes.

primary multiple organ dysfunction Directly related to an insult, such as a major trauma.

prions Protein-containing infectious agents.

process variables Refers to how care is provided, under what circumstances, and how patients are moved into, through, and out of the health care system.

proctocolectomy Surgical removal of the rectum together with part or all of the colon.

prodrome phase The beginning clinical manifestations that a person has for an upcoming illness.

prolactin A hormone from the anterior pituitary that stimulates the breast to cause lactation.

prophylactic Preventing or contributing to the prevention of disease.

proprioception Awareness and coordination of movement and position of the body, head, and limbs.

proptosis Forward placement of the eye.

prostatitis Inflammation of the prostate gland.

prosthesis A replacement of a missing body part, such as an extremity.

protein binding Process in which the drug, once absorbed into the bloodstream, attaches itself to a protein molecule (usually albumin) to be transported to it site of action.

proteinuria Increase in protein in the urine.

pruritus Dermatological symptom described as itching and a desire to scratch.

psoriasis T cell–mediated inflammatory disease characterized by epidermal hyperplasia (overproduction of epidermal tissue) usually localized in certain regions of the body.

psychomotor domain Area of learning that involves performance of motor skills.

psychoneuroimmunoendocrinology (PNIE) A multidisciplinary paradigm involving mind-body medicine that emerged in 1955, and is sometimes referred to as psychoneuroimmunology.

psychoneuroimmunology (PNI) An emerging field of science that studies the complex relationship between the mind and body, specifically the cognitive/affective system in the brain, the neurological system, and the immune system.

ptosis Drooping of the eyelid.

pulmonary artery (PA) catheter A long balloon-tipped catheter that is positioned in the pulmonary artery and monitors different pressures in the heart.

pulse pressure Difference between systolic and diastolic blood pressure.

pulsus alternans Alternating weak and strong heart beats.

pulsus paradoxus Pathological decrease in systolic blood pressure by 10 mm Hg or more on inspiration.

Purkinje fibers Conductive fibers that help to spread the electrical impulses of throughout the ventricular muscle. They have an inherent rate of 15 to 40 beats per minute.

purulent Containing the detritus of white blood cell activity within an infectious process usually.

purulent sputum A light green to yellowish white fluid formed in infected tissue and consists of white blood cells, cellular debris, and necrotic or dead tissue.

pustules Circumscribed elevations containing purulent exudates (pustular psoriasis, bromoderma or small pox).

pyelonephritis Infection of the ureters and kidney.

pyrosis A substernal burning sensation often radiating to the neck; commonly called heartburn.

Q

QRS complex Graphic representation of ventricular depolarization.

QT interval Graphic representation of the amount of time it takes for ventricular depolarization and repolarization.

quadriplegia (tetraplegia) Paralysis involving upper and lower extremities.

R

race A grouping of people based on biological similarities.

racism Form of oppression defined as discrimination directed toward individuals who are misperceived to be inferior because of biological differences.

radiculopathy A term used to specifically describe pain and other symptoms, like numbness, tingling, and weakness, in arms or legs that are caused by a problem with nerve roots.

radioisotope A compound that contains radioactive materials that are used in nuclear scans; the activity of these tagged materials allows the study of substances as they course through the body.

radiotherapy The use of X-rays and other forms of radiation in treatment.

Raynaud's disease Venous disease caused by unilateral vasospasm of the upper and lower extremities. Bilateral vasospasm is identified as Raynaud's disease, usually occurs in the age group over 30 and is equally distributed between genders.

rebound hypertension Rapid increase in blood pressure after abrupt stopping of medication.

receptive aphasia (Wernicke's aphasia) A condition in which a patient is unable to understand what is being said or what is written.

receptor Site on the cell membrane that can be occupied by a drug to cause an effect within the body.

recessive trait A trait that is expressed only when an individual is homozygous for that specific gene.

referred pain The transfer of visceral pain sensations and deep somatic pain via the autonomic nervous system to a body surface at a distance from the actual origin.

refractory ascites Ascites that cannot be effectively managed with normal therapies.

regeneration Replacement of damaged or lost tissue with more of the same tissue. Only the epidermis and superficial dermis are capable of regeneration.

relative hypovolemia A shifting of fluid from the intravascular space to the extravascular space that can result from a loss of intravascular integrity, increased capillary permeability, or a decreased colloidal osmotic pressure.

relaxation response A state of increased arousal of the parasympathetic nervous system, which leads to a relaxed physiological state.

remodeling A continuously occurring process in the bone that maintains the structure and integrity of the bone.

remote assessment Use of technology such as video links or teleconferencing to allow for health care personnel and patients to transmit assessment information over long distances.

renal Pertaining to the kidney.

renal parenchyma The cortex and medulla of the kidney that contain the functioning units and collecting ducts of the kidney.

repolarization Electrical change in the interior of an excitable cell following depolarization in which the inside of the cell becomes more negatively charged.

residual volume (RV) The amount remaining in the lungs and airways after a maximal expiration.

resilience Dynamic process that involves protective factors such as effective problem-solving strategies and adaptability to situations that the person cannot control or change.

resorption The removal of bone tissue by normal physiological process or as part of a pathological process, such as an infection.

resting energy expenditure A measurement of resting metabolic rate expressed as kilocalories per 24 hours.

restorative care Follow-up postoperative care, home care, and rehabilitation.

reticuloendothethial (RE) system Phagocytic system composed of monocytes and macrophages.

retroperitoneal space The space between the peritoneum (the membranous sac that surrounds the organs of the abdominal cavity) and the posterior abdominal wall that contains the kidneys and associated structures, the pancreas, part of the aorta, and inferior vena cava.

review of literature Less rigorous form of summary process used in nursing.

review of systems (ROS) A brief account from a patient of any recent signs of symptoms associated with any of the body systems.

rhabdomyolysis Destruction of skeletal muscle cells that causes the release of myoglobin.

rhinitis A seasonal or year-round immunoglobulin E (IgE)-mediated inflammation of the nasal mucosa; may be infectious, inflammatory, or allergic in nature.

rhinitis medicamentosa Rebound congestion of the nasal mucous membranes caused by overuse of decongestant nasal sprays.

rhinorrhea Thin, watery discharge from the nose.

rhonchi Bubbling or gurgling sounds heard primarily on expiration and indicate fluid in the larger airways.

RICE The acronym used for Rest, Ice, Compression, and Elevation when treating a sprain.

right to die Belief that humans have a basic right to die.

rights-based ethics Proscribes that there are specific human rights to specific human goods.

rigors A muscular tremor caused by a chill.

rotator cuff tears Refers to tears in one or more of the four muscles that form a single tendon in the shoulder. The rotator cuff is responsible for circumduction and internal and external rotation of the shoulder.

rye ergot A fungus from the rye plant causing hallucinations, gastrointestinal upset, and a form of gangrene if ingested.

S

SA node Primary pacemaker of the heart with an inherent rate of 60 to 100 beats per minute.

sacroilitis Inflammation of the sacroiliac joint.

sarcoma A form of cancer that arises in the supportive tissues such as bone, cartilage, fat, or muscle.

sarcomere The contractile unit of the muscle.

sarcopenia Age-related decreases in muscle mass.

schistocytes Fragmented red blood cells.

Schwartze's sign Rosy or reddish-blue color of the tympanic membrane related to vascular changes.

science The most reliable source of knowledge on which to base clinical decisions.

science of research synthesis Field of science that generates evidence summaries to provide state-of-the-science conclusions about knowledge thus far developed.

scoliometer An instrument for measuring curves, especially those in lateral curvature of the spine.

scoliosis An abnormal lateral curvature of the spine.

secondary amenorrhea Cessation of the menstrual cycles after they are established in the absence of pregnancy.

secondary anorgasmia Loss of the ability to achieve orgasm in a woman who was previously orgasmic.

secondary intention Heals by spread of granulation.

secondary multiple organ dysfunction The result of failure of organs that were not affected by the initial insult.

secondary or specific antibody response Includes the activation of B cells and the memory cells (IgG, IgM, IgA, and IgE); and activation of T cells, cytotoxic (killer) cells, lymphokine-producing cells, helper cells, and suppressor cells.

sedation Reduction of anxiety, stress, irritability, or excitement by the administration of a sedative agent or drug.

seizure Brief episode of abnormal electrical activity in the brain.

self-efficacy Perceived capability of mastering difficult situations and the ability to actively control one's own destiny; closely linked to a positive self-esteem and internal locus of control.

self-monitoring of blood glucose (SMBG) A method whereby a patient tests his or her own blood glucose levels.

semipermeable membranes Separation between two areas that allows movement of some fluids or solutes.

sepsis A systemic inflammatory response to an infection.

sequela Any abnormality following or resulting from a disease or injury or treatment.

serum The liquid part of blood after coagulation.

serum sickness A type III hypersensitivity reaction that results from the injection of heterologous or foreign protein or serum.

sex roles Culturally determined patterns associated with being male or female.

sexual dysfunction Unsatisfactory enjoyment of sex or inability to participate in sexual intimacy as desired because of multiple causes, including lack of sexual interest, impaired sexual arousal (erectile dysfunction in the male, lack of lubrication in the female), or inability to achieve orgasm.

sexuality Human characteristic that refers not just to gender but to all the aspects of being male or female, including feelings, attitudes, beliefs, and behavior.

shaman A folk healer priest who uses natural and supernatural forces to heal others, has an extensive knowledge of herbs, is skilled in many forms of healing, and serves as guardian of the spirits.

shamanism A form of spiritual healing that refers to the practice of entering altered states of consciousness with the intent of helping others to enhance healing and well-being. The shaman connects with spiritual guides and seeks healing on behalf of others.

shock syndrome A systemic condition when the peripheral blood flow is inadequate to provide sufficient blood to the heart for normal function and transport of oxygen to all organs and tissues.

short stay surgery Usually preplanned, nonemergency procedures with an expected hospital or surgical center stay of less than 23 hours.

shunting That portion of the cardiac output that does not exchange with alveolar air.

side effects Expected physiological effects of a drug that are not related to the desired drug effect.

sinusoids Specialized capillaries found only in the liver and are identified by specific types of cells.

slow pain Pain originating in the endings of the smaller unmyelinated nerves that has a throbbing or aching quality.

social support The person's perception of, and the degree of satisfaction with, support systems.

solutes Particles contained within the fluid that contribute to the concentration or osmolality of the fluid.

somatic (parietal) pain Pain that originates from the bone, joints, muscles, skin, or connective tissue. Sharp or knife-like in character, usually precisely located to the affected areas.

somesthesia Awareness of body; derived from the Greek words meaning body and sensation.

somnolence Prolonged drowsiness or sleepiness.

spermatocelectomy Surgical removal of the spermatocele.

spermatogenesis Formation of mature functional spermatozoa from the testes, usually beginning during puberty and continuing throughout the life of the adult male.

spinal shock A loss of all motor and sensory function, generally occurring after spinal cord injury.

spirituality Relationship with one's self, a sense of connection with others, and a relationship with a higher power or divine source.

sports medicine The application of professional knowledge to the understanding, prevention, treatment, and rehabilitation of sports- and exercise-related problems.

staging The extent or spread of the tumor within the body from the site of origin.

standard precautions Actions to be used with all patients to reduce risk of transmission of disease.

stapedectomy Removal of the stapes and replacing the stapes with a prosthetic device.

state-of-the-science review Less rigorous form of summary process used in nursing.

status asthmaticus Severe and persistent asthma that does not respond to conventional therapy and that may lead to respiratory failure.

steatorrhea Pale-yellow, greasy, fatty stool, or chronic watery diarrhea.

stereognosis Identify objects by touch.

stereotactic radiotherapy (SRS) Noninvasive use of computers and radiation to target tumor cells within the brain.

stereotyping Expectation that all people within the same racial, ethnic, or cultural group act alike and share the same beliefs and attitudes.

stomatitis The inflammation of the soft tissues in the mouth resulting in mouth sores. It is a common side effect of chemotherapy, radiation therapy, and some biological therapy.

strabismus (tropia) When one muscle is weak resulting in one eye deviating from the other when the eyes are focused on an object.

stress The body's reaction to any stimulus.

stridor Inspiratory wheezing.

structural variables Organizational features or participant characteristics that have an impact on organizational performance.

stye (hordeolum) A localized inflammatory swelling of one or more of the glands of the eyelid.

subarachnoid hemorrhage Blood that leaks into the subarachnoid space.

subclavian steal syndrome Occurs when the subclavian artery is occluded, and blood flow is diminished or obstructed to the upper extremities.

subculture Group of people within the dominant group who are functionally unified by factors, such as status, ethnic background, residence, religion, or education and whose experiences differ from those of the dominant group.

subjective data Data from the patient's point of view that may include feelings, perceptions, and concerns.

superficial burn Also called a first-degree burn; it only involves the epidural layer of the skin.

superficial partial-thickness burn Also called a second-degree burn; it involves the entire epidermis and the upper third of the dermis.

supernumerary nipples Small dark spots on the chest that may indicate undeveloped nipples and areola.

suppurative cholangitis A condition when pus is produced in the biliary tract.

surrogate decision maker Agent or proxy who is legally able to make health care decisions for another who has lost the capacity to do so for himself or herself.

sycosis Inflammation of the entire hair follicle.

sycosis barbae Inflammation of the entire hair follicle that is traumatized by shaving.

synchronized cardioversion Delivering an electrical shock to the heart that is synchronized to the patient's R wave.

synchronized intermittent mandatory ventilation (SIMV) The ventilator delivers preset breaths in coordination with the respiratory effort of the patient. Spontaneous breathing is allowed between breaths.

syndrome X Classic angina symptoms without angiographic evidence of CAD.

syndrome X (insulin resistance syndrome) A group of abnormalities of metabolism that act together to increase the risk of cardiovascular disease.

synergy model Combination of factors that each multiplies the effects of the other(s), rather than merely adding to them.

syngeneic transplant Blood or tissue donated by an identical twin.

synovium A fibrous envelope that produces a fluid to help to reduce friction and wear in a joint.

system Set of parts linked in orderly and logical interdependence that function together as a synergistic unit.

systematic review Newer term for an evidence summary.

systemic inflammatory response syndrome (SIRS) Widespread uncontrolled acute inflammatory response to a severe insult.

systolic blood pressure Blood pressure measured at the moment of contraction.

T

T wave Graphic representation of ventricular repolarization.

tachypnea An abnormally rapid rate of breathing.

Tao Traditional spiritual belief system of the Chinese. The belief that everything is the Tao, and the Tao is everything leads to the understanding of oneness in all things in nature.

target tissues Tissues or organs in the body that are affected by specific hormones.

teaching Active process in which one individual shares information with another as a means to facilitate behavioral changes.

teaching-learning process Planned interaction that promotes a behavioral change that is not a result of maturation or coincidence.

teaching strategies Techniques employed by the teacher to promote learning.

telangiectasia Dilatation of small blood vessels on the cheeks, nose, and ears, as well as pigmental changes, such as freckles from exposure to sun light.

teleology Evaluation of final causes.

tendons Connect muscle to bone and allow bone to move once the muscle has contracted.

tendosynovial Pertaining to the tendon insertion in the joint near the synovial membrane.

tenesmus Distressing but ineffectual urge to evacuate the rectum.

teratogens Agents that produces or increases the incidence of congenital malformations.

terminal illness One in which there is no possibility for a cure, resulting in the decline of the patient's physical condition and then death.

tertiary care Includes acute and complex interventions.

tertiary intention Wound requires suturing of granulation layers.

testicular self-examination (TSE) A method of a male assessing his testicles for any changes as a preventive measure against testicular cancer.

thenar Refers to the palm of the hand or the sole of the foot.

therapeutic range Serum drug level that lies between the minimum effective concentration and the toxic concentration. Level to be maintained to achieve desired affects and avoid symptoms of toxicity.

therapeutic touch (TT) Assessing alterations in a person's energy field and using a hand to direct energy to achieve a balanced energy state.

thermoregulation A patient's status in relation to internal temperature control.

third spacing The accumulation of fluid in the extracellular and intracellular spaces and in a third body, such as the intestine, that does not support circulation.

thrombophlebitis The inflammation of a vein accompanied by the formation of thrombus (blood clot), which can be dislodged and lead to pulmonary emboli. Deep vein thrombosis (DVT) is a term often used for this venous complication, which most commonly occurs in the deep veins of the lower extremities.

thrombus Blood clot that blocks a blood vessel.

thyroid-releasing hormone (TRH) The hormone that stimulates the anterior pituitary to release TSH.

thyroid-stimulating hormone (TSH) A hormone produced from the anterior pituitary that regulates the function of the thyroid.

thyroxine (T_4) The most abundant thyroid hormone; makes up approximately 90 percent of the thyroid hormone secretion.

tic douloureux Trigeminal neuralgia; dysfunction causing pain along the pathway of the fifth cranial nerve.

tidal volume (Vt) The amount of air in and out of the lungs with a normal breath.

tineas Fungal infections.

Tinel's sign A tingling sensation produced by pressing on or tapping the nerve that has been damaged or is regenerating following trauma.

tinnitus A ringing, buzzing, or jingling sound in the ear.

tolerance Occurs when a higher dose of a drug (e.g., an opioid) is required to achieve the desired effect.

tophus A chalky deposit of sodium urate occurring in gout, tophi forms most often around joints in cartilage, bone, bursae, and subcutaneous tissue and in the external ear, producing a chronic foreign body inflammatory response.

total parenteral nutrition (TPN) The intravenous (IV) administration of nutrients to patients through a central venous catheter.

total quality management (TQM) Structured systematic process for organizational planning and implementation of CQI.

toxoid A toxin that has had the active portion removed but can still be recognized by the immune system.

trabecular The porous cavity found inside the compact bone.

tracheostomy Operation of cutting into the trachea usually for insertion of a tube to overcome tracheal obstruction.

tracheostomy tube A tube placed by surgical incision into the trachea and secured by sutures to maintain an open airway or facilitate long-term mechanical ventilation.

transcellular fluid Fluid that is in neither the intracellular nor extracellular space, and includes cerebrospinal fluid, joint fluid, and the fluid within the gastrointestinal tract.

transduction The initiation of the pain stimulus.

transient ischemic attack (TIA) Temporary loss of blood flow to the brain that results in temporary loss of function.

translocation The transfer of a segment of one chromosome to a nonhomologous chromosome. When no material is lost or gained, the translocation is said to be balanced.

transmission The process of carrying the pain information along the axon of a sensory nerve to the CNS.

transmission routes Ways by which microorganisms reach the body.

tremor Rhythmic, purposeless, quivering muscle movement.

trends The general direction or prevailing tendency in following a general course.

triage system A method to rank or classify patient's illnesses or severity of injury.

triggers Cause the release of inflammatory mediators from the bronchial mast cells, macrophages, and epithelial cells and lead to recurrent episodes of wheezing, breathlessness, chest tightness, and coughing.

triiodothyronine (T_3) The most powerful thyroid hormone; 10 percent secreted by thyroid and the remainder converted from T_4 by peripheral tissues.

trisomies Three of a given chromosome instead of the usual pair.

trocar A large-bore abdominal paracentesis needle.

trough drug level Minimum blood serum level of a drug reached immediately before the next scheduled dose.

tubercles Nodules or swelling of lymphocytes and epithelioid cells that forms the lesions seen in tuberculosis.

tumor markers Substances that are expressed by the tumor or by normal tissue in response to a tumor.

tumor necrosis factor Inflammatory biochemical that is produced in response to various stressors.

tumor suppressor gene A gene that can block or suppress the development of cancer.

tumors Larger and deeper circumscribed solid lesions; they can be benign or malignant.

turgor The skin's elasticity, resilience, and hydration.

tympanometry A test performed to detect abnormalities in the middle ear, such as fluid, eustachian tube dysfunction, or problems with the ossicles.

tympanosclerosis Formation of fibrous tissue around the ossicles preventing vibratory movement.

U

upper motor neuron The descending motor pathway, which originates in the brain and synapse with lower motor neurons in the spinal cord.

uremia Accumulation of end-products of protein metabolism in the bloodstream due to renal failure.

ureteral strictures A narrowing of the lumen of the ureter.

urethral strictures A narrowing of the lumen of the urethra.

urethritis Inflammation of the urethra.

urethroplasty A procedure that removes the diseased portion of the urethra and inserts a new urethra constructed from other tissue.

urethrotomy An opening in the urethra.

urinary tract infection (UTI) An infection involving the kidneys, ureters, bladder, or urethra.

urolithiasis (calculi) Refers to stones in the urinary tract.

urticaria A hypersensitive dermatological manifestation in response to the release of histamine in an antigen-antibody reaction.

utilitarian Belief that an action should be of benefit to the greatest number of people affected by the action.

V

vaginitis Inflammation of the vagina.

valgus Bending or twisting outward from the midline of the body.

valvular regurgitation Backward flow of blood through a heart valve.

valvular stenosis A narrowing or constriction of the diameter of a bodily passage or orifice.

valvuloplasty Plastic surgery performed to repair a valve in the body.

varicocele A group of varicose veins within the scrotum.

varicocelectomy Surgical removal of the varicocele.

varicose veins Tortuous varicosities, in which the veins are dilated and lack surrounding muscle support.

varus Bending or twisting inward toward the midline of the body.

vasectomy Surgical sterilization of men through removal, ligation, or destruction of a small portion of the vas deferens to prevent passage of sperm to the urethra.

vector-borne transmission Infectious material carried by living organism tissue from base of wound.

venous stasis ulcers Erosions of the skin because of lack of blood flow to the extremity, which leads to skin necrosis, open wounds, and black, hardened skin known as eschar.

ventilation The movement of air in and out of the lungs.

ventilator weaning The gradual withdrawal of ventilatory support.

ventricular assist device (VAD) A mechanical device designed to eliminate the workload on the left ventricle, right ventricle, or both and is designed for long-term therapy unlike the intra-aortic balloon pump.

vertigo A sensation or feeling of a loss of equilibrium, sometimes referred to as spinning or whirling.

vesicant An intravenous (IV) medication that causes blisters and tissue injury when it escapes into surrounding tissue. Vesicatory refers to causing blisters.

vesicles Sharply circumscribed, elevated fluid-containing vesicle lesions (herpes, dyshidrosis, pompholyx, varicella, or contact dermatitis).

vesicoureteral reflux Backward propulsion of urine through the valve that normally closes the bladder and ureteral junction to backward flow of urine.

vesicular rash A raised, blistering rash.

visceral pain Pain that originates from any of the large interior organs that occupy a body cavity (cranial, thoracic, abdominal, or pelvic).

visual learners Style of learning in which people learn by processing information by seeing.

vital capacity (VC) The volume of air in and out of the lungs with maximal inspiratory effort and maximal expiratory effort.

volume control ventilation Delivers breaths at a preset target volume.

volvulus A twisting of the intestine on itself that causes obstruction.

W

wellness care Care focused on prevention of illness and promotion of health.

wheals Solid superficial elevations usually in response to pruritus conditions (insect bites, urticaria, or allergic reactions).

wheezes Musical sounds heard primarily on expiration and indicate narrowing of the larger airways, with either spasm or secretions.

wheezing A whistling sound when breathing out related to airway constriction.

workforce diversity Differences in attributes or belief system among members of the workforce.

X

xanthelasma A yellow, lipid-rich plaque present on the eyelids.

xenogeneic A genetic relationship between individuals of differing species.

xerosis Abnormal dryness of skin, mucous membranes, or conjunctiva.

xerostomia Dry mouth.

Z

zone of coagulation Area of the burn that has the most contact with the causative agent, causing coagulated cellular necrosis.

zone of hyperemia Area peripheral to the zone of stasis characterized by viable cells with minimal injury.

zone of stasis Area peripheral to the zone of coagulation characterized by injured viable cells with compromised blood flow.

zoophilic Animal source.